Tumors of the Mediastinum

AFIP Atlas
of
Tumor Pathology

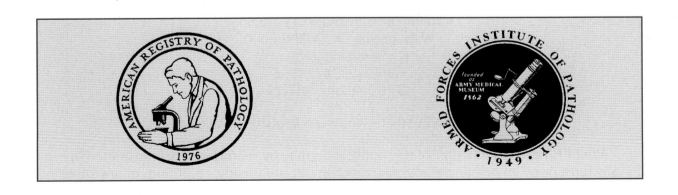

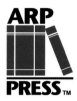

ARP PRESS

Silver Spring, Maryland

Editorial & Production Manager: Mirlinda Q. Caton
Production Editor: Dian S. Thomas
Editorial Assistant: Magdalena C. Silva
Editorial Assistant: Alana N. Black
Copyeditor: Audrey Kahn

Available from the American Registry of Pathology
Armed Forces Institute of Pathology
Washington, DC 20306-6000
www.afip.org
ISBN 1-933477-07-5
978-1-933477-07-7

AFIP ATLAS OF TUMOR PATHOLOGY

Fourth Series
Fascicle 11

TUMORS OF THE MEDIASTINUM

by

Yukio Shimosato, MD
Formerly, National Cancer Center Hospital
Tokyo, Japan

Kiyoshi Mukai, MD
Department of Diagnostic Pathology
Tokyo Medical University
Tokyo, Japan

Yoshihiro Matsuno, MD
Department of Surgical Pathology
Hokkaido University Hospital
Sapporo, Japan

Published by the
American Registry of Pathology
Washington, DC
in collaboration with the
Armed Forces Institute of Pathology
Washington, DC
2010

AFIP ATLAS OF TUMOR PATHOLOGY

EDITOR
Steven G. Silverberg, MD
Department of Pathology
University of Maryland School of Medicine
Baltimore, Maryland

ASSOCIATE EDITOR
William A. Gardner, MD
American Registry of Pathology
Washington, DC

ASSOCIATE EDITOR
Leslie H. Sobin, MD
Armed Forces Institute of Pathology
Washington, DC

EDITORIAL ADVISORY BOARD

Manuscript Reviewed by:
William J. Frable, MD
Saul Suster, MD

EDITORS' NOTE

The Atlas of Tumor Pathology has a long and distinguished history. It was first conceived at a cancer research meeting held in St. Louis in September 1947 as an attempt to standardize the nomenclature of neoplastic diseases. The first series was sponsored by the National Academy of Sciences-National Research Council. The organization of this Sisyphean effort was entrusted to the Subcommittee on Oncology of the Committee on Pathology, and Dr. Arthur Purdy Stout was the first editor-in-chief. Many of the illustrations were provided by the Medical Illustration Service of the Armed Forces Institute of Pathology (AFIP), the type was set by the Government Printing Office, and the final printing was done at the Armed Forces Institute of Pathology (hence the colloquial appellation "AFIP Fascicles"). The American Registry of Pathology (ARP) purchased the Fascicles from the Government Printing Office and sold them virtually at cost. Over a period of 20 years, approximately 15,000 copies each of nearly 40 Fascicles were produced. The worldwide impact of these publications over the years has largely surpassed the original goal. They quickly became among the most influential publications on tumor pathology, primarily because of their overall high quality, but also because their low cost made them easily accessible the world over to pathologists and other students of oncology.

Upon completion of the first series, the National Academy of Sciences-National Research Council handed further pursuit of the project over to the newly created Universities Associated for Research and Education in Pathology (UAREP). A second series was started, generously supported by grants from the AFIP, the National Cancer Institute, and the American Cancer Society. Dr. Harlan I. Firminger became the editor-in-chief and was succeeded by Dr. William H. Hartmann. The second series' Fascicles were produced as bound volumes instead of loose leaflets. They featured a more comprehensive coverage of the subjects, to the extent that the Fascicles could no longer be regarded as "atlases" but rather as monographs describing and illustrating in detail the tumors and tumor-like conditions of the various organs and systems.

Once the second series was completed, with a success that matched that of the first, ARP, UAREP, and AFIP decided to embark on a third series. Dr. Juan Rosai was appointed as editor-in-chief, and Dr. Leslie H. Sobin became associate editor. A distinguished Editorial Advisory Board was also convened, and these outstanding pathologists and educators played a major role in the success of this series, the first publication of which appeared in 1991 and the last (number 32) in 2003.

The same organizational framework applies to the current fourth series, but with UAREP no longer in existence, ARP plays the major role. New features include a hardbound cover, illustrations almost exclusively in color, and an accompanying electronic version of each Fascicle. There is also an increased emphasis (wherever appropriate) on the cytopathologic (intraoperative, exfoliative, and/or fine needle aspiration) and molecular features that are important in diagnosis and prognosis. What does not change from the three previous series, however, is the goal of providing the practicing pathologist with thorough, concise, and up-to-date information on the nomenclature and classification; epidemiologic, clinical, and pathogenetic features; and, most importantly, guidance in the diagnosis of the tumors and tumorlike lesions of all major organ systems and body sites.

As in the third series, a continuous attempt is made to correlate, whenever possible, the nomenclature used in the Fascicles with that proposed by the World Health Organization's Classification of Tumors, as well as to ensure a consistency of style throughout. Close cooperation between the various authors and their respective liaisons from the Editorial Board continues to be emphasized in order to minimize unnecessary repetition and discrepancies in the text and illustrations.

Particular thanks are due to the members of the Editorial Advisory Board, the reviewers (at least two for each Fascicle), the editorial and production staff, and—first and foremost—the individual Fascicle authors for their ongoing efforts to ensure that this series is a worthy successor to the previous three.

Steven G. Silverberg, MD
William A. Gardner, MD
Leslie H. Sobin, MD

PREFACE AND ACKNOWLEDGEMENTS

The Atlas of Tumor Pathology, Fascicle 21, Third Series, *Tumors of the Mediastinum*, authored by Y. Shimosato and K. Mukai, was published in 1997. Since then, the World Health Organization (WHO) published the *Histological Typing of Tumours of the Thymus* in 1999, authored by Juan Rosai in collaboration with L. H. Sobin and pathologists in eight countries, including K. Mukai. In 2004, the WHO published the *Classification of Tumours, Pathology and Genetics of Tumours of the Lung, Pleura, Thymus and Heart*. Y. Shimosato and K. Mukai were members of the working group authoring this work.

In the last 10 years, little progress has been made in the study of tumors of the thymus, although a few new subtypes have been reported. The most significant change was the subtyping by the WHO of tumors of the thymus that do not cause constitutional changes. This classification was a compromise that adopted both the morphologic classification (originally by Bernatz et al.), widely used in the United States, and the histogenetic classification of Müller–Hermelink et al., widely used in Europe and a few institutions in the United States. The WHO classification uses noncommittal terminology, such as alphabet letters and numerals, to designate each subtype. This is supplemented by the morphologic and histogenetic classifications of each subtype in parentheses. The present Fascicle has adopted the WHO system of classification.

Some pathologists may not be familiar with the WHO classification system. We have tried, therefore, to extensively explain and illustrate both the morphologic and histogenetic classification systems that are the bases of the WHO system.

An issue that was not resolved by the WHO histologic classification system was where to place epithelial neuroendocrine tumors. In the lung, carcinoid tumor is considered a malignant epithelial tumor and is placed separately from other types of carcinoma, including small cell carcinoma; large cell neuroendocrine carcinoma is considered a variant of large cell carcinoma. In the WHO classification of thymic tumors, carcinoid tumor, small cell carcinoma, and large cell neuroendocrine carcinoma are considered neuroendocrine carcinomas, and are classified equally with squamous cell carcinoma and other thymic carcinoma subtypes.

Due to the changes in nomenclature, the chapter on thymic epithelial tumors has been considerably revised. The main diagnostic terms are presented along with the previous conventional morphologic and histogenetic terms, for the readers' sake. Newly recognized tumor entities, new cytologic and genetic findings, and recent references have been added. Tables have been revised to reflect new data on survival, staging, and classification.

Most of the cases in this Fascicle are from the pathology files at the National Cancer Center Hospital, Tokyo, and consultation material that was sent to us. Cases with which we had no personal experience and material that was not in our possession were generously supplied by pathologists from Japan, the United States, and Europe, and included original data published in scientific journals as well as photographs used in the Fascicles of the First, Second, and Third series.

Regarding germ cell, hematopoietic, neurogenic, and mesenchymal tumors, readers are referred to corresponding Fascicles for general descriptions; features that are peculiar to the mediastinum only are stressed. Only minor changes were made on the chapters on anatomy, non-neoplastic conditions, tumor-like lesions of the thymus, ectopic tissue and tumors, and tumors and cysts of the mediastinum excluding the thymus, heart, and great vessels.

We would like to express our gratitude for the cases supplied (in alphabetical order) by Drs. Yoshiro Ebihara, Tadaaki Eimoto, Tsunekazu Hishima, Toru Kameya, Tetsuro Kodama, Kazuya Kondo, Shojiroh Morinaga, Junichi Shiraishi, and Tamiko Takemura in Japan; Drs. Cesar A. Moran, Saul Suster, and William D. Travis in the United States; Drs. H. Konrad Müller-Hermelink and Alexander Marx in Germany; and Dr. Juan Rosai in Italy.

Our gratitude is extended also to Shunji Osaka and Shigeru Tamura, who prepared hundreds of gross and microscopic photographs and to Professor J. Patrick Barron for reading and correcting the manuscript. Finally, we wish to acknowledge the contributions and kindest help of our colleagues, both chest physicians/surgeons and pathologists, particularly Drs. Ryosuke Tsuchiya, Hisao Asamura, and Setsuo Hirohashi at the National Cancer Center Hospital and Research Institute in Tokyo. The opinions and assertions this Fascicle contains are the personal views of the authors and are not to be construed as entirely reflecting the view of the Chest Group at the National Cancer Center Hospitals.

Yukio Shimosato, MD
Kiyoshi Mukai, MD
Yoshihiro Matsuno, MD

Permission to use copyrighted illustrations has been granted with kind permission by:

American Journal of Pathology
Am J Pathol 1988;133:618-20. For figures 2-101 and 2-102.

Bunkodo Co., Ltd.
Byori to Rinsho [Pathology and Clinical Medicine] 2002;20:609-11. For figures 2-77, 2-80A–C, 2-81, and 3-34A&B.

Elsevier Limited
Ackerman's Surgical Pathology, 8th ed. St Louis: CV Mosby; 1996:436. For figure 1-2.
Anderson's Pathology, 9th ed. St Louis: CV Mosby; 1990:1493. For figure 1-3.
Ann Thorac Surg 2003;76:879. For figure 3-36.
J Thorac Cardiovasc Surg 2003;126:1136-8. For table 2-6, and figures 2-71 and 2-106.

IARC Press
World Health Organization Classification of Tumours. Pathology and Genetics of Tumours of the Lung, Pleura, Thymus and Heart. Lyon; 2004:153. For table 2-8.

Lippincott Williams & Wilkins
Am J Surg Pathol 1991;15:390. For figure 8-8A.
Am J Surg Pathol 1990;14:163. For figure 4-29.
Am J Surg Pathol 1989;13:491-4. For figures 11-11A&C.
Am J Surg Pathol 1987;11:984. For figure 3-7.
Histology for Pathologists. New York: Raven Press; 1992:274. For table 9-3.
Neoplastic Hematopathology, 2nd ed. Philadelphia; 2001:178. For figure 1-19.
Sternberg's Diagnostic Surgical Pathology, 4th ed. Philadelphia; 2004:2170. For table 5-1.

McGraw-Hill Companies
Review of Gross Anatomy, 6th ed. New York; 1996;359. For figures 1-1 and 1-5.

Springer Verlag
Cell Tissue Res 1984;237:229-233. For table 1-2 and figures 1-10B–D.
Curr Top Pathol 1986;75:216. For table 1-1.
Microenvironments in The Lymphoid System. Advances in Experimental Medicine and Biology, vol 186. New York: Plenum Press; 1985:292-5. For figures 1-10A, E, & F.

Wiley-Blackwell
Histopathology 2000;36:405-10. For tables 1-3, 1-4, and 2-7.
Histopathology 1992;21:506. For table 9-1.
Jpn J Cancer Res 1992;83:129. For figure 3-39.
Pathol Int 1994;44:506. For table 2-12.

Wiley-Liss, Inc., a subsidiary of John Wiley & Sons, Inc.
Cancer 2002;94:628. For figures 2-70 and 2-105.
Cancer 1994;74:613. For figure 2-69.
Cancer 1991;68:1986. For table 2-11.
Cancer 1987;60:2737. For figure 2-68.
Cancer 1981;48:2485. For table 2-10.
TNM Supplement: A Commentary on Uniform Use, 3rd ed. New York; 2003:118-9. For table 2-13.

CONTENTS

1. Anatomy and Anatomic Compartments of the Mediastinum 1
   The Mediastinum 1
   Normal Thymus Gland 1
      Embryology 2
      Anatomic Location 3
      Gross Findings 4
      Microscopic Findings 4
      Maturation of Thymocytes 15
      Involution 16
2. Thymoma 19
   Classification of Thymic Tumors 19
   Thymoma 19
      General Features 23
      Clinical Features 24
      Diagnostic Approach 25
      Gross Findings 29
      Microscopic Findings 33
      Cellular Subtypes 41
      Histologic Subtypes 48
      Histogenetic Subtypes 55
      Controversies Surrounding Histogenetic and WHO Histologic Subtypes 56
      Variants and Uncommon Histologic Subtypes 58
      Histologic Factors Associated with Degree of Malignancy 67
      Frozen Section Findings 77
      Cytologic Findings 77
      Immunohistochemistry and Functional Correlation 84
      Ultrastructural Findings 89
      Molecular and Other Special Techniques 94
      Differential Diagnosis 97
      Conditions and Diseases Associated with Thymoma 99
      Spread and Metastases 101
      Staging 102
      Treatment 105
      Prognosis 105
3. Thymic Carcinoma 115
   General Features 115

Clinical Features 116

Gross Findings 118

Microscopic Findings and Histologic Subtypes 118

    Squamous Cell Carcinoma 120

    Basaloid Carcinoma 127

    Mucoepidermoid Carcinoma 127

    Adenosquamous Carcinoma 129

    Adenocarcinoma 131

    Carcinoma with Adenoid Cystic Carcinoma-Like Features 135

    Lymphoepithelioma-Like Carcinoma 135

    Clear Cell Carcinoma 135

    Large Cell Carcinoma (Undifferentiated Carcinoma in the WHO Classification) . . 137

    Sarcomatoid Carcinoma 138

    Carcinoma with t(15;19) Translocation 139

Cytologic Findings 139

Immunohistochemical Findings 141

Molecular and Other Special Techniques 143

Prognostic and Malignancy-Associated Factors 144

    TNM and Stage 144

    Histologic Types 144

    Degree of Histologic Differentiation and Cell Atypia 145

    Immunohistochemical Prognostic Factors 146

    Nuclear DNA Content and Histograms 146

Differential Diagnosis 146

Tumor Spread and Metastasis 149

Treatment 149

Prognosis 150

Association of Epstein-Barr Virus with Development of Thymic Epithelial Tumors . . 150

4. Thymic Neuroendocrine Carcinomas 157

   Well-Differentiated Neuroendocrine Carcinoma (Carcinoid Tumor) 157

    Histogenesis 158

    Clinical Findings 159

    Gross Findings 160

    Microscopic Findings 160

    Histologic Variants 166

    Ultrastructural Findings 168

    Cytologic Findings 168

    Immunohistochemical Findings (Including Functional Correlation with
      Paraneoplastic Syndrome) 168

Molecular and Other Special Diagnostic Techniques 176

Differential Diagnosis. 176

Treatment and Prognosis 177

Poorly Differentiated Neuroendocrine Carcinomas 178

Large Cell Neuroendocrine Carcinoma 178

Small Cell Carcinoma of Neuroendocrine Type 179

Histogenesis 184

Cytologic Findings 184

Immunohistochemical Findings 184

Molecular and Other Special Diagnostic Techniques 185

Differential Diagnosis. 185

Prognosis and Malignancy-Associated Factors 185

Treatment 185

Combined Thymic Epithelial Tumors (Including Neuroendocrine Carcinomas) 185

5. Germ Cell Tumors 193

Definition and Classification 193

Incidence and Clinical Features 193

Diagnostic Approach 196

Tumors of One Histologic Type 201

Teratoma. 201

Seminoma (Germinoma) 208

Embryonal Carcinoma 211

Yolk Sac Tumor (Endodermal Sinus Tumor) 211

Choriocarcinoma 212

Tumors of More Than One Histologic Type: Mixed Germ Cell Tumors 212

Teratoma with Nongerminal Malignant Tumor 212

Molecular and Other Special Techniques. 216

Malignant Germ Cell Tumors of Infants and Young Children 216

Malignant Germ Cell Tumors of Adolescents and Adults 216

Pure Teratoma (Immature and Mature) 216

Tumor Spread and Staging 216

Treatment and Prognosis 216

6. Malignant Lymphomas and Hematopoietic Neoplasms 225

B-Cell Lymphomas 225

Primary Mediastinal Large B-Cell Lymphoma. 225

Thymic Extranodal Marginal Zone B-Cell Lymphoma of Mucosa-Associated
Lymphoid Tissue 231

T-Cell Lymphomas 237

Precursor T-Lymphoblastic Leukemia/Lymphoblastic Lymphoma (Precursor T-Cell Acute Lymphoblastic Leukemia/Precursor T-Cell Lymphoblastic Lymphoma) . . 237

Anaplastic Large Cell Lymphoma and Other Rare Mature T- and NK-Cell Lymphomas of the Mediastinum 241

Hodgkin Lymphoma 241

Histocytic and Dendritic Cell Tumors 245

   Langerhans Cell Histiocytosis and Sarcoma 246

   Histiocytic Sarcoma 246

   Follicular Dendritic Cell Tumor/Sarcoma 246

   Interdigitating Dendritic Cell Tumor/Sarcoma 246

   Myeloid Sarcoma and Extramedullary Acute Myeloid Leukemia 247

7. Secondary Involvement of the Thymus by Carcinoma and Mesothelioma 253

   Secondary Carcinoma Involving the Thymus 253

      Distinction between Thymic and Pulmonary Carcinomas 254

   Mesothelioma Involving the Thymus 255

8. Other Tumors and Tumor-Like Lesions of the Thymus 257

   Thymolipoma 257

   Ectopic Hamartomatous Thymoma 260

   Malignant Melanoma 262

   Thymic Cyst 262

      Congenital Thymic Cyst 262

      Acquired Multilocular Thymic Cyst 263

   Other Tumor-Like Lesions 265

9. Non-Neoplastic Conditions of the Thymus 271

   Thymus in Immunodeficiency 271

      Thymus in Primary Immunodeficiencies 272

      Thymus in Secondary Immunodeficiencies 274

   Thymic Hyperplasia 274

      True Thymic Hyperplasia 274

      Lymphoid Hyperplasia 276

10. Ectopic Tissue and Tumors in the Anterosuperior Mediastinum 281

   Thyroid Lesions 281

   Parathyroid Lesions 281

11. Mesenchymal and Neurogenic Tumors of the Mediastinum Excluding the Heart and Great Vessels 285

   Mesenchymal Tumors 285

      Benign Mesenchymal Tumors and Tumor-Like Lesions 285

      Mesenchymal Tumors of Intermediate Malignancy 288

      Malignant Mesenchymal Tumors 292

Neurogenic Tumors and Tumors of Paraganglia 295

    Immunohistochemistry of Neurogenic Tumors and Paraganglioma 301

12. Mediastinal Cysts (Other Than Thymic Cyst) 305

    Bronchogenic Cyst 305

    Esophageal Cyst 307

    Gastroenteric Cyst 307

    Celomic Cyst (Pericardial Cyst and Mesothelial Cyst) 307

    Thoracic Duct Cyst 308

    Cyst-Like Lesions Other Than True Cysts 308

13. Other Mediastinal Tumor-Like Conditions 309

    Castleman Disease 309

      Hyaline-Vascular Type Castleman Disease 310

      Plasma Cell Type Castleman Disease 311

    Index 315

1 ANATOMY AND ANATOMIC COMPARTMENTS OF THE MEDIASTINUM

THE MEDIASTINUM

The mediastinum is a large compartment in the thoracic cavity, bounded laterally by the pleurae, anteriorly by the sternum, posteriorly by the vertebral column, superiorly by the thoracic inlet, and inferiorly by the diaphragm. It contains a large number of organs and structures. In clinical practice, the mediastinum is divided into four arbitrary portions: the superior, anterior, middle, and posterior compartments (fig. 1-1). This division enables radiologists to localize lesions with accuracy and is valuable in the differential diagnosis of mediastinal lesions, since certain cystic lesions and neoplasms occur preferentially in one compartment (fig. 1-2) (15,15a). The anatomy and normal histology of organs and structures in the mediastinum, other than the thymus gland, are referred to in corresponding monographs and other Fascicles of this series.

NORMAL THYMUS GLAND

The thymus gland, one of the central lymphoid organs, plays an important role in cellular immunity by generating circulating T lymphocytes. Histologically, it is the prototype lymphoepithelial organ in that it consists of an intimate mixture of epithelial cells and lymphocytes (20), as well as other cell types important

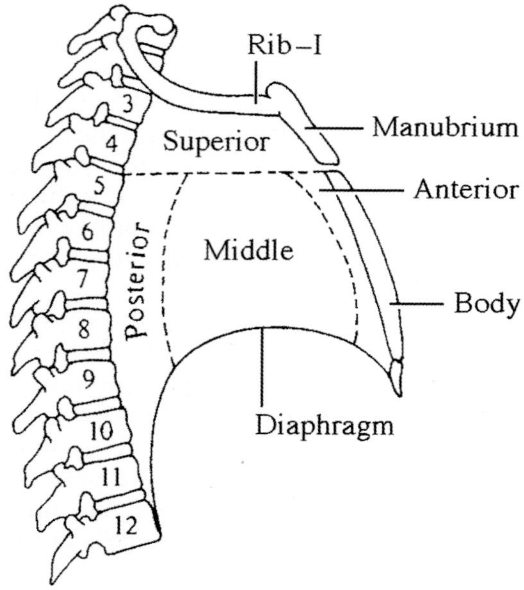

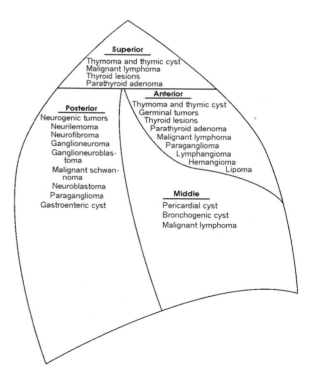

Figure 1-1

ANATOMIC COMPARTMENTS OF THE MEDIASTINUM

(Fig. from Pansky B. Review of gross anatomy, 6th ed. New York: McGraw-Hill; 1996:359.)

Figure 1-2

LOCATION OF MOST COMMON LESIONS OF THE MEDIASTINUM

(Fig. 8-1 from Rosai J. Ackerman's surgical pathology, 8th ed. St. Louis: CV Mosby; 1996:436.)

1

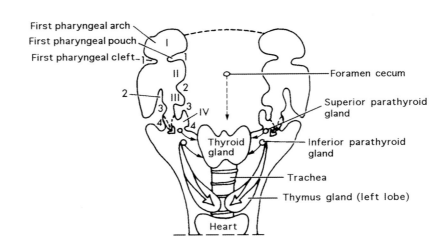

Figure 1-3

SCHEMATIC REPRESENTATION OF THYMIC EMBRYOGENESIS

The thymus gland originates from the pouch and cleft of the third pharyngeal structure. (Fig. 29-1 from Griffith RC. Thymus gland. In: Kissane JM, ed. Anderson's pathology, 9th ed. St. Louis: CV Mosby; 1990:1493.)

for the function of this organ. Advances in immunology, especially in the development of the immune system, have enhanced knowledge of the function of the thymus and, to a certain extent, thymic tumors.

Embryology

In humans, thymic epithelium arises bilaterally from the third and probably fourth branchial pouches, which contain elements derived from all three germinal layers. Different clefts and pouches contribute to the thymus in other animals. Development begins in the 6th gestational week when paired cellular proliferations emerge from the third branchial cleft and from the endoderm of the ventral wing of the third pharyngeal pouch (fig. 1-3). The inferior parathyroid gland arises similarly from the dorsal wing of the pharyngeal pouch. Both primordia separate from the pharyngeal wall and begin their caudal migration into the anterosuperior mediastinum as epithelial tubules or cords. During this process, the ectoderm of the third branchial cleft covers the endodermally derived epithelium. The mesoderm provides vascular stroma and mesenchymal cells (3,12,20).

During the 8th gestational week, the thymic primordia elongate caudally, forming two epithelial bars that fuse along the midline to occupy their final position within the anterosuperior mediastinum. During this migration, small fragments may separate from the primordia and persist postnatally along the migratory route, often connected to the inferior parathyroid gland (fig. 1-4) (16,17). When the migration ends at

the base of the heart, the thymus lies anteriorly to the great vessels in the superior mediastinum, with its upper poles extending laterally along the trachea into the base of the thyroid gland.

Until the 9th gestational week, the embryonic thymus remains as a purely epithelial organ. By the 10th week, small lymphoid cells that originate in the fetal liver and bone marrow begin to migrate into the epithelial organ (3,6,20). Lobulation also occurs by the 10th week as a result of ingrowth of the capsule of the gland. The influx of lymphoid stem cells into the thymus occurs in successive waves. This is an active phenomenon that depends on the maturational state of the thymic epithelium. Differentiation of the thymus into cortex and medulla occurs as the lymphoid cells migrate into the thymic anlage. Inductive tissue interactions between the epithelial and mesenchymal components are necessary for the thymus to develop normally.

At this developmental stage, the epithelial cells at the periphery of the lobules become rounded, whereas those in the center appear more spindle shaped. Adjacent epithelial cells are connected by well-developed desmosomes. Other large mesenchymal cells are present at this time in the septa of the lobules and among the central epithelial cells. These cells are histogenetically and functionally related to the interdigitating reticulum cells of thymus-dependent regions of peripheral lymphoid tissue. Macrophages colonize the thymus at the same stage as the lymphoid progenitors. Rare cells containing myofilaments, called myoid cells, are present in the central anlage as early as the 8th week. Erythroblasts, representing residua from earlier hematopoiesis in the primordial gland, may also be found.

Small tubular structures composed of epithelial cells are present in the central portion of the primordial lobule. They become Hassall corpuscles at a later stage (20).

The development of the cortex and medulla is completed between the 14th and 16th gestational weeks. This morphologic differentiation is accompanied by phenotypic characterization of the epithelial cells and lymphocytes.

Anatomic Location

The thymus gland is located predominantly in the anterosuperior mediastinum (fig. 1-5). Its base lies upon the pericardium and the great vessels. The upper pole of each lobe extends into the neck and is joined to the lower pole of the corresponding lobe of the thyroid gland by the thyrothymic ligament. The lower poles of the thymic lobes extend down over the pericardium for a variable distance, usually to the level of the fourth costal cartilage.

The upper poles are closely applied to the trachea. The posterior boundary of the thymus is the pretracheal fascia, which separates it from the great vessels. Anteriorly, it is in contact with cervical fascia, strap muscles of the neck, the sternum, costal cartilages, and intercostal muscles. Reflections from the parietal pleura partially cover the lateral aspects of the gland.

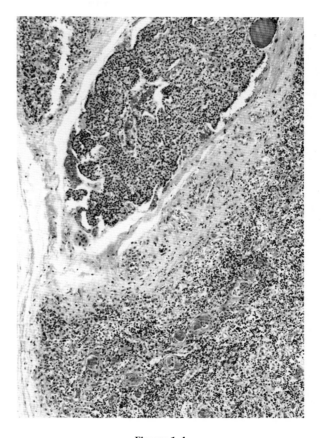

Figure 1-4

**ECTOPIC THYMIC TISSUE
SURROUNDING PARATHYROID GLAND**

This may be called a parathymus: parathyroid tissue on the upper side is surrounded by thymic tissue in which Hassall corpuscles are seen.

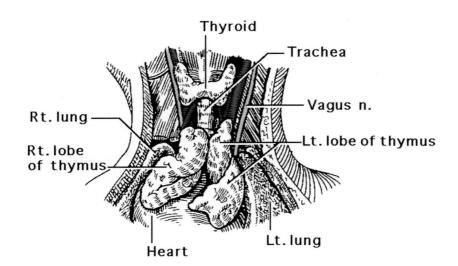

Figure 1-5

LOCATION OF THYMUS

(Fig. from Pansky B. Review of gross anatomy, 6th ed. New York: McGraw-Hill; 1996:359.)

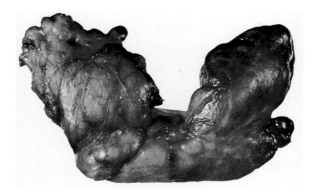

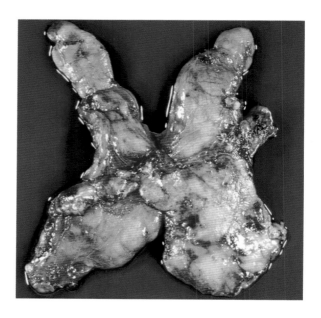

Figure 1-6

NORMAL THYMUS

Above: Infant thymus. Two separate lobes join at the lower poles

Right: Adult thymus (27-year-old male). The thymus often shows an X- or H-shaped configuration (same case as that in fig. 1-8). (Fig. 1-6, Fascicle 21, Third Series.)

Gross Findings

The thymus gland is a pyramid-shaped organ composed of two fused lobes (fig. 1-6); each is completely covered by a fibrous capsule (16). The fully developed thymus is pink, becoming gray following formalin fixation. It turns yellow with the involution of aging, reflecting an increased deposition of mature fat. The vascularization of the thymus gland derives from branches of the inferior thyroid arteries, the internal mammary arteries, and the pericardiophrenic arteries. The innervation, which is minimal and probably restricted to blood vessels, originates from the vagus nerve and cervical sympathetic nerves.

The size of the human thymus gland varies greatly. There have been several studies in which the weight of the thymus was measured, but most were done many years ago and may not be valid today. The weight of the normal thymus gland is mainly related to age: it is greatest in relation to body weight at the time of birth, weighing an average of 15 g. It continues to increase in size and weight until puberty to reach an average weight of 30 to 40 g (3,7,12,16,20). Subsequently, thymic weight declines during the process of aging involution and at 60 years of age is 10 to 15 g (fig. 1-7). Many conditions contribute to involution or enlargement of the thymus. Chronic stressful conditions cause involution.

Death from asphyxia (largely in young persons) and several cardiovascular conditions are associated with higher than normal thymic weight (7) including myocardial fibrosis; coronary thrombosis, myocardial infarction, and ruptured myocardium; cor pulmonale; hypertensive heart disease with congestive heart failure; and coronary occlusion due to atheroma. The causal relationship between these conditions and increased thymic weight is unknown.

Microscopic Findings

The thymus is divided into many small lobules by fibrous septa extending from the capsule (fig. 1-8). Each lobule measures from 0.5 to 2.0 mm and constitutes the basic structural unit of the gland. Each lobule is composed of two areas that can be clearly distinguished in histologic sections: cortex and medulla. The cortex appears darker because of its population of lymphocytes, traditionally known as thymocytes (20). The thymocytes are admixed with a few epithelial and mesenchymal cells. Conversely, the medulla is lighter due to fewer lymphocytes and more epithelial cells. The medullary portions are continuous from lobule to lobule, resulting in a highly branched stalk configuration.

Epithelial Cells. The epithelial cells of the thymus form the framework of the organ and are functionally essential for the maturation of T lymphocytes. They have been traditionally

4

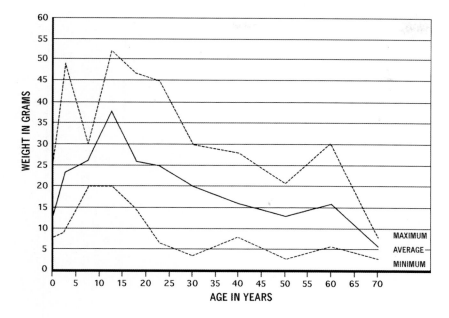

Figure 1-7

WEIGHT OF HUMAN THYMUS

Average and range of the weight of normal thymuses at any given age. (Fig. 1-7 from Fascicle 21, Third Series.)

Figure 1-8

NORMAL THYMUS

Thymic parenchyma from a 27-year-old male shows lobulation by fatty tissue. Each lobule contains a dark cortex and pale medulla.

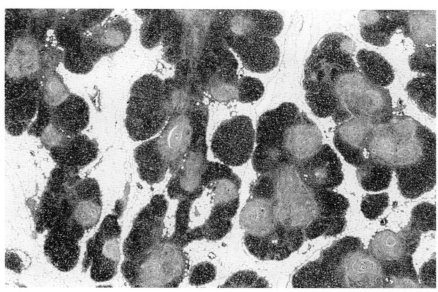

divided into cortical and medullary types on the basis of their location. Their cytologic features are distinct enough to be recognized by light microscopy (Table 1-1; fig. 1-9) (13).

Van de Wijngaert et al. (22) identified six types of thymic epithelial cells based on their ultrastructural features (Table 1-2; fig. 1-10). Types 2 and 3 are characterized by a special pattern of epithelium-lymphocyte interaction ("thymic nurse cells"), as demonstrated by the intracytoplasmic presence of lymphocytes.

Immunohistochemical studies using various monoclonal antibodies against different antigens have demonstrated heterogeneity of human thymic epithelial cells (1,13,21). Recently, using various cytokeratin subtypes (Table 1-3), Kuo (10) demonstrated that epithelial cells of the thymus can be classified into four subtypes according to their location and cytokeratin profiles. These include subcapsular, cortical, and medullary epithelial cells and cells of Hassall corpuscle (Table 1-4; fig. 1-11). Studies of

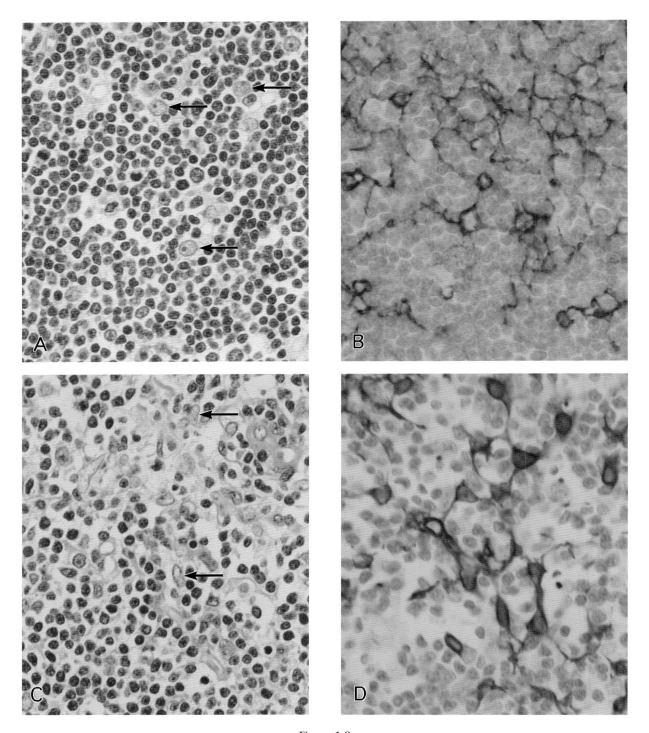

Figure 1-9

THYMIC EPITHELIAL CELLS

A: Epithelial cells of cortical type have large, round to oval and clear nuclei and a conspicuous nucleolus (arrows).
B: Immunohistochemistry for cytokeratin 19 depicts stellate cell body with thin cytoplasmic processes.
C: Medullary epithelial cells (arrows) have a spindle-shaped nucleus and interconnecting cell processes.
D: Immunohistochemistry for cytokeratin 19 shows interconnecting spindle-shaped epithelial cells.

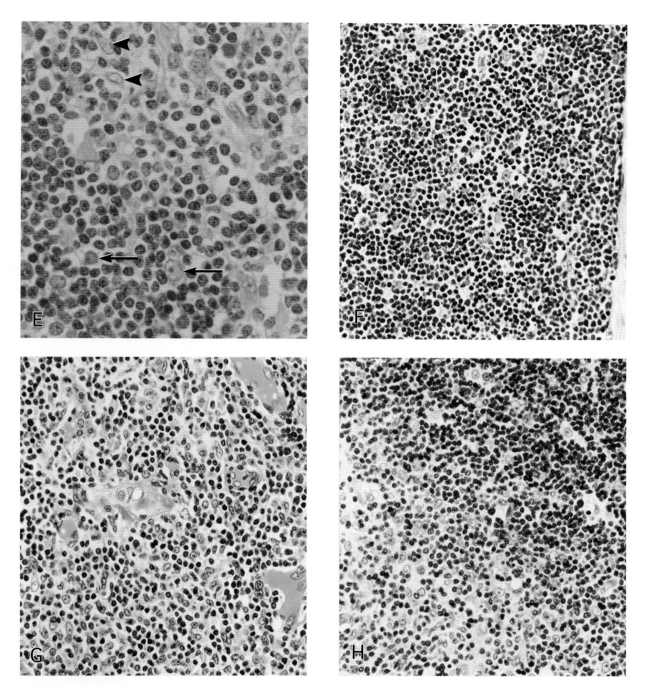

Figure 1-9 (Continued)

E: At corticomedullary junction, epithelial cells of cortical type (arrow) and medullary type (arrowheads) are intermingled.

F: Cortex: epithelial cells of cortical type, which are scattered in a background consisting of lymphocytes, have a large, round to oval, clear nucleus and a distinct nucleolus.

G: Medulla: fusiform epithelial cells have a spindle-shaped nucleus, coarse chromatin structure, and interconnecting cell processes. A portion of a Hassall corpuscle is seen in the center.

H: Corticomedullary junction: cortex with epithelial cells of the cortical type is in the left upper corner, and medulla with epithelial cells of the medullary type in the right lower corner, where a few epithelial cells of the cortical type are intermingled. (F–H from CD-ROM of the Third Series, Fascicle 21.)

Table 1-1

**DIFFERENTIAL CHARACTERISTICS OF CORTICAL AND
MEDULLARY THYMIC EPITHELIAL CELLS UNDER LIGHT MICROSCOPY[a]**

	Cortical	Medullary
Shape	Stellate	Spindle with cytoplasmic processes
Nucleus		
Shape	Oval-round	Oval-spindle, often with irregular contour
Size	Medium-large	Small-medium
Character	Thin and distinct nuclear membrane, very loose chromatin (clear nucleus)	Distinct nuclear membrane, finely distributed heterochromatin
Nucleolus	1, often prominent, round, central	+/−, little, not prominent
Cytoplasm	Scant, clear, or faintly eosinophilic	Scant, eosinophilic, mostly seen in the cellular process
Cytoplasmic processes	Very thin, faintly eosinophilic	Long, thin, eosinophilic

[a]Table 3 from Müller-Hermelink HK, Marino M, Palestro G. Pathology of thymic epithelial tumors. In: Müller-Hermelink HK, ed. The human thymus. Current Top Pathol 1986;75:216.

Figure 1-10

**ELECTRON MICROSCOPY OF
THYMIC EPITHELIAL CELLS**

Six types of cells are identified.

A: Type 1 "subcapsular-perivascular" epithelial cell (6 1/2-year-old donor). R: cisternae of rough endoplasmic reticulum (RER); G: a Golgi complex; d: desmosomes; bl: basal lamina; tf: tonofilaments. Inset: Higher magnification shows micropinocytotic vesicles facing the basal lamina.

B: Type 2 "pale" epithelial cell in the outer cortex. R: profiles of RER; G: a Golgi complex; arrow: multivesicular body.

C: Type 4 "dark" epithelial cell in the deep cortex. A nuclear cisternum is dilated. vac: vacuoles; arrow: swollen mitochondria; arrowhead: residual bodies.

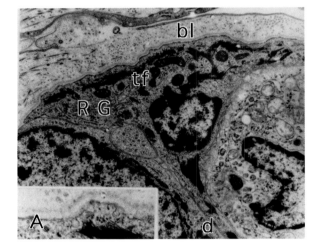

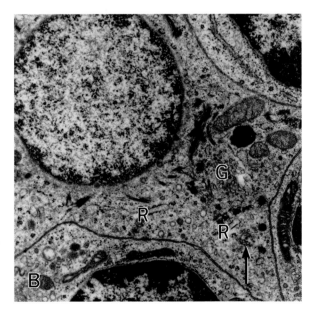

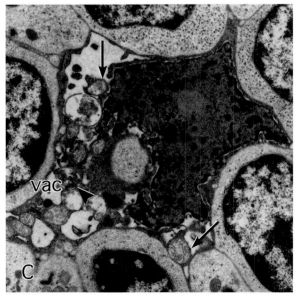

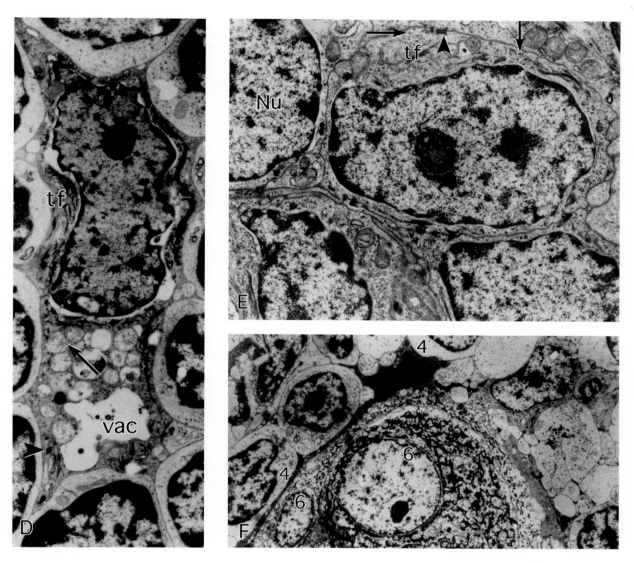

Fig. 1-10 (continued)

D: Type 3 "intermediate" epithelial cell in the outer cortex. A dilated nuclear cisternum is seen. tf: tonofilaments; vac: vacuoles; arrowhead: desmosome; arrow: swollen mitochondria.

E: Type 5 "undifferentiated" epithelial cell in the corticomedullary region. Nu: nucleus; tf: tonofilaments; arrowhead: desmosome; arrow: polyribosome.

F: Two type 6 "large medullary" epithelial cells (6) adjacent to a Hassall corpuscle and two type 4 epithelial cells (4) in the medulla. (A, E, F: Figs. 2, 4, 5 from Kendall MD, van de Wijngaert FP, Shuurman HJ, Rademakers LH, Kater L. Heterogeneity of the human epithelial microenvironment at the ultrastructural level. In: Klaus GG, ed. Microenvironments in the lymphoid system. Advances in experimental medicine and biology, vol 186, New York: Plenum Press; 1985;292-5. B, C, D: Figs 5, 6, 8 from van de Wijngaert FP, Kendall MD, Shuurman HJ, Rademakers LH, Kater L. Heterogeneity of epithelial cells in human thymus. An ultrastructural study. Cell Tissue Res 1984:237:231-3.)

thymomas have revealed that they can also be classified by cytokeratin profiles. Although further study is needed, combining cytokeratin profiles and lymphocyte phenotype will make histogenetic classification of thymomas a reality. This is discussed in detail in chapter 2.

Hassall Corpuscles. Hassall corpuscles are characteristic structures of the thymus gland (fig. 1-12). They are present exclusively in the medulla and are recognized as round, keratinized formations. They show a concentric arrangement of mature epithelial cells and a

Table 1-2

MORPHOLOGIC CHARACTERISTICS AND LOCATION OF TYPES OF EPITHELIAL CELLS IN THE HUMAN THYMUS[a]

	Morphologic Characteristics	Location
Type 1 "subcapsular-perivascular"	Basal lamina, heterochromatic nucleus, long cisternae of RER[b], well-developed Golgi complex, micropinocytotic vesicles	Beneath capsule, around capillaries in cortex and corticomedullary region
Type 2 "pale"	Round euchromatic nucleus, well-developed Golgi complex, short profiles of RER, electron-dense granules, tubular structures	Scattered in cortex and medulla, predominant in outer cortex
Type 3 "intermediate"	Spectrum in morphology between type 2 and type 4, euchromatic or heterochromatic irregularly shaped nucleus, dilated cisternae of nucleus and RER	Midcortex, deep cortex, medulla
Type 4 "dark"	Heterochromatic, electron-dense, irregularly shaped nucleus; dilated cisternae of nucleus and RER; residual bodies; swollen mitochondria	Deep cortex, scattered in medulla and around Hassall corpuscles
Type 5 "undifferentiated"	Rounded nucleus with some heterochromatin, polyribosomes, small bundles of tonofilaments, small desmosomes	In groups in corticomedullary region, scattered in medulla
Type 6 "large medullary"	Large, rounded nucleus, either euchromatic or heterochromatic; sometimes RER well developed; abundant tonofilaments; tubular structures	Scattered in medulla, adjacent to large Hassall corpuscles, part of small Hassall corpuscles

[a]Table 1 from van de Wijngaert FP, Kendall MD, Schuurman HK, Rademakers LH, Karter L. Heterogeneity of epithelial cells in the human thymus. An ultrastructural study. Cell Tissue Res 1984;237:229.
[b]RER = rough endoplasmic reticulum.

Table 1-3

ANTIBODIES USED FOR ANALYSIS OF THYMIC EPITHELIAL CELLS[a]

Specificity (Clone)[b]	Type of Cytokeratin
CK7 (OV-TL 12/30)	Simple epithelium
CK8 (C-51)	Simple epithelium
CK18 (DC10)	Simple epithelium
CK19 (RCK 108)	Simple epithelium
CK20 (IT-Ks20.8)	Simple epithelium
CK10 (DE-K10)	Keratinized squamous epithelium
CK13 (AE8)	Nonkeratinized squamous epithelium
CK14 (LL002)	Basal cell
Involucrin (Sy5)	Squamous cell

[a]Section taken from Table 2 from Kuo TT. Cytokeratin profiles of the thymus and thymomas: histogenetic correlations and proposal for a histological classification of thymomas. Histopathology 2000;36:405.
[b]Source of cytokeratin antibodies: BioGenex, San Ramon, CA; source of involucrin: YLEM, Rome, Italy.

keratinized center, which is often calcified. The periphery of the corpuscle is continuous with the medullary epithelial cells from which it is derived. Hassall corpuscles may show secondary changes such as central cystic degeneration, with accumulation of cellular debris and inflammatory cells (fig. 1-13) (20). Marked cystic de-generation may result in "multilocular thymic cyst," a condition which had been regarded as a congenital abnormality previously but may be instead the result of cystic enlargement of Hassall corpuscles resulting from acquired inflammatory changes in the thymus. The presence of columnar epithelium-lined cysts may also be related to cystic degeneration of Hassall corpuscles (20). This columnar epithelium probably is derived from the remnant of the pharyngeal pouch from which the thymus originates.

Thymic Hormones. The production of thymic hormones by the epithelial cells of the thymus gland has been a subject of extensive research (2,4,5). Recent investigations have demonstrated that none of the "thymic hormones/factors" are thymus-specific but are produced by nerve cells and other cell types. Nonetheless, these molecules are biologically important because of their diverse intracellular and extracellular functions. Some of these molecules have been shown to be effective in restoring immune functions and others are used for the treatment of viral hepatitis (11). One hormone, thymosin, has been shown to rectify an immunodeficient state.

Lymphocytes (Thymocytes). The thymic cortex is densely populated by lymphocytes of various

Table 1-4

CYTOKERATIN PROFILE AND EXPRESSION OF INVOLUCRIN
IN DIFFERENT COMPARTMENTS OF THE NON-NEOPLASTIC THYMUS[a]

Thymus	Cytokeratins								IVL[b]
	CK7	CK8	CK10	CK13	CK14	CK18	CK19	CK20	
Subcapsular cell	+[c]	–	–	–	+	–	+	–	–
Cortex	–	–	–	–	–	–	+	–	–
Medulla	+	+	–	–	+	+	+	–	–
Hassall corpuscle	+	+	+	+	+	+	+	–	+

[a]Modified from Table 4 from Kuo TT. Cytokeratin profiles of the thymus and thymomas: histogenetic correlations and proposal for a histological classification of thymomas. Histopathology 2000;36:407.
[b]IVL = involucrin.
[c]+ = majority of cases are focally and/or diffusely stained; – = negative or minority of cases are focally and/or diffusely stained.

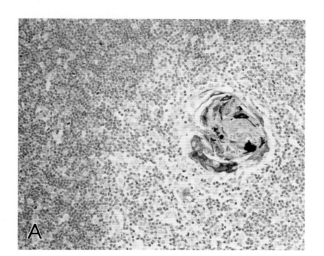

Figure 1-11

EXPRESSION OF CYTOKERATINS 10,
14, AND 19 IN HUMAN THYMUS

A: Cytokeratin (CK) 10 is positive only in the epithelial cells of Hassall corpuscles.

B: CK14 is positive in the subcapsular and medullary epithelial cells, epithelial cells of Hassall corpuscles, and rare cortical epithelial cells (cortical cells were negative in most areas).

C: Epithelial cells of the cortex and medulla, including those of a Hassall corpuscle, are equally positive for CK19.

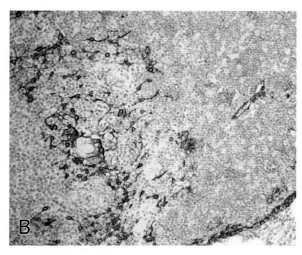

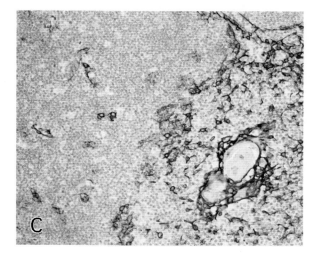

sizes. Mitotically active prothymocytes or large lymphoblasts comprise about 10 to 15 percent of the lymphoid cells in the thymus; they are found predominantly in the subcapsular portion of the outer cortex (13,20). A gradient of smaller, less mitotically active lymphocytes is seen in the outer cortex, into the deep cortex, into the cortical medullary junction, and into

Figure 1-12

HASSALL CORPUSCLE

A Hassall corpuscle with a granular layer, present in the medulla, displays keratinization.

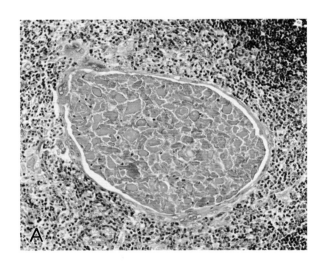

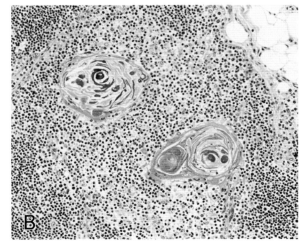

Figure 1-13

DEGENERATIVE CHANGE IN HASSALL CORPUSCLES

A: Cystic dilatation with accumulation of cellular debris and a few inflammatory cells.

B: Dystrophic calcification.

C: Accumulation of mucoid substances with microcystic changes.

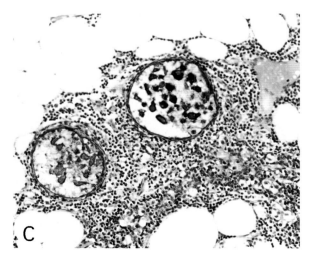

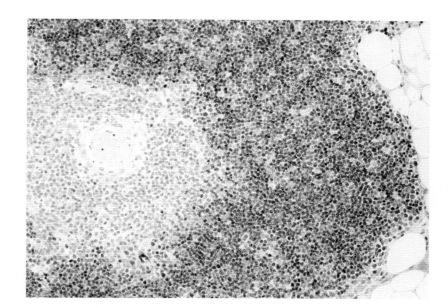

Figure 1-14

TERMINAL DEOXYNUCLEOTIDYLTRANSFERASE IN THYMOCYTES

The large majority of lymphocytes in the thymic cortex stain for terminal deoxynucleotidyltransferase (TdT). None of lymphocytes in the medulla are positive.

the medulla. The term thymocyte was used originally to designate all lymphocytes in the thymus. Currently, the term is restricted to indicate immature T lymphocytes in the thymus, which are positive for terminal deoxynucleotidyltransferase (TdT) (fig. 1-14), CD1a, and CD99 (with the anti-MIC2 antibody, O13).

In the cortex, intense lymphopoiesis, lympholysis, and active phagocytosis are indicative of extensive ineffective lymphopoiesis (probably 99 percent of thymocytes die in situ). This results in a prominent "starry sky" appearance in the active thymus (20).

Other Cell Types. In addition to epithelial cells and lymphocytes of T-cell lineage, the thymus contains a variety of other cell types (20,23). B lymphocytes are found either as lymphoid follicles with germinal centers in the septa or scattered in the medulla (fig. 1-15). The presence of germinal centers in the perivascular space led to the proposal that the thymus may be divided into two major compartments: the cortex and medulla composing the true thymic parenchyma and the extraparenchymal compartment consisting of the perivascular spaces of the thymus (20). Germinal centers occur in the thymuses of 2 to 40 percent of normal individuals. This wide variation may be related to a sampling factor or to the age of the patients. Germinal centers are especially common in children and adolescents.

Macrophages are mainly present in the cortex but also occur in the medulla (fig. 1-16) (19). They are functionally active and show strong lysosomal enzyme activity. Interdigitating reticulum cells are numerous in the medulla and at the corticomedullary junction (fig. 1-17) (9,19). They are positive for S-100 protein and have little lysosomal enzyme activity. Both of these cells express class I and class II major histocompatibility (MHC) antigens, have attributes of antigen-presenting cells, and play an important role in the clonal expansion of T lymphocytes.

Langerhans cells have also been identified in the thymic medulla. Eosinophils, mast cells, and plasma cells are present in the connective tissue septa of the thymus.

Myoid or striated cells are located in the medulla (fig. 1-18) (3,20). They are prominent in the thymus of birds and reptiles but are also found in the human thymus. They are located in small groups adjacent to Hassall corpuscles and are more frequent in newborns. Myoid cells are identical to striated muscle cells by immunohistochemical and ultrastructural criteria. The histogenesis of myoid cells remains a subject of debate. Although the myoid cells are in close proximity to thymic epithelial cells, evidence that these cells are derived from epithelial cells is lacking. Some investigators favor a neural crest origin for this cell type (14). Myoid cells are of great interest because of their potential

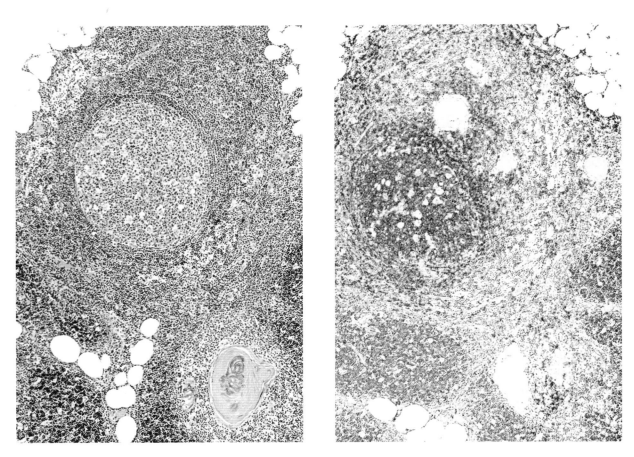

Figure 1-15

PRESENCE OF B-CELL FOLLICLE WITH GERMINAL CENTER

Hematoxylin and eosin (H&E) stain (left) and immunohistochemical stain for CD20 (right). B cells are also scattered in the medulla.

Figure 1-16

DISTRIBUTION OF MACROPHAGES

Most lysozyme-positive macrophages are present in the cortex, especially in the sub-capsular or subseptal region. A few macrophages are also present in the medulla (immunohistochemical stain for lysozyme).

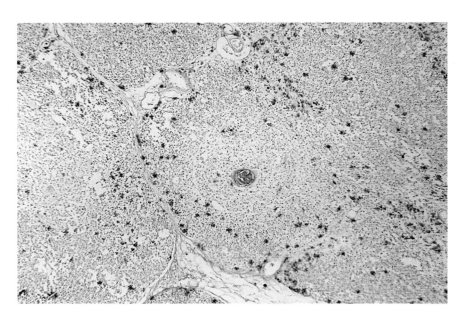

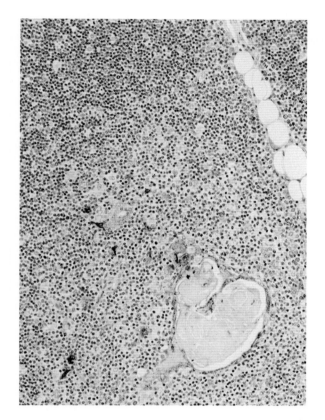

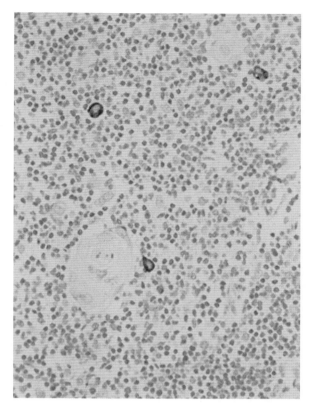

Figure 1-17

DISTRIBUTION OF INTERDIGITATING RETICULUM CELLS

S-100 protein–positive reticulum cells are present in the medulla (immunohistochemical stain for S-100 protein).

Figure 1-18

MYOID CELLS IN THE MEDULLA

Desmin-positive myoid cells are in close proximity to Hassall corpuscles (immunohistochemical stain for desmin).

role in the pathogenesis of myasthenia gravis (18). Connective tissue elements of the thymus include vessels, fibrous tissue, nerves, and fat.

Maturation of Thymocytes

The thymus provides the essential microenvironment for the differentiation and expansion of T-lymphocyte subpopulations. The process of T-lymphocyte expansion is an essential component of the complex network of immunoregulatory and cell-mediated effector functions.

The lymphoid population of the thymus has been shown to exhibit marked immunophenotypic heterogeneity, reflecting its functional diversity. The process of T-cell differentiation begins after hematopoietic progenitor cells, the prothymocytes, migrate from the bone marrow to the subcapsular area of the thymus, and involves an intrathymic migration through a theoretical cellular microenvironment from the cortex to

the medulla (8). During this process, interactions between the developing thymocytes and stromal thymic epithelial cells occur. Thymic nurse cell-thymocyte interaction is believed to be an essential step in this process (6). At the end of this maturation gradient, thymocytes with essentially mature phenotypes exit through the thymus to the peripheral lymphatic compartment, where functional diversification is completed.

The intrathymic portion of T-cell maturation has been divided empirically into three stages (fig. 1-19) (8,20). As the thymocytes encounter the various inductive, hormonal, and proliferative signals from various subpopulations of subcortical and cortical epithelial cells and interdigitating reticulum cells, genes, enzymes, and surface receptor molecules are activated. This differential expression of genes identifies thymocytes in each developmental stage. Although the molecular events operative at the

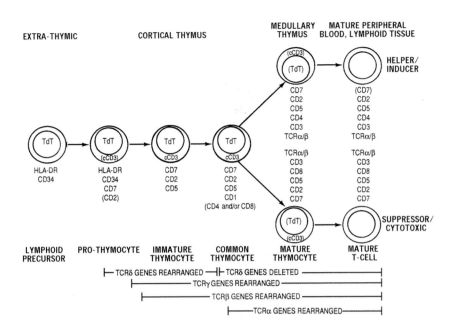

Figure 1-19

SCHEMATIC REPRESENTATION OF T-CELL ONTOGENY

The parentheses indicate that only a subpopulation of these cells expresses this marker. (Fig. 3.57 from Knowles DM. Immunophenotypic markers useful in the diagnosis and classification of hematopoietic neoplasms. In Knowles DM, ed. Neoplastic hematopathology, 2nd ed. Philadelphia: Lippincott Williams & Wilkins; 2001:178.)

early stage of thymocyte development are not completely understood, it is now appreciated that genes that encode the T-cell antigen receptors and other important surface molecules of the thymocytes interact with epithelial MHC antigens. The result of these interactions is a clonal selection for the T-lymphocyte antigen receptors that distinguishes self from nonself.

Involution

The thymus gland normally decreases in size and weight with advancing age. This process of involution starts at puberty, at which time the organ reaches its maximum absolute weight (3,12,16,20). Involution is accompanied by gradual changes in thymocyte populations relative to different rates of involution of the cortical and medullary epithelium. The thymus continues to serve as the site of T-cell differentiation and maturation throughout life.

In the young adult, the parenchymal loss is primarily due to a decreasing number of cortical thymocytes, with relative sparing of the epithelial elements. With advancing age, the epithelial component atrophies, and the gland consists of islands of spindle-shaped epithelial cells, with partially cystic, closely arranged Hassall corpuscles and scattered small lymphocytes in abundant adipose tissue (fig. 1-20). This gradual decrease in the volume of the thymus is fol-lowed by a more gradual decrease in the volume of the peripheral T-lymphocyte compartment.

The most striking microscopic changes seen in connection with involution relate to the distribution, architectural arrangement, and cytologic appearance of the epithelial cells (fig. 1-21) (20). Some epithelial cells have a spindle-shaped, mesenchymal-like appearance, while others arrange themselves in rosette-like formations devoid of central lumens. Sometimes, the thymic remnant may be mistaken for a neoplastic process due to the formation of round, solid epithelial nests or elongated strands of epithelial cells. These architectural formations may be present within lymphomas or seminomas and may be misinterpreted as evidence of the epithelial nature of the neoplasm (20).

Thymic remnants are often made up almost exclusively of lymphocytes, thus simulating lymph nodes (20). The involuted lymphoid tissue of the thymic remnant in fatty tissue, unlike the ordinary lymph node, does not have a capsule. In addition, with careful search of the periphery of the nests, epithelial cells may be seen encircling the nests, representing the residual coat of subcapsular cortical cells of the normal organ. Although the thymus in elderly individuals may appear totally replaced by adipose tissue, microscopic thymic remnants are almost always recognizable.

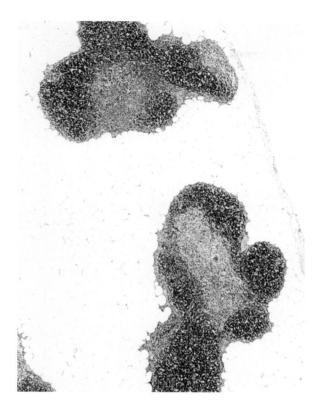 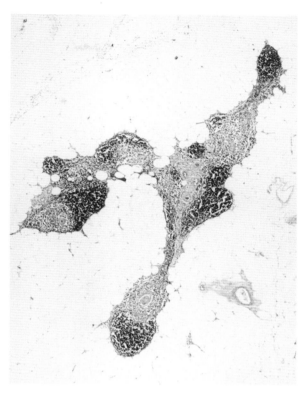

Figure 1-20

INVOLUTING THYMUS

The adult thymuses from a 56-year-old woman (left) and a 48-year-old man (right) show involution with fat replacement.

REFERENCES

1. Fukai I, Masaoka A, Hashimoto T, Yamakawa Y, Mizuno T, Tanamura O. Cytokeratins in normal thymus and thymic epithelial tumors. Cancer 1993;71:99-105.
2. Goldstein AL, Badamchian M. Thymosins: chemistry and biological properties in health and disease. Expert Opin Biol Ther 2004;4:559-73.
3. Griffith RC. Thymus gland. In: Kissane JM, ed. Anderson's pathology, 9th ed. St. Louis: CV Mosby; 1990:1493-516.
4. Hannappel E, Huff T. The thymosins. Prothymosin alpha, parathymosin, and beta thymosins: structure and function. Vitam Horm 2003;66:257-96
5. Huff T, Muller CS, Otto AM, Netzker R, Hannappel E. Beta-thymosins, small acidic peptides with multiple functions. Int J Biochem Cell Biol 2001;33:205-20
6. Kendall MD. Functional anatomy of the thymic microenvironment. J Anat 1991;177:1-29.
7. Kendall MD, Johnson HR, Singh J. The weight of the human thymus gland at necropsy. J Anat 1980;131:483-97.
8. Knowles DM. Immunophenotypic markers useful in the diagnosis and classification of hematopoietic neoplasms. In Knowles DM, ed. Neoplastic hematopathology, 2nd ed. Philadelphia: Lippincott Williams & Wilkins; 2001:93-226.
9. Kondo K, Mukai K, Sato Y, Matsuno Y, Shimosato Y, Monden Y. An immunohistochemical study of thymic epithelial tumors. III. The distribution of interdigitating reticulum cells and S-100 beta-positive small lymphocytes. Am J Surg Pathol 1990;14:1139-47.
10. Kuo T. Cytokeratin profiles of the thymus and thymomas: histogenetic correlations and proposal for a histological classification of thymomas. Histopathology 2000;36:403-14.
11. Liaw YF. Thymalfasin (thymosin-alpha 1) therapy in patients with chronic hepatitis B. J Gastroenterol Hepatol 2004;19:S73-5.

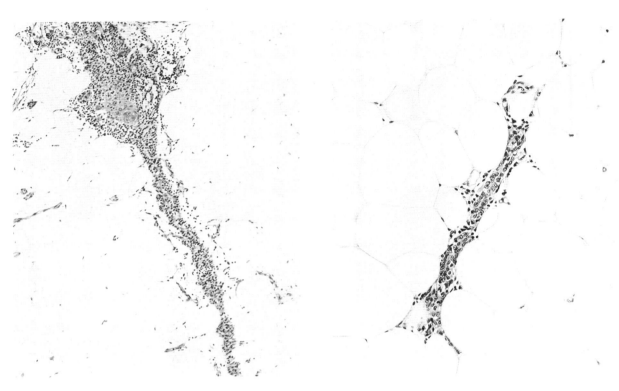

Figure 1-21

INVOLUTED THYMUS OF A 71-YEAR-OLD MAN

Left: Abortive Hassall corpuscles are surrounded by small lymphocytes and inconspicuous epithelial cells.
Right: Strands of epithelial cells are surrounded by a few small lymphocytes within the fat.

12. Marchevsky AM, Kaneko M. Surgical pathology of mediastinum, 2nd ed. New York: Raven Press; 1992.
13. Müller-Hermelink HK, Marino M, Palestro G. Pathology of thymic epithelial tumors. Curr Top Pathol 1986;75:207-68.
14. Nakamura H, Ayer-Le Lievre C. Neural crest cell and thymic myoid cells. Curr Top Dev Biol 1986;20:111-5.
15. Rosai J. Mediastinum. In Rosai J, ed. Ackerman's surgical pathology, 8th ed. St. Louis: CV Mosby; 1996:435-91.
15a. Rosai J. Mediastinum. In Rosai J, ed. Rosai and Ackerman's surgical pathology, 9th ed. New York: Mosby; 2004:459-513.
16. Rosai J, Levine GD. Tumors of the thymus. Atlas of Tumor Pathology, 2nd Series, Fascicle 13, Washington D.C.: Armed Forces Institute of Pathology; 1975.
17. Rosai J, Sobin LH. World Health Organization Histological Classification of Tumours, Histological Typing of Tumours of the Thymus, 2nd ed. Berlin-Heidelberg: Springer-Verlag; 1999.
18. Roxanis I, Micklem K, McConville J, Newsom-Davis J, Willcox N. Thymic myoid cells and germinal center formation in myasthenia gravis; possible role in pathogenesis. J Neuroimmunol 2002;125:185-97.
19. Ruco LP, Rosati S, Monardo R, Pescarmona E, Rendina EA, Baroni CD. Macrophages and interdigitating reticulum cells in normal thymus and in thymoma: an immunohistochemical study. Histopathology 1989;14:37-45.
20. Suster S, Rosai J. Thymus. In Sternberg SS, ed. Histology for pathologists, 2nd ed. Philadelphia: Lippincott-Raven; 1997:687-706.
21. Travis WD, Brambilla E, Müller-Hermelink HK, Harris CC, eds. World Health Organization Classification of Tumours. Pathology and genetics of tumours of the lung, pleura, thymus and heart. Lyon: IARC Press; 2004.
22. van de Wijngaert FP, Kendall MD, Schuurman HJ, Rademakers LH, Kater L. Heterogeneity of epithelial cells in the human thymus. An ultrastructural study. Cell Tissue Res 1984;237:227-37.
23. Wirt DP, Grogan TM, Nagle RB, et al. A comprehensive immunotopographic map of human thymus. J Histochem Cytochem 1988;36:1-12.

2 THYMOMA

CLASSIFICATION OF THYMIC TUMORS

In the second series Fascicle on thymic tumors published in 1976 (7), Rosai and Levine analyzed and summarized the classification systems for thymic tumors proposed by various investigators up to 1968, and pointed out the presence of "inconsistencies, inaccuracies, and in some instances mistaken concepts" (Table 2-1). According to them, tumors of the thymus included thymoma, thymolipoma, carcinoid tumors, germ cell tumors, malignant lymphoma, and secondary involvement of the thymus by carcinoma.

Other classification schemes have been proposed since then, mainly representing modifications of those presented in the second series Fascicle. These schemes are summarized in Table 2-2 (2,3,10–15). New entities have been recognized, such as large B-cell lymphoma with sclerosis and a variety of thymic carcinomas (5,12–15). In addition, a histogenetic classification of thymic epithelial tumors was proposed, using an approach different from that of the classification schemes widely used at that time (1,4,6)

Despite this cumulative work, there was still controversy regarding the classification of thymoma, thymic carcinoma, and carcinoid tumor (9). This was understandable because the origin of certain tumors and their interrelationships were not fully clarified. Therefore, in the third series Fascicle, published in 1997, we proposed a classification that was most widely used, easily understandable, and readily applicable at that time (Table 2-2) (11). The classification schemes of Lewis et al. (3) and Rosai and Levine (2,7) were modified further. In their schemes, factors considered for the morphologic typing of thymic tumors were epithelial cell morphology and the functional aspects of the epithelial cells, such as maturation of T cells, association of myasthenia gravis, and disease outcome. Although thymoma presents a variety of histologic features, no more detailed subtyping was attempted, except for listing the tumor by the predominant cell component, i.e., epithelial, lymphocytic, or mixed, and by the epithelial cell type, i.e., polygonal or spindle cell type, with or without cell atypia. Thymomas with a special morphology were described separately. In contrast, thymic carcinoma was divided into several subtypes.

In 1999, the second edition of the World Health Organization (WHO) *Histologic Typing of Tumors of the Thymus* (8) was published. Thymic tumors had not been included in the first edition, because knowledge of thymic tumors was woefully inadequate at the time. In the second edition classification, tumors of the thymus consist of epithelial tumors (thymoma and thymic carcinoma), neuroendocrine tumors (carcinoid tumor and small cell and large cell neuroendocrine carcinomas), germ cell tumors, lymphoid tumors, stromal tumors, metastatic tumors, and others (Table 2-3). Major changes were made in the classification of epithelial and neuroendocrine tumors as a result of a compromise proposal employing both the morphologic classification widely used in the United States and many other countries (2,3,10–15) and the histogenetic classification of Müller-Hermelink et al. (1,4) mainly used in Europe. This system is described in the chapters on thymoma, thymic carcinoma, and neuroendocrine carcinoma. Readers are referred to *Pathology and Genetics of Tumors of the Lung, Pleura, Thymus and Heart* published by the WHO in 2003 (14), which is more detailed in describing thymic tumors than the second edition (8).

THYMOMA

In a generic sense, *thymoma* means a tumor of the thymus, irrespective of cell of origin or degree of malignancy. This definition includes tumors of thymic epithelial cells, lymphocytes, fibrous tissue, vessels, fat, and any other constituents of the thymus. From the 1950s, thymoma was vaguely understood to be a benign or low-grade malignant tumor of thymic epithelial cell origin (24), although the concept that thymic epithelial cells and thymic lymphocytes had a common origin persisted. In the second series

Table 2-1

PROPOSED CLASSIFICATION OF THYMIC TUMORS I (up to 1968)[a]

Ewing (1916)
  Lymphosarcoma or thymoma
  Carcinoma (arising from the reticulum cells)
  Spindle cell sarcoma or myxosarcoma

Symmers (1932)
  Perithelioma
  Lymphosarcoma
  Epithelioma
  Spindle cell sarcoma
  Hodgkin disease

Hellwig (1914)
  Lymphosarcoma
  Leukosarcoma
  Hodgkin disease
  Carcinoma

Lowenhaupt (1948)
  Carcinoma of primitive epithelial reticulum
  Carcinoma of variegated cell pattern
  Carcinoma of granulomatous pattern
  Carcinoma of thymic round cell (lymphoepithelioma)
  Encapsulated thymoma (lymphosarcoma)
  Carcinoma of adamantinomatous pattern

Effler and McCormack (1956)
  Lymphomatous
    Lymphocytic
    Hodgkin disease
  Carcinomatous
    Lymphoepithelioma
    Epithelial

Thomson and Thackray (1957)
  Epithelial
    Differentiated or epidermoid
    Oval or spindle cell
    Lymphoepithelioma
    Granulomatous
    Undifferentiated
  Lymphoid
  Teratomatous

Andritsakis and Sommers (1959)
  Epithelial
    Undifferentiated
    Reticular
      Spindle cell
      Clear cell
    Trabecular
    Epidermoid
    Glandular
    Adenoacanthomatous
  Lymphoid
  Embryonic
  Fatty
  Cystic
  Hyperplastic

Bernatz et al. (1961)
  Predominantly lymphocytic
  Predominantly epithelial
  Predominantly mixed
  Predominantly spindle cell

Böhm and Strauch (1962)
  Epithelioma
    Spindle cell
    Reticular
    Solid to adenoid
    Mixed
  Carcinoma

Lattes (1962)
  Predominantly lymphoid
  Predominantly spindle cell
  Predominantly epithelial
  Predominantly rosette forming (pseudorosette type)
  Atypical epithelial thymoma with granulomatous foci
  Granulomatous thymoma
  Seminoma-like tumor of the thymus

Leg and Brady (1965)
  Small cell
  Protoplasmic
  Spindle cell

Watanabe (1966)
  Lymphocytic
  Mixed
    Even mixture
    Predominantly lymphocytic
    Predominantly epithelial
  Epithelial
    Polygonal
    Spindle

Friedman (1967)
  Lymphoepithelial
    Thymoma
    Lymphoepithelioma
    Thymocarcinoma
  Teratoid
    Germinoma
    Teratoma
    Teratocarcinoma
    Embryonal and choriocarcinoma
  Lymphomas
    Lymphosarcoma
    Hodgkin disease
  Myoid tumors
    Myosarcoma

Fisher (1968)
  Lymphocytic
  Epithelial
  Mixed lymphocytic and epithelial (lymphoepithelioma)
  Granulomatous
  Seminoma-like
  Squamous cell carcinoma
  Thymolipoma

[a]Table 3-1 from Fascicle 21, 3rd Series.

Table 2-2

PROPOSED CLASSIFICATION OF THYMIC TUMORS II (1976 to 1997)[a]

Rosai and Levine (1976)
  Thymoma
    By cell type: round-oval cell, spindle cell, mixed
    By degree of lymphocytic infiltration: absent, scant, moderate, predominant
    By extent: encapsulated, invasive
  Thymolipoma
  Carcinoid tumor
  Germ cell tumors
  Malignant lymphoma
  Tumor-like conditions

Levine and Rosai (1978)
  Thymoma
    Circumscribed
    Malignant:
      Type I (invasive thymoma with no or minimal atypia)
      Type II (cytologically malignant = thymic carcinoma)
        Squamous cell carcinoma
        Lymphoepithelioma-like carcinoma
        Clear cell carcinoma
        Sarcomatoid carcinoma
        Undifferentiated carcinoma

Wick et al. (1982) and Lewis et al. (1987)
  Composed of thymic epithelial cells
    Thymoma (cytologically benign)
      By extent: encapsulated, invasive, metastasizing
      By cell type: predominantly lymphocytic, mixed lympho-epithelial, predominantly epithelial, spindle cell
    Thymic carcinoma (cytologically malignant)
      Lymphoepithelioma-like poorly differentiated carcinoma
      Spindling squamous cell carcinoma
      Sarcomatoid carcinoma
      Small cell neuroendocrine carcinoma
  Composed of other elements
    Thymic carcinoid and neuroendocrine tumors
    Germ cell tumors
    Malignant lymphomas
    Thymolipoma and thymoliposarcoma

Snover et al. (1982)
  Thymic carcinoma
    Squamous cell carcinoma
    Lymphoepithelioma-like carcinoma
    Undifferentiated carcinoma
    Small cell undifferentiated (oat cell) carcinoma
    Mixed small cell undifferentiated squamous cell carcinoma
    Basaloid carcinoma
    Mucoepidermoid carcinoma
    Clear cell carcinoma
    Sarcomatoid carcinoma

Suster and Rosai (1991)
  Thymic carcinoma
    Low-grade histology
      Well-differentiated (keratinizing) squamous cell carcinoma
      Well-differentiated mucoepidermoid carcinoma
      Basaloid carcinoma
    High-grade histology
      Lymphoepithelioma-like carcinoma
      Small cell/neuroendocrine carcinoma
      Undifferentiated/anaplastic carcinoma
      Sarcomatoid carcinoma
      Clear cell carcinoma

Müller-Hermelink et al. (1985, 1992)
  Thymoma
    Medullary
    Mixed (medullary and cortical)
    Predominantly cortical
    Cortical
  Well-differentiated thymic carcinoma (organotypical, low grade)
  Thymic carcinoma
    Epidermoid
    Undifferentiated
    Endocrine carcinoma-carcinoid
  Germ cell tumors
  Malignant lymphomas

Shimosato and Mukai (Tumors of the Mediastinum, 1997)
  Thymolipoma and hamartomatous tumor
  Tumors of thymic epithelium
    Thymoma
      By extent: circumscribed: encapsulated, non-encapsulated (invasive but confined to within thymus); invasive (invading neighboring organs) with implantation or metastasis
      By histology: lymphocyte-predominant mixed lymphocytic and epithelial cell predominant
      By cell type: spindle cell, mixed spindle cell and polygonal cell, and polygonal-oval cell
      By cell atypia: absent, slight, moderate, and marked
    Thymic carcinoma
      Squamous cell carcinoma (well, moderately, and poorly differentiated)
      Basaloid carcinoma
      Mucoepidermoid carcinoma
      Adenosquamous carcinoma
      Adenocarcinoma
      Small cell/neuroendocrine carcinoma
      Lymphoepithelioma-like carcinoma
      Large cell carcinoma
      Clear cell carcinoma
      Sarcomatoid carcinoma
    Tumors composed of other elements
      Carcinoid tumor
      Germ cell tumors
      Malignant lymphomas

[a]Modified from Table 3-2 from Fascicle 21, Third Series.

of this Fascicle, Rosai and Levine (120) proposed that the designation of thymoma be restricted to neoplasms of thymic epithelial cells.

Until 1976, when the second series Fascicle was published, the lack of knowledge regarding thymic epithelial cells and lymphocytes resulted in many

Table 2-3

HISTOLOGIC CLASSIFICATION OF THE TUMORS OF THE THYMUS (WORLD HEALTH ORGANIZATION [WHO])[a]

Epithelial Tumors
Thymoma
  Type A (spindle cell, medullary)
  Type AB (mixed)
  Type B1 (lymphocyte-rich, lymphocytic, predomin-
    antly cortical, organoid)
  Type B2 (cortical)
  Type B3 (epithelial, atypical, squamoid, well-differ-
    entiated thymic carcinoma)
  Rare other thymomas
  Micronodular thymoma
  Metaplastic thymoma
  Microscopic thymoma
  Sclerosing thymoma
  Lipofibroadenoma
Thymic carcinoma (including neuroendocrine epithe-
  lial tumors of the thymus)
  Squamous cell carcinoma
  Basaloid carcinoma
  Mucopidermoid carcinoma
  Lymphoepithelioma-like carcinoma
  Sarcomatoid carcinoma
  Clear cell carcinoma
  Adenocarcinoma
    Papillary carcinoma
    Other adenocarcinoma
  Carcinoma with t(15;19) translocation
  Neuroendocrine carcinoma
    Well-differentiated neuroendocrine carcinoma
      (carcinoid tumor)
      Typical carcinoid
      Atypical carcinoid
    Poorly differentiated neuroendocrine carcinoma
      Small cell carcinoma, neuroendocrine type
      Large cell neuroendocrine carcinoma
  Undifferentiated carcinoma
Combined thymic epithelial tumors, including
  neuroendocrine carcinomas

Germ Cell Tumors (GCT) of the Mediastinum
GCTs of one histological type (pure GCTs)
  Seminoma
Embryonal carcinoma
Yolk sac tumor
Choriocarcinoma

Teratoma (mature, immature)
GCTs of more than one histological type (mixed GCTs)
  Variant: polyembryoma
GCTs with somatic-type malignancy
GCTs with associated hematologic malignancy

Mediastinal Lymphomas and Hematopoietic Neoplasms
B-cell lymphoma
  Primary mediastinal large B-cell lymphoma
  Thymic extranodal marginal zone B-cell lymphoma of
    mucosa-associated lymphoid tissue (MALT)
T-cell lymphoma
  Precursor T-lymphoblastic lymphoma/leukemia (LBL)
  Anaplastic large cell lymphoma and other rare mature
    T- and NK-cell lymphomas of the mediastinum
Hodgkin lymphoma of the mediastinum
"Gray zone" between Hodgkin and non-Hodgkin lymphoma
Histiocytic and dendritic cell tumors
  Langerhans cell histiocytosis/sarcoma
  Histiocytic sarcoma and malignant histiocytosis
  Follicular dendritic cell tumor/sarcoma
  Interdigitating dendritic cell sarcoma/tumor
Myeloid sarcoma and extramedullary acute myeloid leukemia

Mesenchymal Tumors of the Thymus and Mediastinum,
  including Thymolipoma
Thymolipoma
Lipoma of the mediastinum
Liposarcoma of the mediastinum
Solitary fibrous tumor
Synovial sarcoma
Vascular neoplasms
Rhabdomyocarcoma
Leiomyomatous tumors
Tumors of the peripheral nerves
Miscellaneous soft tissue neoplasms of the mediastinum

Rare Tumors of the Mediastinum
Ectopic tumors of the anterior mediastinum
  Ectopic thyroid tumors
  Ectopic parathyroid tumors

Metastasis to Thymus and Anterior Mediastinum

Other Rare Tumors

[a]With minor modifications and additions of recently recognized tumor entities for this Fascicle by the authors.

misnomers used to indicate thymoma, such as mixed tumor, perithelioma, benign lymphocytic lymphoma, lymphosarcoma, reticulum cell sarcoma, and granulomatous thymoma. According to the definitions of Levine and Rosai (73) and Rosai and Sobin (121), thymic carcinoma is included in thymoma (type II malignant thymoma of Levine and Rosai and type C thymoma of the WHO classification); germ cell tumors and malignant lymphomas are excluded. Many terms are used to indicate a variety of thymic carcinomas (146,152,159), which are detailed in the section dealing with thymic carcinoma.

We define thymoma as a benign or low-grade malignant tumor of the thymic epithelium with characteristic histologic features, frequently associated with a variable population of immature but non-neoplastic T cells (57,58,127,133,135). We consider thymic carcinoma to be an entity different from the more commonly encountered "thymoma," because of the marked differences in the morphologic and functional properties that exist between these two tumor types. We define thymic carcinoma as a tumor composed of nests and diffuse growth of obviously atypical cells of an invasive nature, as seen in carcinomas of other organs, although completely encapsulated in rare instances. There are no immature (or cortical) T cells, and the phenotype of the infiltrating lymphocytes is similar to that of carcinomas of other organs (127,135).

In the most recent 2004 WHO classification (151), thymomas are defined as "neoplasms arising from or exhibiting differentiation towards thymic epithelial cells with no overt cell atypia, and thymic carcinomas as malignant epithelial tumors with overt cytologic atypia, almost invariable invasiveness and lack of thymus-like features." In this Fascicle, the WHO Classification of Tumours, Pathology and Genetics of Tumours of the Lung, Pleura, Thymus and Heart (151) is used supplemented by the widely used, morphologic and histogenetic classification.

General Features

The clinical manifestations, diagnosis, pathologic features, staging, and treatment of thymoma have been reviewed by Morgenthaler et al. (89), who also discussed prognosis.

Thymoma is the most common and most frequently occurring neoplasm not only in the anterior mediastinal compartment but also in the entire mediastinum, if solid tumors with surgical indications are considered. There appears to be no predilection for race or sex, or geographic distribution, although females predominate over males in many published series. Table 2-4 indicates the histologic types and number of cases of mediastinal tumors resected surgically at the National Cancer Center, Tokyo, during a 21-year period from 1962 to 1992 (no complete data after 1993 are available at present). The number of patients with thymoma initially treated at this institute during the previous 42 years (from 1962 to 2003) was 130 (54 males, 76 females); on average three thymomas were resected per year. During the same period, about 5,500 lung cancers were resected. During the year 2004, 465 primary lung cancers, 17 thymomas, and 1 thymic carcinoma were resected. In a 45-year period (1949 to 1993) at the Memorial Sloan-Kettering Cancer Center, the number of thymomas resected was 118 (22), and in a 30-year period (1942 to 1971) at the Johns Hopkins Hospital, the number was 49 (124). In a 41-year period (1941 to 1981) 283 thymomas were resected at the Mayo Clinic (75).

Table 2-4

SURGICALLY RESECTED MEDIASTINAL TUMORS AND TUMOR-LIKE CONDITIONS[a]

Histologic Types	Number	
Cyst	55	
Bronchogenic cyst		26
Thymic cyst		16
Coelomic cyst		13
Mediastinal goiter	6	
Thymic lesions	114	
Hyperplasia		8
Thymoma		79
Squamous cell carcinoma		17
Undifferentiated carcinoma		5
Carcinoid tumor		5
Germ cell tumor	60	
Teratoma, benign		45
malignant (combining malignant germ cell tumors)		12
Seminoma		1
Choriocarcinoma		2
Neurogenic tumor	67	
Paraganglioma		3
Schwannoma, benign		44
malignant		3
Neurofibromatosis		5
Ganglioneuroma		8
Neuroblastoma		2
Ganglioneuroblastoma		2
Mesenchymal tumor	6	
Lipoma		2
Liposarcoma		1
Mesenchymal chondrosarcoma		1
Malignant fibrous histiocytoma		1
Angiosarcoma		1
Malignant lymphoma[b]	12	
Non-Hodgkin lymphoma[c]		9
Hodgkin disease		3
Others	6	
Fat necrosis		2
Giant lymph node hyperplasia (Castleman disease)		4
Total	326	

[a]National Cancer Center Hospital, 1962-1992; no detailed data on resected mediastinal tumors by histologic type during the period of 1993-2003 are available. The numbers of mediastinal tumors of major histologic types such as thymoma, germ cell tumors, etc. are described in the text.
[b]Including cases diagnosed by biopsy only.
[c]Including four cases of B-cell type diffuse large cell lymphoma and one case of probable low-grade B-cell lymphoma of mucosa-associated lymphoid tissue.

Although thymoma occurs in children (115), it is much more frequent in adults, particularly during the 5th and 6th decades. The median age reported is about 50 years, and in our series the mean age was 54 ± 13 years. Seven thymomas

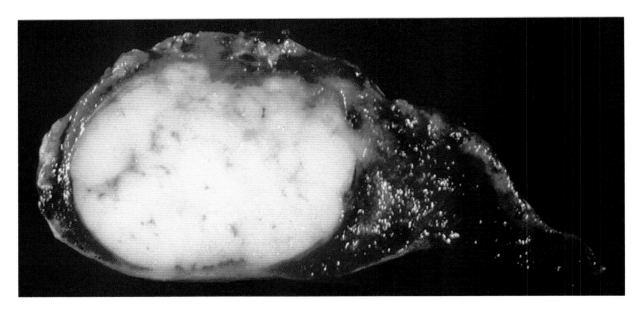

Figure 2-1

ECTOPIC THYMOMA IN THE LUNG

A 3.5 x 2.7 x 2.0 cm tumor in the posterior segment of the right upper lobe of the lung was resected by segmentectomy. The cut surface of the intrapulmonary thymoma is pale yellow and lobulated. Computerized tomography (CT) of the thorax 1 year after surgery revealed neither recurrence of the tumor nor any lesion in the mediastinum. (Courtesy of Dr. Masashi Fukayama, Tokyo, Japan.)

in children under the age of 16, including four cases with "unusual features," were reported by Cajal and Suster (23); five cases of thymoma in children aged 11 to 15 years treated at three different institutions were reported by Pescarmona et al. (105). None of the cases were associated with myasthenia gravis but one was complicated by hypoplastic anemia. Most patients had a good outcome. There is one report of thymoma associated with regenerative and aplastic anemia in a 5-year-old (147). It should be noted that thymic carcinoma also occurs in children, and almost always has a rapidly aggressive course.

Clinical Features

The majority of thymomas are found in the normal location of the thymus, i.e., the anterior mediastinum, sometimes extending to the superior compartment. Ectopic occurrence of thymoma includes the neck as high as the submandibular region and the middle or inferior mediastinum, close to either the main bronchi or diaphragm (26,75,124). Such locations result from failure of the thymus to descend or from excessive descent. The presence of thymic tissue

near or attached to the thyroid gland is often noted in surgical specimens obtained at the time of thyroid surgery. Rarely, ectopic thymoma is present in the posterior mediastinum, the parietal or visceral pleura, or even inside the lung parenchyma (fig. 2-1) (38,47,86,88). In such cases, however, the alternative possibility of a solitary metastasis from a small undetected primary tumor in the thymus should always be considered.

Symptoms and signs related to the presence of thymoma include cough, chest pain, dyspnea, weight loss, unexplained fever, dysphagia, hoarseness, swollen neck lymph nodes, superior vena cava syndrome, and pleural effusion. The most common complication associated with thymoma is myasthenia gravis, which has been reported to occur in 30 to 50 percent of patients seen in general hospitals (75,124). In contrast, 20 to 30 percent of patients with myasthenia gravis have thymoma. Myasthenia gravis occurs when neuromuscular transmission is blocked by an antibody against the acetylcholine receptor at the neuromuscular junction; the antibody is produced mainly in the thymus (55,71).

Thymoma is less frequently associated with pure red cell aplasia or hypoplasia, hypogammaglobulinemia, and collagen diseases such as systemic lupus erythematosus and rheumatoid arthritis; pure red cell aplasia is seen in 5 percent of patients with thymoma in general hospitals and half of the patients with pure red cell aplasia have associated thymomas (122). The thymoma is often of spindle cell or medullary type (type A); however, the five thymomas associated with pure red cell aplasia studied by Kuo and Shih (67) showed various histologic features and none was a spindle cell thymoma. They concluded that the pathogenesis of pure red cell aplasia associated with thymoma does not seem to be related to a particular histologic type. Although pure red cell aplasia is an autoimmune disease, its exact cause is not yet known.

The frequency of thymoma complicated by such paraneoplastic syndromes was much lower in a cancer hospital; here, the frequency of asymptomatic thymoma found incidentally by routine chest X-ray examination accounted for over 40 percent of all cases (20). At the National Cancer Center Hospital in Tokyo, only 16 of 130 thymomas (12.3 percent) were associated with myasthenia gravis (95) and only 1 with pure red cell hypoplasia (57).

Diagnostic Approach

The presence of thymoma in the anterior mediastinum is revealed by plain posterior-anterior and lateral chest roentgenograms in most instances, although tumors less than 2 cm in diameter may not be evident (40). Oval or round, often homogeneous densities with distinct borders project from the mediastinum into the right or left pleural cavity with equal frequency, and in some instances, project into both pleural spaces (fig. 2-2). The tumor may have a multinodular contour.

Slightly less than half of all thymomas are located in the upper and middle thirds of the mediastinum and the remainder in the lower third. Calcification may be present (fig. 2-3). Computerized tomography (CT) confirms the location and may reveal some characteristics of the tumor, such as cystic changes and involvement of surrounding structures such as the great vessels, bronchi, or lungs, or may reveal small tumors undetectable by plain chest X-ray

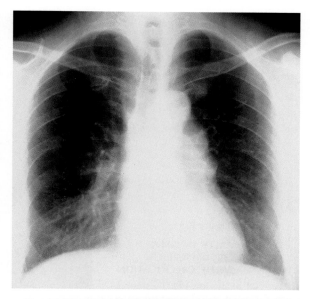
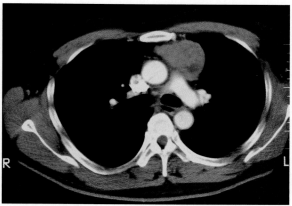

Figure 2-2

NONINVASIVE THYMOMA

Top: Plain chest X ray shows a well-defined, tumorous density superimposed on the left pulmonary hilus and superior portion of the cardiac border.

Bottom: CT at the level of the tracheal carina reveals a clearly defined tumor of nonhomogeneous density between the sternum, ascending aorta, and truncus of the pulmonary artery, enhanced by radiopaque material. Note the smooth border facing the left lung. (Fig. 3-7 from Fascicle 21, Third Series.)

examination (figs. 2-4, 2-5) (94,123). These findings, however, are not specific for thymoma, and may be seen in other mediastinal tumors such as germ cell tumor, carcinoid tumor, and malignant lymphoma. Thymomas invading the lung may be difficult to differentiate from lung cancer invading the mediastinum, and

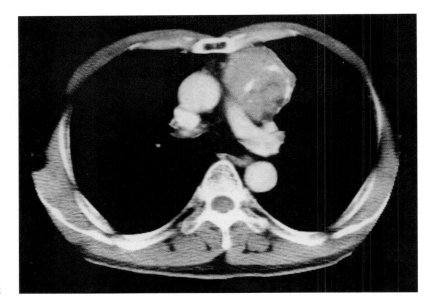

Figure 2-3

**MINIMALLY INVASIVE
BUT CIRCUMSCRIBED
THYMOMA WITH CALCIFICATION**

Top: CT at the level of the tracheal carina reveals a well-defined tumorous density enhanced by radiopaque material about 5 cm in diameter on the left side of the ascending aorta and adjacent to the left side of the pulmonary artery truncus. The nonhomogeneous tumor displaces the superior division of the left upper pulmonary lobe, and contains a ring-shaped calcification.

Bottom: The cut surface of the tumor reveals hemorrhage, cystic change, and invasive growth through a thick calcified capsule.

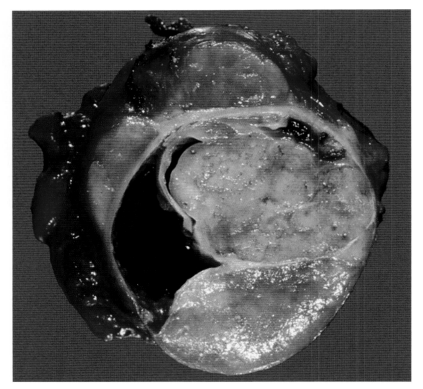

thymomas located along the main bronchus may show radiographic features similar to those of mediastinal giant lymph node hyperplasia (Castleman disease). The diagnosis of thymoma can be established almost with certainty when myasthenia gravis, red cell hypoplasia, or hypogammaglobulinemia is associated.

The cytologic and histologic diagnosis of thymoma can be made either by percutaneous needle biopsy or biopsy through a mediastinoscope or a thoracoscope. Percutaneous needle biopsy under CT guidance is an excellent diagnostic approach, particularly for anterior mediastinal tumors. With mediastinoscopy,

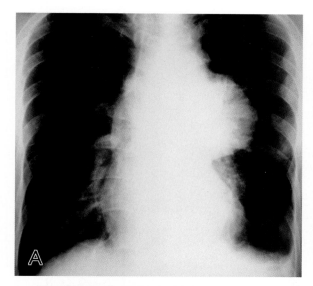

Figure 2-4

INVASIVE THYMOMA WITH PLEURAL IMPLANTATIONS

A: A tumor 7 cm in diameter projects into the left lung field and widens the mediastinal density. Tumors convex toward the lung are scattered in the left lateral pleura, and effusion is seen.

B: CT at the level of the tracheal carina discloses the irregular invasive growth of an anterior mediastinal tumor into the superior division of the left upper pulmonary lobe. Implanted tumors are on the left parietal pleura with effusion.

C: CT 11 cm below the level of the tracheal carina reveals an irregular, nonhomogeneous anterior mediastinal tumor enhanced by radiopaque material, which displaces posteriorly the ascending aorta, pulmonary artery truncus, and left pulmonary vein.

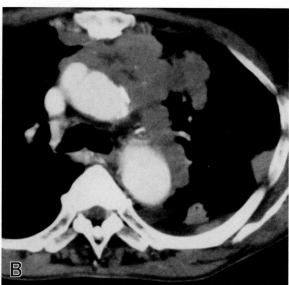

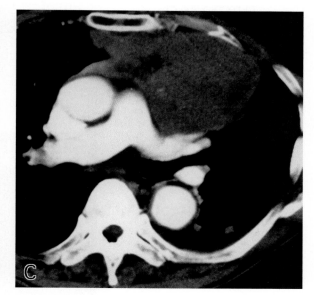

lesions in the superior and anterior mediastinum and around the trachea up to the level of tracheal bifurcation can be directly reached. Compared with the mediastinoscopic approach, the thoracoscopic approach enables easier and safer biopsy with a wide visual field, but there is a risk of tumor implantation. If sufficient material is obtained, a diagnosis is possible in most cases (figs. 2-6, 2-7). Yonemori et al. (164b) reported that CT-guided percutaneous cutting needle biopsy (PCNB) is a reliable method for diagnosing thymic tumors and that there is a good concordance with the WHO histologic classification between the diagnosis based on

a CT-guided PCNB specimen and that based on a surgically resected specimen. Material obtained by aspiration for cytologic examination with Papanicolaou stain should be fixed immediately to avoid any effect of drying on the cells. The correct cytologic diagnosis can be made by examination of properly prepared aspiration cytology smears together with chest X-ray findings (see Cytologic Findings).

Transbronchial biopsy should be attempted for tumors invading the lung and bronchi (fig. 2-8) (16,134). The cytology of the pleural effusion may disclose the phenotypic characteristics of the thymoma cells. If possible, part of the

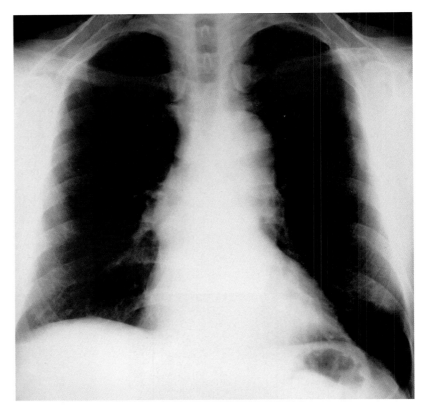

Figure 2-5

**A SMALL THYMOMA
DETECTED BY CT**

Top: The ascending aorta protrudes toward the right lung, but there is no abnormal density in the mediastinum. The lateral view revealed no abnormal density behind the sternum.

Bottom: CT at the level of the tracheal carina discloses a tumorous density 1.5 cm in diameter in the fatty tissue of the anterior mediastinum, anterior to the pulmonary artery truncus.

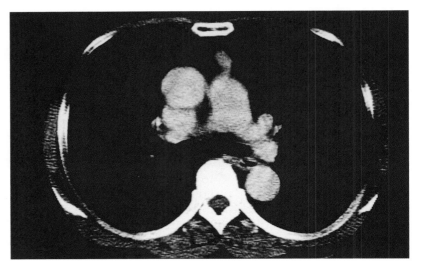

material obtained should be kept frozen or fixed in cold acetone (at 4°C) and embedded in paraffin for preservation of antigens, particularly the surface antigens of the constituent cells, both epithelial cells and lymphocytes (127).

The presence of epithelial cells, which are always positive for cytokeratin and frequently for CD57, and immature (cortical) T cells, which are positive for terminal deoxynucleotidyltransferase (TdT), CD1a, CD3, CD4, CD8, and CD99, is diagnostic of both encapsulated and invasive thymoma (27,33,127). Immature T cells are absent in thymic carcinoma, in which epithelial cells show variable immunohistochemical

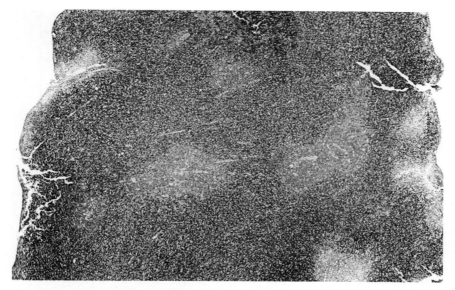

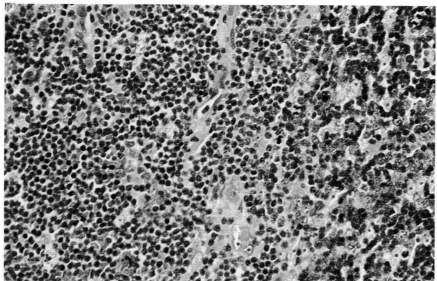

Figure 2-6

LYMPHOCYTE-PREDOMINANT (TYPE B1) THYMOMA DIAGNOSED BY PERCUTANEOUS NEEDLE BIOPSY

Top: The entire width of needle-biopsied tissue shows several lighter-stained areas of medullary differentiation.

Bottom: The border of the area of medullary differentiation reveals uniform, small mature lymphocytes and epithelial cells with or without prominent nucleoli in the "medullary" zone (left half of the figure). An increased number of epithelial cells with distinct, round nucleoli and active lymphocytes is seen in the "cortical" zone (right half of the figure). Immunohistochemistry for cytokeratin in epithelial cells is shown in figure 2-84.

profiles depending on the histologic subtype (see Thymic Carcinoma). For germ cell tumors, tests should be made for the presence of placental alkaline phosphatase, alpha-fetoprotein (AFP), and beta-human chorionic gonadotropin (β-hCG); for lymphoma, leukocyte common antigen (LCA), and B-cell and T-cell markers should be checked.

Serum assays for tumor markers and phenotype analyses of circulating lymphocytes are not useful in establishing a diagnosis of thymoma. AFP and β-hCG should be checked when a malignant germ cell tumor is suspected.

Gross Findings

About one to two thirds of all thymomas are reported to be "encapsulated" or well circumscribed, with "no gross invasion of adjacent structures or implants" (20,47,75,124). Of 130 evaluable surgically resected thymomas seen at the National Cancer Center Hospital in Tokyo, 40 were completely encapsulated, 54 were minimally invasive (thymoma surrounded by a capsule that is focally infiltrated by tumor growth or that invades the mediastinal fat), 25 were widely invasive (thymoma spreading by

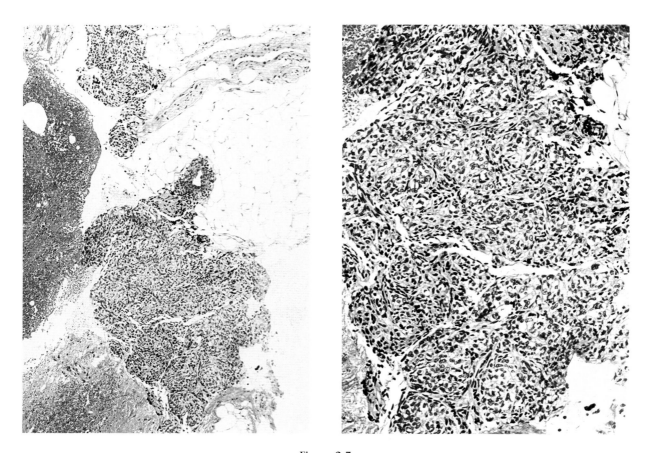

Figure 2-7

**PREDOMINANTLY EPITHELIAL, SPINDLE CELL (TYPE A)
THYMOMA DIAGNOSED BY PERCUTANEOUS NEEDLE BIOPSY**

Left: Low-power magnification shows fragments of tumor, fat, and blood.
Right: The tumor is composed of small lobules of oval to short spindle-shaped epithelial cells with bland nuclei and inconspicuous nucleoli. Lymphocytes are few.

direct extension into adjacent structures such as pericardium, large vessels, or lung), 10 had pleural or pericardial implants, and 1 had a distant metastasis (lung) (see Table 2-6) (95). The size of the grossly visible tumor varied from 1.2 to 28.0 cm in diameter. Microscopically, the smallest were less than 1 mm in diameter; these were invisible to the naked eye and were found incidentally in thymuses removed at the time of lung or cardiac surgery or at autopsy (these microscopic lesions are considered by some as nodular hyperplasia rather than thymoma [see Microscopic Thymoma]). In one instance, three microscopic thymomas were found in the thymus of a single individual. Similar cases of multiple microscopic thymomas have been reported (108). Thymomas associated with myasthenia gravis

are smaller than those unassociated with this disease. Spindle cell (type A) thymoma is larger than polygonal cell type thymoma.

Thymoma may be round or oval with a smooth external surface, sometimes with attached fatty thymic tissue, or it may be irregularly nodular or bosselated resulting from division of the thymoma into various-sized lobules by fibrous tissue (figs. 2-9–2-11). Calcification and, less frequently, ossification may be present in the fibrous capsule or septa dividing the lobules. Rarely, a plaque-like tumor extends from the thymus inferiorly along the anterior thoracic rib cage. The tumor should be carefully examined grossly for evidence of transcapsular invasion, direct invasion of neighboring organs or tissue, and areas of tumor exposure due to incomplete removal.

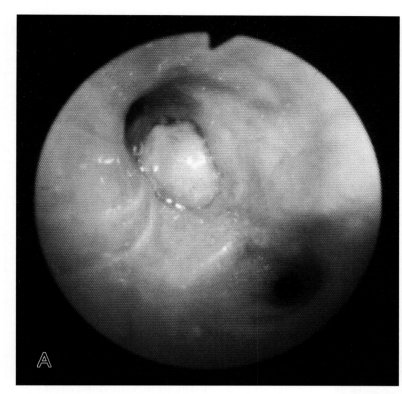

Figure 2-8

THYMOMA INVADING THE LUNG DIAGNOSED BY TRANSBRONCHIAL BIOPSY

A: Fiberoptic bronchoscopy reveals a polypoid tumor projecting into the left B3 bronchus.

B: Transbronchial biopsy specimen consists of lymphoid cells and larger, lighter-stained epithelial cells with a few perivascular spaces showing hyalinization. A diagnosis of mixed lymphocytic and epithelial (type B2) thymoma was made.

C: Surgically resected specimen (see fig. 2-14) reveals a tumor projecting into the bronchial lumen. Immunostaining of frozen sections revealed frequent CD1a-, CD3-, and CD4- or CD8-positive lymphocytes, confirming the diagnosis of thymoma. (Figs. 2-8 and 2-14 are from the same patient.)

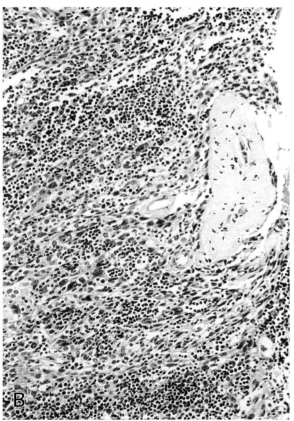

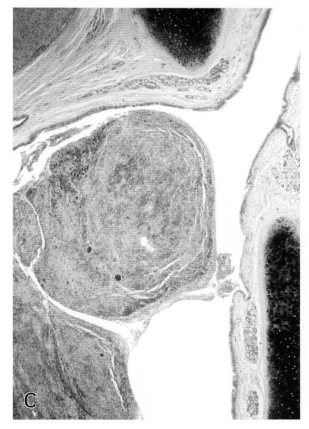

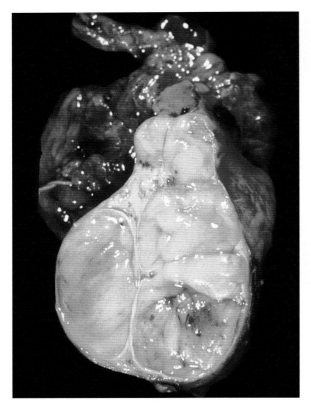

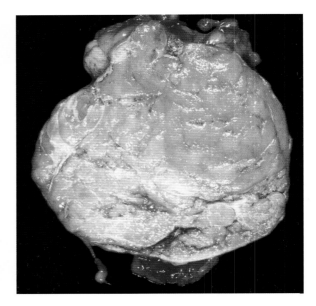

Figure 2-10

ENCAPSULATED THYMOMA (PREDOMINANTLY EPITHELIAL, SPINDLE CELL [TYPE A])

An oval tumor is completely encapsulated. The cut surface is pale tan, bulging, and irregularly lobulated. (Figs. 2-10, 2-37, 2-88, and 2-90 are from the same patient.)

Figure 2-9

ENCAPSULATED THYMOMA (MIXED LYMPHOCYTIC AND EPITHELIAL [TYPE B2])

A bottle-shaped tumor is encapsulated. It has a bulging, homogeneous, faintly lobulated, ivory colored cut surface.

The cut surface of thymoma is pale tan or gray-pink and is often lobulated. Lobulation is the most characteristic feature of thymoma and is present in most cases; however, lobulation is absent in a few thymomas regardless of the degree of lymphocytic infiltration. Cystic changes are frequently seen. Cysts vary from very small and barely recognizable, containing clear fluid, to large cysts filled with blood or yellowish brown grumous material (figs. 2-12, 2-13). In rare cases, almost the entire tumor may become cystic with irregular trabeculae on the inner surface (145). A cystic lesion should always be examined for any remnant of thymoma. Examination of multiple blocks may be necessary to prove the cystic nature of the lesion.

Foci of coagulation necrosis may be seen, but are infrequent. Twenty-five cases of thymoma with prominent cystic and hemorrhagic changes and areas of necrosis and infarction were studied by Moran and Suster (85). In 23 cases, the tumors were well circumscribed and encapsulated; areas of infarction were always intimately associated with vasoocclusive and thrombotic phenomena (see fig. 2-103) and were not associated with an adverse outcome. The presence of coagulation necrosis does not necessarily indicate a malignant nature, although it is more frequent and more extensive in thymic carcinoma than in invasive thymoma. The hemorrhage seen in some thymomas is due to surgical manipulation of the tumor in most instances.

Two or more separate nodules of thymoma may be found in a thymus. The authors have seen a case with multiple nodules of both thymoma and thymic carcinoma, with some nodules showing transitional features between the two (see figs. 3-7, 3-17) (90). Some cases of multiple thymoma have been reported, and this raises the question of the possibility of multicentricity (21,50a,97a,164a).

Thymoma invading the lung or other adjacent structures may be lobulated and even partly encapsulated at the site of invasion, although

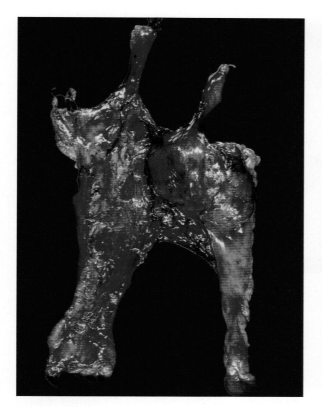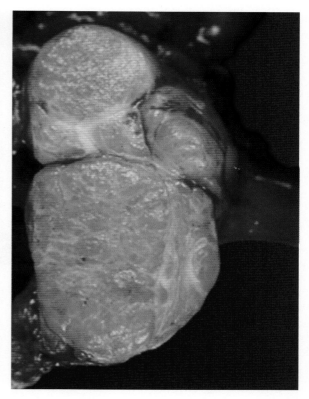

Figure 2-11

MINIMALLY INVASIVE, CIRCUMSCRIBED THYMOMA (MIXED LYMPHOCYTIC AND EPITHELIAL, AND MIXED POLYGONAL AND SPINDLE CELL [TYPE AB])

Left: The tumor is in the left lobe of the thymus.

Right: The cut surface bulges, is pale tan, and is faintly lobulated. The tumor invaded the capsule at a few points but still remained within the thymus.

the advancing borders are not always distinct, and even at times blurred (figs. 2-14, 2-15). Tumors implanted on the pleura, pericardium, and diaphragm are grossly similar to the primary tumor, as are metastatic foci in lymph nodes and distant organs. Lobulation may be less distinct than in the primary tumor, due probably to a reduction in the amount of fibrous tissue (fig. 2-16).

Microscopic Findings

The majority of thymomas are either completely or partially encapsulated by a fibrous capsule of varying thickness, which connects with the dense fibrous bands within the tumor that divide it into lobules (fig. 2-17). The capsule may contain calcium deposits, but ossification is rare (fig. 2-18). Since a capsule is absent in microscopic thymomas found incidentally in routine sections of the thymus taken at the

time of lung and cardiac surgery or at autopsy (see figs. 2-65–2-67) (108,135), it is assumed that capsule formation is the result of the host's defense mechanism and reflects the growth properties of the tumor. That is, the slower the tumor growth, the thicker and more complete the capsule. A capsule is also found at the advancing border of tumors invading the lung and in implantation metastases (fig. 2-19). Lack of a capsule at the advancing border may indicate a tumor with accelerated growth, since it appears more frequently in thymoma of the predominantly polygonal (round or oval) epithelial cell type (fig. 2-20). At times, the thick fibrous capsule is invaded by the tumor, which may bud outside the capsule into non-neoplastic thymic tissue (fig. 2-21) and extend into the lobules of the non-neoplastic thymus (fig. 2-22). Encapsulation of such budding occurs occasionally (fig. 2-23). For staging

33

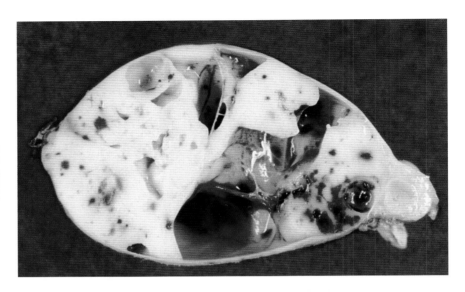

Figure 2-12

ENCAPSULATED CYSTIC THYMOMA (PREDOMINANTLY LYMPHOCYTIC [TYPE B1])

Postformalin-fixed cut surface reveals an ivory colored tumor with multiple cystic spaces varying from pinhead sized to several centimeters in diameter. Small hemorrhages are also seen.

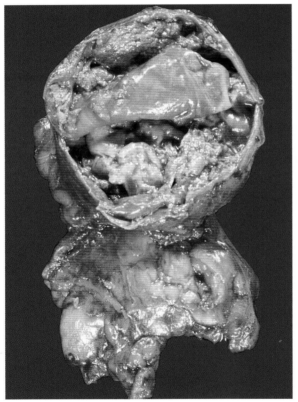

Figure 2-13

ENCAPSULATED CYSTIC THYMOMA (PREDOMINANTLY LYMPHOCYTIC [TYPE B1])

A tumor encapsulated by a thick capsule contains brown liquid and necrotic material. The lining is partly smooth and partly irregular with excrescences of necrotic and viable tumor tissue.

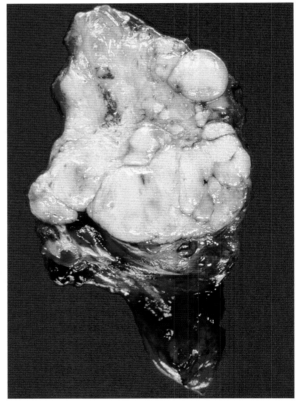

Figure 2-14

THYMOMA, MIXED LYMPHOCYTIC AND EPITHELIAL (TYPE B2), INVADING THE LUNG PARENCHYMA AND A BRONCHUS

An irregularly shaped tumor is partly lobulated and partly nodular, with a distinct border at the margin invading the lung tissue. A small polypoid projection into the left B3 bronchus is noted in the left lower corner.

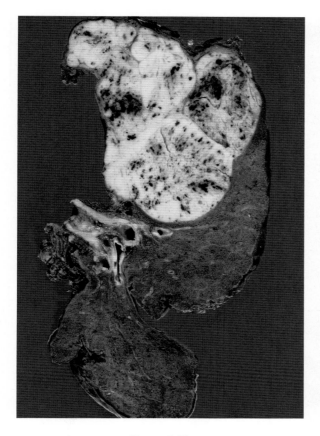

Figure 2-15

**INVASIVE THYMOMA (LYMPHOCYTE
PREDOMINANT [B1/B2 TYPE])**

About half of the tumor is in the mediastinum and the rest in the upper lobe (S1+2, S5) of the left lung. The cut surface shows faint lobulation, areas of hemorrhage, and nodular infiltrative borders. The borders are sharply defined in large areas and blurred in small areas.

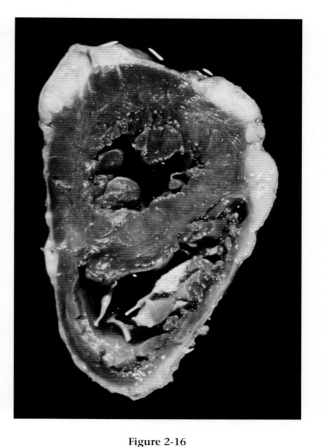

Figure 2-16

**THYMOMA IMPLANTED ON
THE PERICARDIUM (AUTOPSY CASE)**

This ivory colored, faintly lobulated tumor obliterated the pericardial sac and invaded the myocardium at the anterior and posterolateral border of the left ventricle. Histologically, it was mixed lymphocytic and epithelial and polygonal cell type (type B2).

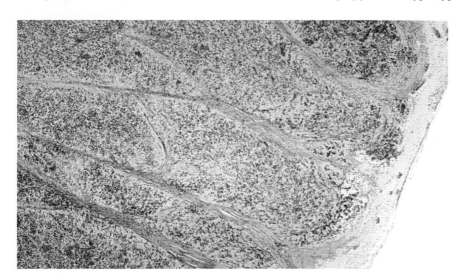

Figure 2-17

ENCAPSULATED THYMOMA

The tumor is encapsulated by thick collagenous tissue and subdivided into irregular lobules by fibrous tissue.

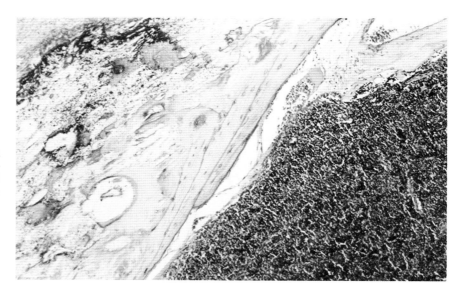

Figure 2-18

OSSIFICATION IN THE CAPSULE OF THYMOMA

Ossification with calcification is evident in the capsule of lymphocyte-predominant (type B1) thymoma of polygonal cell type.

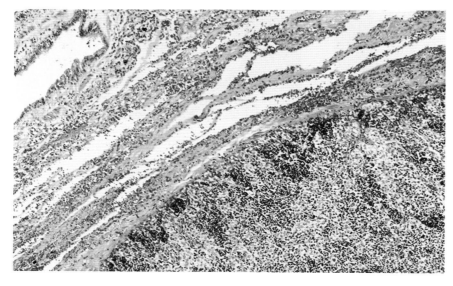

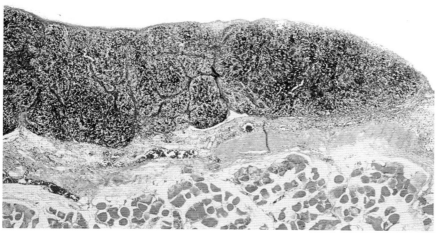

Figure 2-19

THYMOMA WITH INVASION INTO THE LUNG AND IMPLANTATION METASTASIS TO THE DIAPHRAGM

Top: Thymoma of the mixed lymphocytic and epithelial cell type (type B2) has invaded the lung, where a thin collagenous capsule has formed.

Bottom: The tumor implanted on the diaphragm is lobulated and has a thin capsule.

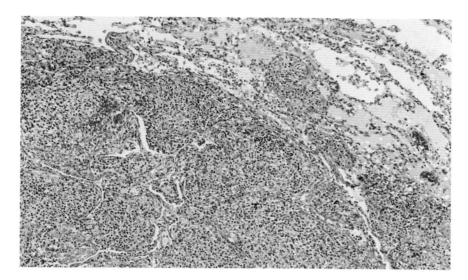

Figure 2-20

THYMOMA INVADING THE LUNG

At the advancing front of a thymoma of predominantly epithelial and polygonal cell type with mild nuclear atypia (type B3), tumor nests are floating in alveoli without forming a fibrous capsule. (Figs. 2-20 and 2-36 are from the same patient.)

Figure 2-21

THYMOMA INVADING THE CAPSULE

A mushroom shape results when the tumor invades its own thick capsule. Invasive tumor involves non-neoplastic thymic tissue with a Hassall corpuscle at its apex.

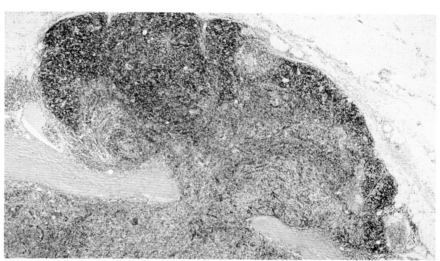

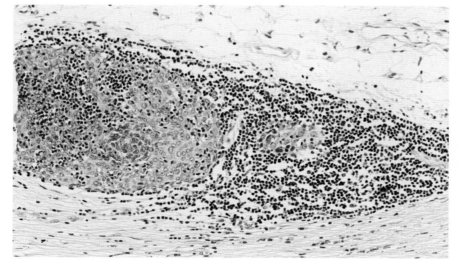

Figure 2-22

THYMOMA INVADING THYMIC TISSUE OUTSIDE THE THICK CAPSULE

Thymic tissue attached to the fibrous capsule of a thymoma has been invaded by a thymoma of the polygonal cell type with distinct nucleoli, identical in histology to the largely encapsulated thymoma.

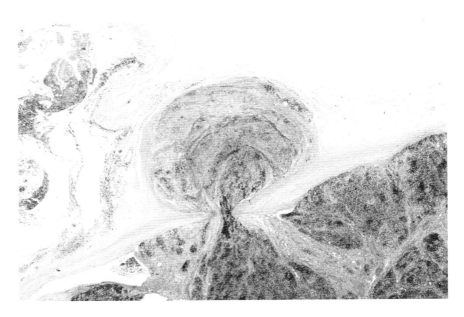

Figure 2-23

THYMOMA INVADING THE CAPSULE

A round tumor formed outside the thymoma capsule is also encapsulated.

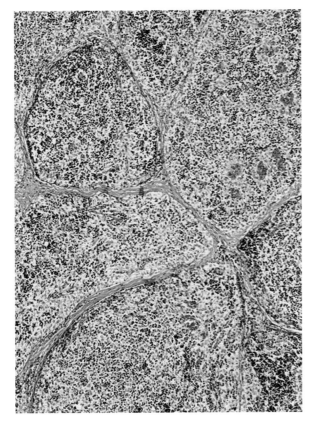

Figure 2-24

THYMOMA (MIXED LYMPHOCYTIC AND EPITHELIAL [TYPE B2])

The tumor shows distinct lobulation due to bands of collagenous tissue.

purposes, tumors with encapsulated buds must be determined in the future to be either encapsulated or minimally invasive.

The lobules of a thymoma subdivided by fibrous trabeculae vary in size and shape, are often irregular in outline, and have distinctive borders in many instances (fig. 2-24). The boundaries may be blurred, however, particularly in cases of mixed thymoma (mixed spindle cell and oval or polygonal cell [type A] thymoma), where the fibrous trabeculae themselves are composed of spindle-shaped neoplastic epithelial cells with a fibroblast-like appearance (fig. 2-25).

Another characteristic histologic feature seen in about two thirds of thymomas is the formation of perivascular spaces. These are formed and bordered at times by palisading epithelial cells with a basement membrane. They contain mature lymphocytes of both B-cell and T-cell types, plasma cells, mast cells, and plasma fluid. They vary in size from minute lesions, recognizable only by careful observation, to those as large as 1 mm in diameter. Near the center, a small vessel, probably a capillary or postcapillary venule, can be identified (figs. 2-26–2-28). The spaces may contain foamy macrophages and show a tendency to hyalinize. Hyalinization usually begins with the exudation of fibrinous materials into the spaces, followed by gradual hyalinization and obliteration of the spaces (figs. 2-29–2-31).

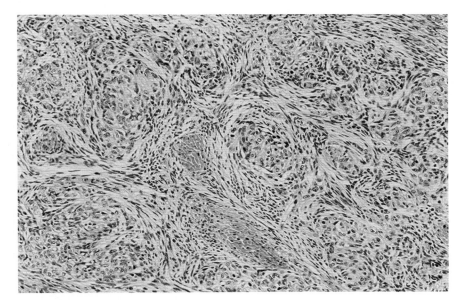

Figure 2-25

THYMOMA OF MIXED OVAL/POLYGONAL AND SPINDLE CELL TYPE (TYPE A)

The tumor is subdivided into lobules consisting of oval/polygonal cells by bands of fibroblast-like spindle-shaped tumor cells.

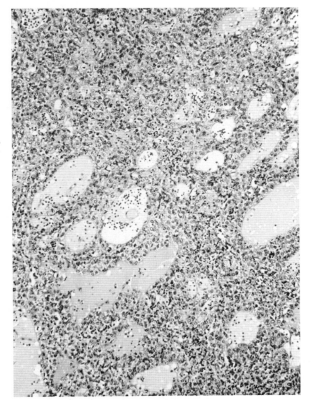

Figure 2-26

PERIVASCULAR SPACES IN THYMOMA

There are many small to medium-sized perivascular spaces in this predominantly epithelial, polygonal cell (type B3) thymoma. The spaces contain a central fine blood vessel, lymphoid cells, and serous fluid, and are lined by cuboidal epithelial cells.

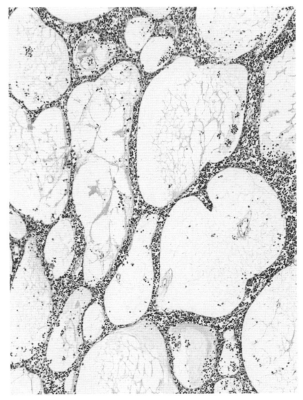

Figure 2-27

PERIVASCULAR SPACES IN THYMOMA

The perivascular spaces are cystically dilated and lined by inconspicuous epithelial cells. Central blood vessels may be difficult to find.

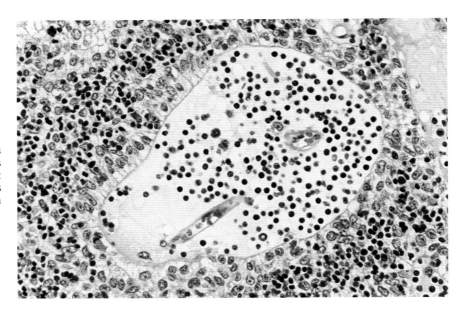

Figure 2-28

PERIVASCULAR SPACES IN THYMOMA

The perivascular spaces contain not only lymphoid cells and serous fluid but also mast cells. The lining epithelial cells are columnar with basal lamina (type B2).

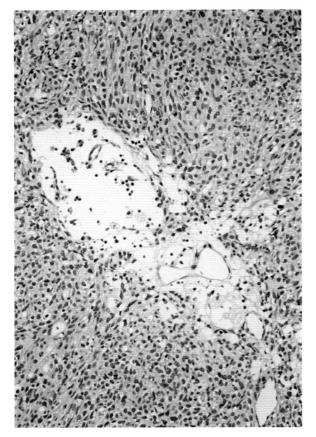

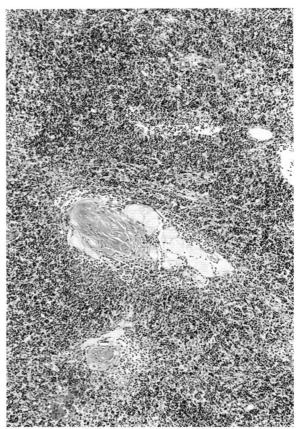

Figure 2-29

PERIVASCULAR SPACE IN THYMOMA

A perivascular space shows features of early organization with the appearance of fibroblasts (type B3 thymoma).

Figure 2-30

PERIVASCULAR SPACES IN THYMOMA

A perivascular space is being obliterated by fibrinous material and collagen (type B1 thymoma).

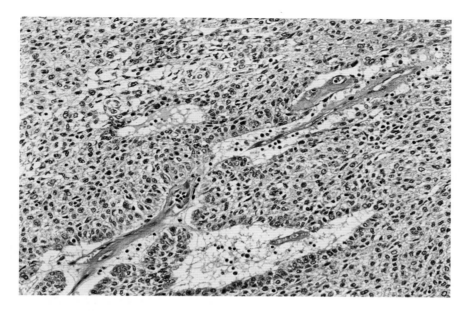

Figure 2-31

PERIVASCULAR SPACES IN THYMOMA

The walls of the blood vessels are hyalinized. The tumor is predominantly epithelial (polygonal cell type [type B3]) with a suggestion of an epidermoid arrangement.

Perivascular spaces can be seen in both spindle/oval cell (type A) and polygonal/round cell (type B) thymomas, but are much more frequent in the latter. In the spindle/oval cell (type A) thymoma, palisading of epithelial cells is not apparent, and spaces are rarely seen, although the reason for this is not clear. The presence of perivascular spaces in a mediastinal tumor is strongly suggestive of thymoma, particularly of the predominantly cortical, lymphocyte-predominant (type B1); cortical, mixed lymphocytic and epithelial (type B2); and epithelial cell-predominant (type B3) types. The presence of perivascular spaces is an important feature for excluding the alternative diagnosis of malignant lymphoma; however, perivascular spaces are not a specific feature of thymoma, and may be seen in thymic carcinoma, although rarely (see chapter 3). Structures similar to perivascular spaces in thymoma can also be seen in thymic carcinoid tumor, but most are simply artifacts since they are empty and do not contain blood plasma or lymphocytes. Perivascular spaces were at one time considered to be perivascular lymphatic spaces, but endothelial cells cannot be identified.

Cellular Subtypes

Thymoma is composed of a mixture of neoplastic epithelial cells and non-neoplastic lymphocytes in varying proportions (52). At one end of the spectrum, the tumor appears to consist almost entirely of lymphocytes, mimicking diffuse malignant lymphoma; at the other end, it is made up of a diffuse growth of polygonal epithelial cells or haphazardly arranged short spindled epithelial cells, which may create difficulties in the distinction from thymic carcinoma, solitary localized fibrous tumor, and other benign mesenchymal tumors. Between these two extremes is mixed epithelial and lymphocytic thymoma.

Epithelial Cell Subtypes. The epithelial cells of thymoma vary in shape and size, but they have been customarily divided into polygonal (round or oval) (figs. 2-32–2-36) and spindle shaped (figs. 2-37–2-39). Although it is common to classify thymomas histologically by the amount of epithelial component and lymphocytes, Müller-Hermelink and associates proposed a classification of thymic epithelial tumors based on histogenesis (53,54,78,91). They divided the epithelial cells of thymoma into medullary and cortical types (Table 2-5) (78). Elongated spindle-shaped cells may resemble fibroblasts, but their epithelial nature is supported by positive cytokeratin immunostaining (fig. 2-39).

Separation of thymoma by epithelial cell type may be difficult at times, due partly to the presence of intermediate categories and partly to a mixture of two cell types. In a series of 130 thymomas at the National Cancer Center Hospital in Tokyo, 43 percent were polygonal cell type (types B1, B2, and B3 of the WHO classification), 43 percent were mixed cell type

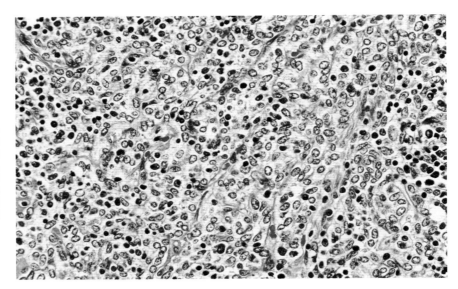

Figure 2-32

TYPE "B2-LIKE" THYMOMA WITH SMALL POLYGONAL (OVAL) EPITHELIAL CELLS

The epithelial cells are small, with oval nuclei showing a fine chromatin pattern, inconspicuous or small nucleoli, scanty cytoplasm, and ill-defined cell borders. These cells are difficult to classify as "medullary" or "cortical" type, and correspond to the small polygonal cells of Kuo (64).

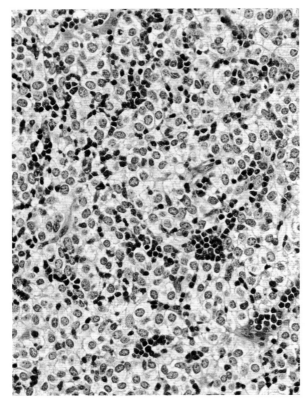

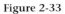

Figure 2-33

TYPE "B2-LIKE" THYMOMA WITH SMALL POLYGONAL (OVAL) EPITHELIAL CELLS

The epithelial cells are small to medium sized, with oval nuclei, a thin nuclear membrane, a fine chromatin pattern, some small nucleoli, and pale-staining cytoplasm. These cells are difficult to classify, and correspond to the small polygonal cells of Kuo (64).

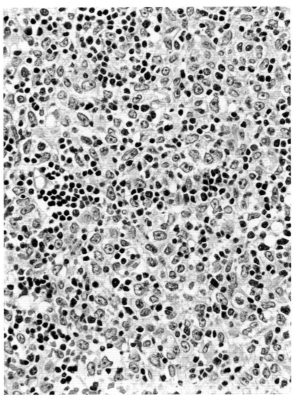

Figure 2-34

THYMOMA WITH POLYGONAL EPITHELIAL CELLS

The epithelial cells are medium sized and have oval vesicular nuclei and moderately prominent nucleoli. These cells are the cortical type of type B2 thymoma.

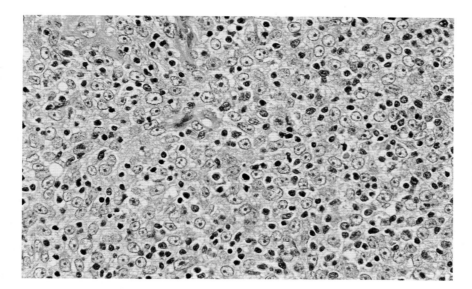

Figure 2-35

THYMOMA WITH POLYGONAL EPITHELIAL CELLS

The epithelial cells vary in size, tending to be large, with large vesicular clear nuclei and prominent round nucleoli. Mitotic figures are rare. These cells are the cortical type epithelial cells of type B2 thymoma.

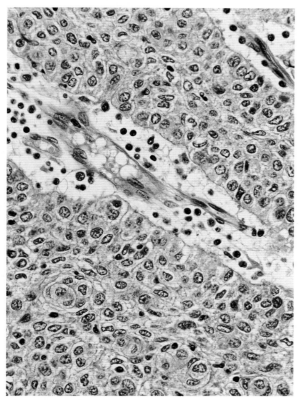

Figure 2-36

THYMOMA WITH POLYGONAL EPITHELIAL CELLS AND AN EPIDERMOID ARRANGEMENT

The epithelial cells are moderately large and slightly atypical, with hyperchromatic nuclei and a few small nucleoli. They are arranged in whorls at a few points and in palisades around the perivascular space (type B3 thymoma).

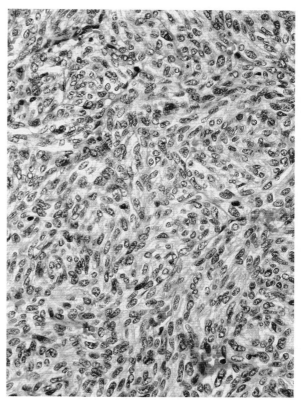

Figure 2-37

THYMOMA OF SPINDLE CELL TYPE

The epithelial cells are of the short spindle cell type, with oval to slightly elongated nuclei, granular chromatin, and inconspicuous nucleoli. The cells are arranged in irregular ill-defined bundles. The tumor somewhat resembles mesenchymal tumor or monomorphic fibrous mesothelioma (type A thymoma).

Figure 2-38

THYMOMA OF THE SPINDLE CELL TYPE

Fibroblast-like long spindle cells have a storiform pattern. Although this resembles benign mesenchymal tumor (fibrous histiocytoma), a few spindle cells contained cytokeratin, and bundles of collagen are noted within the tumor, which are probably parts of the stroma subdividing the tumor into lobules (type A thymoma).

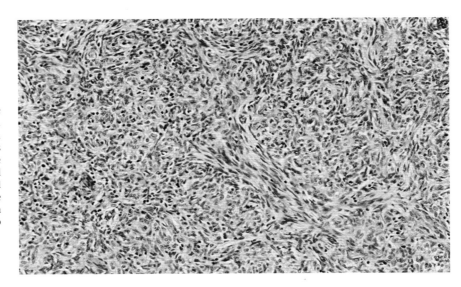

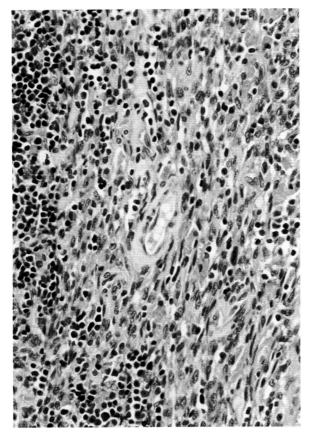
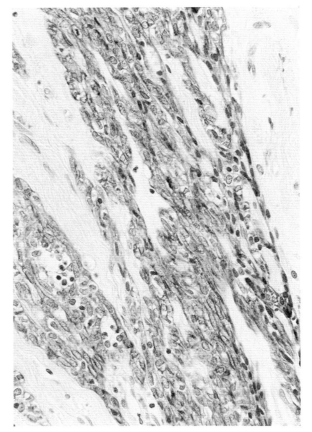

Figure 2-39

THYMOMA OF THE SPINDLE CELL TYPE

Left: Loosely arranged spindle cells resembling mesenchymal cells are diffusely infiltrated by lymphocytes (type AB thymoma).

Right: Immunostaining for cytokeratin discloses a positive reaction in the cytoplasm of almost all the tumor cells, indicating their epithelial nature.

Table 2-5

**RELATIONSHIP BETWEEN WORLD HEALTH ORGANIZATION (WHO),
HISTOGENETIC, AND MORPHOLOGIC CLASSIFICATIONS[a]**

WHO	Histogenetic	Morphologic	Malignancy
Type A	Medullary	Spindle cell; predominantly oval cell with rosettes and glands	Benign
Type AB	Mixed (medullary and cortical)	Mixed spindle (oval) cell and polygonal cell	
Type B1	Predominantly cortical	Lymphocyte predominant with medullary differentiation	Intermediate
Type B2	Cortical	Mixed lymphocyte and polygonal epithelial cell	
Type B3	Well-differentiated thymic carcinoma	Polygonal cell predominant with or without atypia (atypical thymoma, with squamoid features)	Borderline
Type C	Thymic carcinoma	Thymic carcinoma	Malignant

[a]Some individual terms are explained in the text.

(type AB), and 14 percent were spindle/oval cell type (type A) (95); the incidence of spindle cell type is higher than reported in other studies, but lower than the 22 percent in Taiwan reported by Pan et al. (104). The higher incidence of spindle cell type thymoma may be partly due to the lower incidence of thymoma associated with myasthenia gravis in a cancer hospital, or to geographic or ethnic factors.

The cortical type epithelial cells of Müller-Hermelink and associates (78,91,92), which are almost synonymous with the polygonal (round) cell type of the morphologic classification, are characterized by a stellate outline with large, clear, round nuclei; conspicuous nucleoli; and long prominent cellular processes (figs. 2-34, 2-35). Polygonal (round) epithelial cells are small to medium sized, with normochromatic bland nuclei, small nucleoli, and indistinct cytoplasmic processes. This morphology probably corresponds to the small polygonal cells of Kuo (64), and these cells are difficult to classify as cortical type cells (figs. 2-32, 2-33).

Medullary type epithelial cells correspond roughly to the spindle cell type of the morphologic classification, with fusiform nuclei having dispersed or coarser chromatin, inconspicuous nucleoli, scanty eosinophilic cytoplasm, and thin cellular processes (figs. 2-37–2-39). Occasionally, however, medullary type epithelial cells possess round to oval but bland nuclei and inconspicuous nucleoli, and may be arranged in hemangiopericytoma-like, rosette-like, and glandular patterns. Squamous differentiation and Hassall corpuscles are rarely seen.

Spindle cell thymoma tends to remain localized in the anterior mediastinum, but medullary thymoma with rosette-like structures or glandular structures may metastasize to the lung, although displaying an indolent clinical course (135). Therefore, spindle cell type thymoma and medullary thymoma are not exactly the same. In contrast, the majority of thymomas invading neighboring organs or presenting with metastases are of the polygonal (cortical) or mixed cell type. Mitotic figures may be seen in the epithelial cells of the polygonal cell type, but are rare in the spindle cell type. Their frequency appears to be increased in tumors with increased nuclear atypia and nucleolar prominence, reaching up to 10 per 10 high-power fields in aggressive invasive thymoma of the polygonal cell type (atypical thymoma) (fig. 2-40). There is a special form of polygonal (cortical) epithelial cell that shows an epidermoid arrangement or squamoid features with whorls, and borders the perivascular spaces (fig. 2-36). Tumors with such a cell type (type B3 thymoma) consist in part of areas with a cortical type, and are called "well-differentiated (organo-typical, low-grade) thymic carcinoma" by Müller-Hermelink and associates (54). The occurrence of such tumors has been known to pathologists, who have designated them as atypical (aggressive) epithelial cell-predominant thymoma, or invasive thymoma with cell atypia (59).

The division of thymoma into polygonal and spindle-shaped epithelial cell types, or cortical and medullary epithelial cell types is important and useful because of their differences in aggressiveness (75,113). Table 2-6 lists the disease

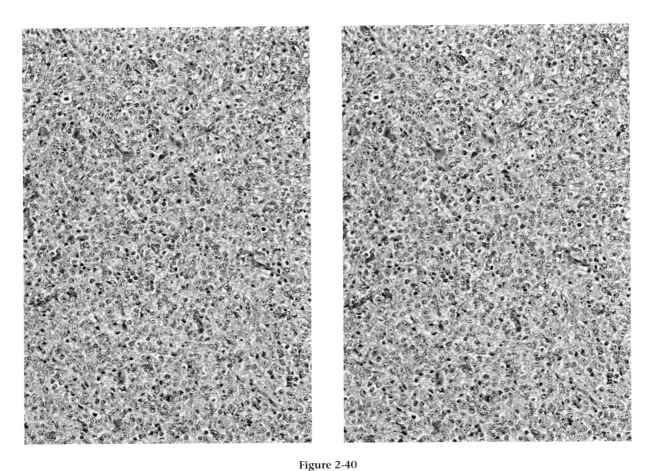

Figure 2-40

ATYPICAL PREDOMINANTLY EPITHELIAL THYMOMA WITH INCREASED MITOTIC ACTIVITY

Left: There is diffuse growth of polygonal cells with vesicular nuclei and prominent nucleoli.

Right: Higher magnification reveals that the constituent cells are of cortical type. Scattered mitotic figures (type B3 thymoma) are seen.

Table 2-6

RELATIONSHIP BETWEEN HISTOLOGIC SUBTYPE AND STAGE[a]

Histologic Subtype	No. of Patients	I	II	III	IVa	IVb
A	18	8	7	2		1
AB	56	28	22	6		
B1	15	2	9	4		
B2	29	2	14	6	7	
B3	12		2	7	3	
Total	130	40	54	25	10	1

[a]Table 2 from Nakagawa K, Asamura H, Matsuno Y, et al. Thymoma: a clinicopathological study based on the new World Health Organization classification. J Thorac Cardiovasc Surg. 2003;126:1136.

stages and thymomas of various histologic types. Thymomas of the spindle cell (medullary) type are more frequently detected at an early stage than polygonal (cortical) cell type thymomas.

The nuclei of the epithelial cells may be large and bizarre. Such a nuclear configuration, not associated with mitotic activity, is often found in patients with a history of radiotherapy (fig. 2-41). It is most likely due to a degenerative process, and may be present in untreated tumors showing degeneration.

Lymphocyte Subtypes. The lymphocytes accompanying thymoma are non-neoplastic (52), usually with small, dark-stained nuclei and an almost invisible cytoplasm. Occasionally, they have an "active" appearance: increased size, a recognizable chromatin pattern, a cytoplasmic rim,

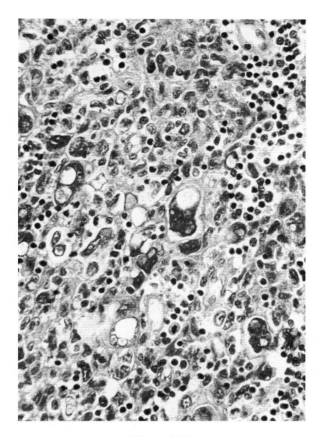

Figure 2-41

THYMOMA WITH GIANT EPITHELIAL CELLS

Scattered in mixed lymphocytic and epithelial thymoma are mononucleated and multinucleated giant epithelial cells with hyperchromatic or vacuolated nuclei. These nuclear changes are due to irradiation and antitumor chemotherapy (autopsy case of type B2 thymoma).

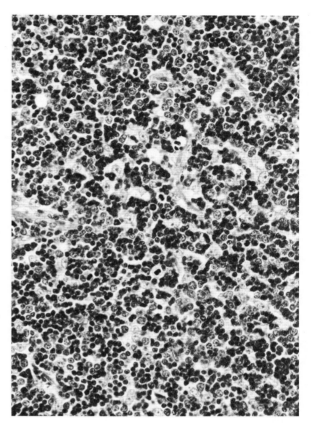

Figure 2-42

LYMPHOCYTE-PREDOMINANT (TYPE B1) THYMOMA

Many lymphocytes are active and moderately large. They have a recognizable nuclear chromatin pattern, small nucleoli, and several mitotic figures. Epithelial cells are polygonal (cortical) with clear nuclei and distinct nucleoli.

and mitotic activity (fig. 2-42). These features are always present in association with epithelial components, even in implanted and distant metastatic foci. Whether the cells undergoing mitosis are epithelial cells or lymphocytes can be distinguished roughly by the cell size and by immunostaining for cytokeratin and surface markers of lymphocytes.

Lymphocytes associated with medullary type epithelial cells are largely mature (positive for CD3, and CD4 or CD8) and small, and those associated with cortical type epithelial cells are of both mature and immature types; the latter are medium sized with granular nuclei active in appearance (positive for TdT, CD1a, CD99, and CD3, and double positive for CD4 and CD8).

According to Okumura et al. (98), who counted the number of tumor-associated CD4- and CD8-positive cells in thymoma cell suspensions, predominantly cortical (lymphocyte-predominant or type B1) thymoma retained the ability to induce CD4 and CD8 double-positive cells at a level compatible to that of the normal thymic cortical epithelial cells, followed by mixed (type AB) and cortical (predominantly lymphocytic and mixed lymphocytic and polygonal epithelial [type B2] thymoma. Spindle cell (medullary or type A) thymoma and organotypical well-differentiated thymic carcinoma (atypical or type B3 thymoma) had this function at a barely detectable level; thymic carcinoma was nonfunctional.

The presence of immature T cells, even in implanted and distant metastatic foci of thymoma, indicates that the epithelial cells of thymoma are capable of attracting immature T cells from the bone marrow; the presence of medullary differentiation in thymoma indicates that immature T cells have the ability to mature in the environment of the thymoma. These phenomena suggest that thymoma is a functional tumor with regard to T-cell maturation. In contrast, thymic carcinoma has lost this property (127,135).

Histologic Subtypes

WHO Classification. In 1999, *The Histological Typing of Tumours of the Thymus* was published for the first time by the WHO (121) and its revised edition, *Pathology and Genetics of Tumours of the Lung, Pleura, Thymus and Heart,* was published in 2004 (Table 2-5) (151). The WHO Histological Classification was intended to promote the adoption of uniform terminology to facilitate communication among cancer workers. It has, therefore, also been adopted in this Fascicle. This classification uses noncommittal terminology such as alphabetical letters and numerals to designate each subtype (types A, AB, B1, B2, and B3), supplemented with corresponding subtypes by morphologic classification (75,135) and by histogenetic (or functional) classification (54,78,113) in parentheses. It is assumed mnemonically that "A" stands for atrophic (i.e., the effete thymic cell of adult life), "B" for bioactive (i.e., the biologically active organ of the fetus and infant), and "C" for carcinoma (121). A compromise was made concerning thymic epithelial tumors, adopting both the morphologic classification which is widely used in the United States and many other countries and the histogenetic classification of Müller-Hermelink et al. (53,54,78,91). It is mandatory to fully understand both morphologic and histogenetic classifications. The definitions of each subtype as delineated by the WHO are presented with some modification.

Type A Thymoma (Spindle Cell, Medullary). Type A thymoma is composed of a population of neoplastic thymic epithelial cells having a spindle/oval shape, lacking nuclear atypia, and accompanied by few or no non-neoplastic lymphocytes. The tumor cells can form a va-

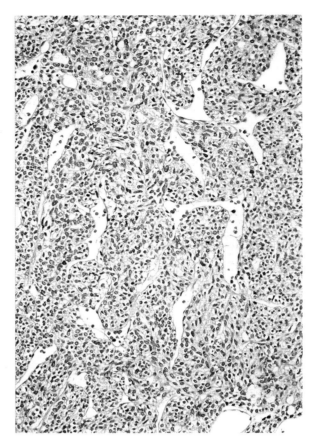

Figure 2-43

THYMOMA WITH HEMANGIOPERICYTOMATOUS FEATURES (TYPE A)

Diffuse growth of polygonal and short spindle cells is associated with dilated sinusoidal vasculature, reminiscent of hemangiopericytoma. (Figs. 2-43, 2-47, and 2-48 are from the same patient.)

riety of histologic structures (figs. 2-37–2-39, 2-43–2-49).

Type AB Thymoma (Mixed). This tumor is composed of a mixture of a lymphocyte-poor type A thymoma component and a lymphocyte-rich type B-like (B1-like or B2-like) component. The type B-like component is composed predominantly of small polygonal epithelial cells with the small round, oval, or short spindle-shaped pale nuclei showing dispersed chromatin and inconspicuous nucleoli, which correspond to the small polygonal cells described by Kuo (64). There is a great variation in the proportion of the two components (figs. 2-39, 2-50).

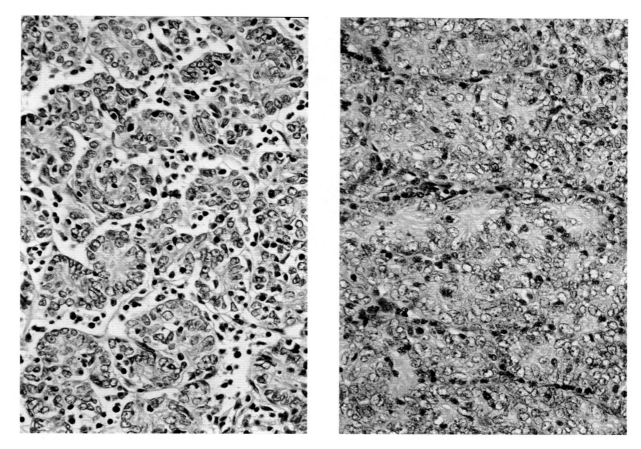

Figure 2-44

ROSETTE-FORMING (TYPE A) THYMOMA

Top: This tumor, metastatic to the lung, was found 3 years after surgical resection of thymoma. The pyramidal tumor cells with basal nuclei form rosettes without central lumens. The cells have a back-to-back arrangement with lymphocytic infiltration between. (Figs. 2-44 and 2-72 are from the same patient.)

Bottom: Rosettes without artificial spaces.

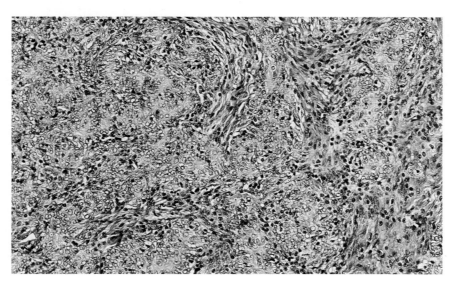

Figure 2-45

THYMOMA (TYPE A) COMPOSED OF ROSETTES AND FIBROBLAST-LIKE SPINDLE-SHAPED EPITHELIAL CELLS

Aggregates of rosettes are subdivided by bundles of long spindle-shaped epithelial cells.

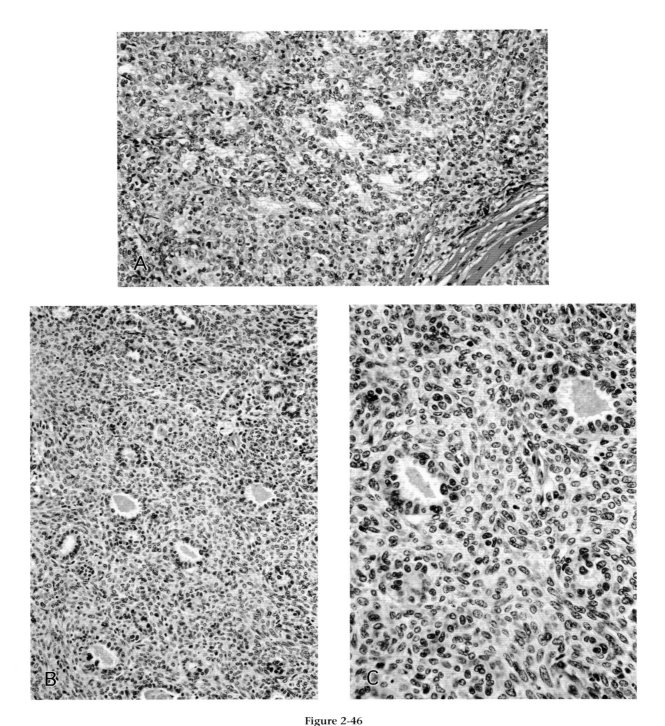

Figure 2-46

THYMOMA (TYPE A) WITH GLANDS

A: Cuboidal epithelial cells with basal nuclei and pale cytoplasm form small glandular spaces.

B: In other areas, scattered glands show secretory activity with eosinophilic material in glandular lumens. This material was periodic acid–Schiff (PAS) positive and Alcian blue negative. Interposing oval cells were cytokeratin positive, although to a lesser extent than the glandular cells (see fig. 2-86).

C: Higher-power view shows cellular details and cytoplasmic snouts of glandular epithelial cells. (Figs. 2-46 and 2-86 are from the same patient.)

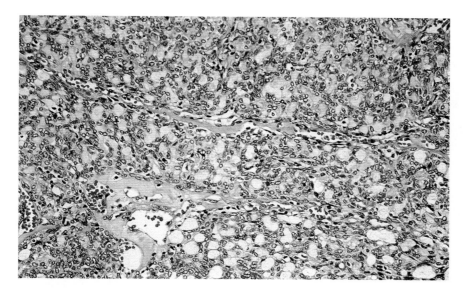

Figure 2-47

THYMOMA (TYPE A) WITH PSEUDOGLANDULAR SPACES

Many microcystic spaces are lined by flat epithelial cells in an epithelial cell–predominant (type A) thymoma. The microcystic lumen contains amorphous material. Individual tumor cells possess oval vesicular nuclei, inconspicuous nucleoli, and scanty cytoplasm.

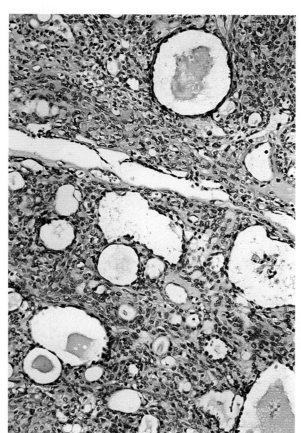

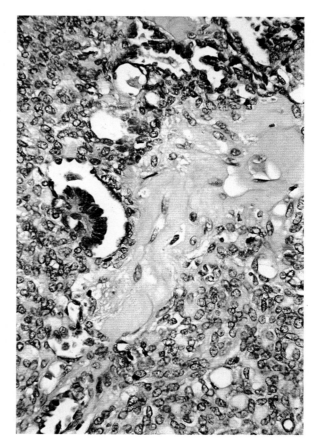

Figure 2-48

THYMOMA (TYPE A) WITH PSEUDOGLANDULAR SPACES AND A GLOMERULOID STRUCTURE

Left: Scattered cystic spaces of various sizes are lined by flattened or cuboidal cells. The spaces contain amorphous material.

Right: A single glomeruloid structure is present in a microcystic space.

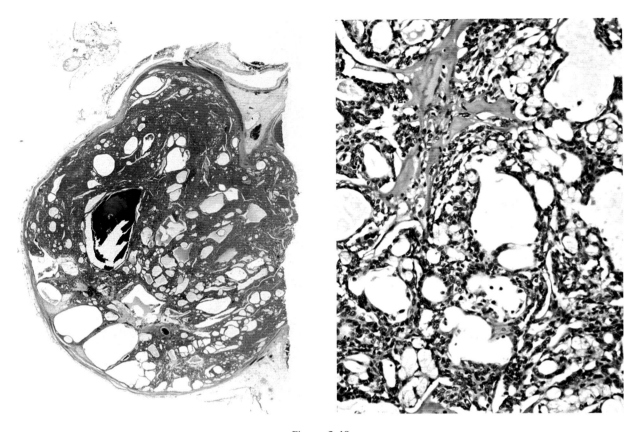

Figure 2-49

THYMOMA (TYPE A) WITH MUCIN–PRODUCING GLANDS

Left: Encapsulation and multiple cysts.
Right: In addition to variably sized cystic spaces, there are several small glands lined by cuboidal and round cells which have basal or eccentric nuclei and foamy cytoplasm. Some signet ring cells contained PAS- and Alcian blue–positive epithelial mucin.

Figure 2-50

MIXED POLYGONAL AND SPINDLE CELL (TYPE AB) THYMOMA

An area composed of mixed lymphocytic and polygonal epithelial cell (type B1-like) thymoma merges into an area consisting of predominantly spindle cell (type A) thymoma.

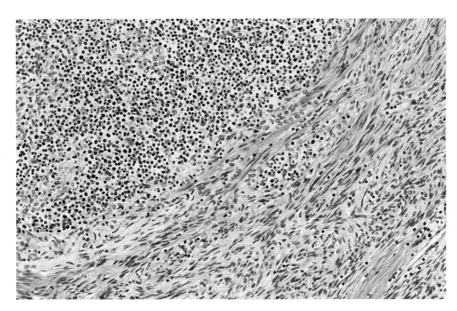

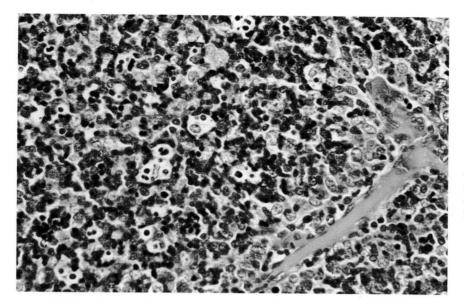

Figure 2-51

LYMPHOCYTE-PREDOMINANT (TYPE B1) THYMOMA WITH STARRY SKY APPEARANCE

The scattered large clear cells within this lymphocyte-rich thymoma are macrophages. They contain a few lymphocytes with pyknotic nuclei.

Type B1 Thymoma (Lymphocyte-Rich, Lymphocytic, Predominantly Cortical, Organoid). Type B1 thymoma resembles the normal functional thymus. It is composed predominantly of areas resembling the thymic cortex, with epithelial cells scattered in a prominent population of immature lymphocytes and areas of medullary differentiation, with or without Hassall corpuscles, similar to normal thymic medulla (figs. 2-6, 2-51–2-53).

Type B2 Thymoma (Cortical). This tumor is composed of large polygonal cells with vesicular nuclei and prominent nucleoli that closely resemble the predominant epithelial cells of the normal thymic cortex. The tumor cells are arranged in a loose network. Immature T cells are always present and outnumber the neoplastic epithelial cells. The tumor may be described as mixed lymphocytic and polygonal epithelial thymoma without medullary differentiation (figs. 2-34, 2-35). Perivascular spaces are common and sometimes prominent. Perivascular arrangement of tumor cells results in a palisading effect.

Type B3 Thymoma (Epithelial, Atypical, Squamoid, Well-Differentiated Thymic Carcinoma). Type B3 thymoma is composed predominantly of medium-sized round or polygonal epithelial cells with mild atypia. The epithelial cells are mixed with a minor component of intraepithelial lymphocytes, resulting in a sheet-like growth of the neoplastic epithelial cells (fig. 2-40). A squamoid arrangement of epithelial cells, without intercellular bridges, is often seen. Individual cells often possess folded or grooved nuclei and smaller and less distinct nucleoli than in B2 thymoma, which frequently coexists with B3 thymoma (figs. 2-31, 2-36, 2-54). Other rare types of thymoma are discussed separately.

"Traditional" Morphologic Classification. Thymoma has been customarily divided into predominantly lymphocytic, mixed lymphocytic and epithelial, predominantly epithelial, and spindle cell types according to the amount of the predominant cell type and epithelial cell morphology present (Table 2-5) (75,135,159), although defining "predominant" is often difficult and arbitrary.

Lymphocyte-predominant thymoma corresponds to type B1 and some of type B2 thymomas in the WHO classification, depending on the presence of foci of medullary differentiation; *mixed lymphocytic and epithelial thymoma* to some of type AB and B2 thymomas; *predominantly epithelial thymoma* to type B3 and some of type A thymomas; and *spindle cell thymoma* to some of type A thymomas. Type A thymomas include thymomas predominantly composed of small to medium-sized polygonal cells with round to oval nuclei, finely dispersed chromatin, and inconspicuous nucleoli. These cells are arranged in sheets or in a perithelial pattern, with or without rosette-like or glandular structures, since these cells are considered to be medullary type epithelial cells by Müller-Hermelink et al. (53,78). In the third series

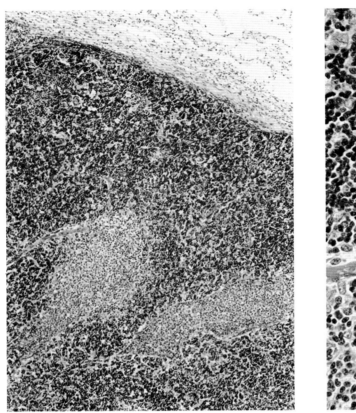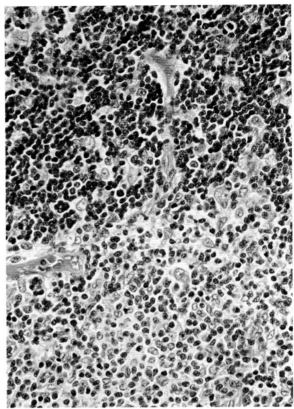

Figure 2-52

LYMPHOCYTE- PREDOMINANT (TYPE B1) THYMOMA WITH MEDULLARY DIFFERENTIATION

Left: The tumor metastatic to the lung reveals two oval-shaped, fairly well-defined, lighter-stained areas of medullary differentiation, where lymphocytes are less densely packed.

Right: Higher magnification of the border of medullary differentiation discloses a different epithelial morphology, i.e., epithelial cells at the periphery of and in areas surrounding medullary differentiation are larger, with more prominent nucleoli than those in central areas of medullary differentiation, where nucleoli are inconspicuous.

Fascicle, however, we categorized tumors of such a cell type into predominantly epithelial thymomas and distinguished them from spindle cell thymomas, since some of these thymomas metastasize to the lung. They usually display indolent progression and patients can survive for years with tumor (135). Some of these tumors correspond to thymomas of small round epithelial cells of Kuo (64).

Foci of medullary differentiation are fairly well-defined, round or slightly irregular zones with a clear and lighter-stained appearance than the surrounding tissue (figs. 2-6, 2-52). Superficially they resemble germinal centers, but their clear appearance is due to lower numbers of lymphocytes than in surrounding areas.

They resemble the medulla of the thymus, with occasional epithelial cell aggregates similar to Hassall corpuscles (fig. 2-53). Immunohistochemically, the foci are composed of mature or medullary T cells, characterized by TdT-, CD1a-, and CD99-negative, CD3-, CD4-, or CD8-positive phenotypes (see fig. 2-91) (127,135).

Mixed lymphocytic and epithelial thymomas (type B2 thymoma) can be diagnosed with relative ease: epithelial cells and lymphocytes are intimately associated in most instances (figs. 2-34, 2-35). In a single tumor, the proportions of epithelial cells and lymphocytes vary among the lobules; a lobule with mixed cellularity may be present adjacent to an epithelial cell–predominant lobule, with fibrous bands between them. Lobules

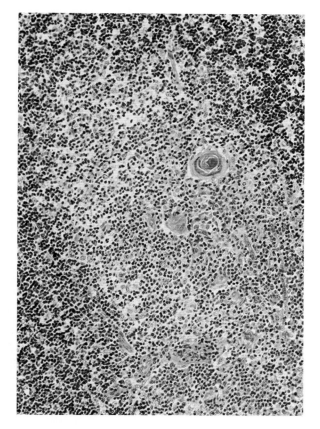

Figure 2-53

HASSALL CORPUSCLES IN LYMPHOCYTE-PREDOMINANT (TYPE B1) THYMOMA

A focus of medullary differentiation with Hassall corpuscles looks like normal thymic tissue. Hassall corpuscles most likely represent differentiation in thymoma but inclusion of normal thymic tissue cannot be overlooked.

are often clearly bordered by a rim of epithelial cells and supported by the fibrous bands.

The histologic features of epithelial cell–predominant (type A) thymoma vary greatly. Short spindle cells may be arranged haphazardly (reminiscent of those seen in benign solitary [localized] fibrous tumor) or elongated spindle cells may be arranged in a storiform pattern (resembling benign fibrous histiocytoma) (figs. 2-37, 2-38). Lymphocytes are scanty and may be barely detectable. This form of thymoma is classified separately from predominantly epithelial (type B3) thymoma and categorized as a spindle cell or medullary (type A) thymoma, since it is often localized within the thymus and patients have an excellent prognosis. Small to

medium-sized polygonal/oval epithelial cells with bland nuclei and inconspicuous nucleoli arranged diffusely in a perithelioma-like pattern or forming rosette-like structures or glands are also seen in medullary (type A) thymoma, although individual cells are not spindle shaped (figs. 2-43–2-49).

The cells of epithelial cell–predominant (type B3) thymoma may be arranged in a squamoid or epidermoid pattern (figs. 2-31, 2-36, 2-54, left). This thymoma overlaps with the well-differentiated thymic carcinoma (an organotypical and low-grade malignant carcinoma) described by Kirchner and associates (54). They chose to call it carcinoma because it appears to be aggressive, with an increased number of mitotic figures and frequent invasion of surrounding organs or tissues. However, it still retains the organoid features of thymoma, attracts immature T cells, and combines, at times, with cortical (or type B2) thymoma. Furthermore, it is often associated with myasthenia gravis. In contrast, a lack of immature T cells and no association with myasthenia gravis are noted in the tumor traditionally classified as thymic carcinoma (see chapter 3).

Histogenetic Subtypes

Müller-Hermelink and associates divided thymoma initially into four, and later into five, histologic subtypes (53,54,78), a practice that has been adopted by other investigators (45,66, 106,113,114). These five subtypes are medullary thymoma (type A thymoma), mixed medullary and cortical thymoma (type AB thymoma), predominantly cortical (organoid) thymoma (type B1 thymoma), cortical thymoma (type B2 thymoma), and well-differentiated thymic carcinoma (type B3 thymoma) (Tables 2-2, 2-5) (54,78,114).

Medullary thymoma (type A thymoma) is composed of medullary type epithelial cells with few or some mature lymphocytes. There may be a storiform pattern, hemangiopericytoma-like pattern, rosette-like structures, or even glandular formation of flat, cuboidal to cylindrical epithelial cells resulting in an adenoma-like pattern. Microcystic and macrocystic changes may be seen (figs. 2-37, 2-38, 2-44–2-49). Since some medullary thymomas are composed of nonspindle cells, the term "spindle cell" cannot be used as a substitute for "medullary."

Mixed thymoma (type AB thymoma) is composed of a mixture of medullary thymoma and cortical thymoma. It is divided into three major patterns: 1) lobules of medullary type epithelial cells mixed with lymphocyte-rich lobules with cortical type epithelial cells; 2) nests of medullary type epithelial cells surrounded by sheets of lymphocyte-rich predominantly cortical components (figs. 2-39, 2-50); and 3) tight intermingling of both components.

Predominantly cortical (organoid) thymoma (type B1 thymoma) is composed of lymphocyte-rich lobules bordered by thin, delicate fibrous tissue. There are fewer cortical type epithelial cells than in the cortical type thymoma (type B2 thymoma), and they possess smaller and less prominent nucleoli. Areas of medullary differentiation may be seen, which may contain Hassall corpuscles (figs. 2-52, 2-53). A "starry sky" appearance with macrophages may be found (fig. 2-51). Perivascular spaces are present and may be dilated (fig. 2-30).

Cortical thymoma (type B2 thymoma) is composed of cortical epithelial cells, often arranged in a loose network, with larger nuclei and more prominent nucleoli than those of predominantly cortical thymoma (type B1 thymoma). These cells are usually outnumbered by non-neoplastic lymphocytes (figs. 2-34, 2-35). There is a well-organized lobular architecture resembling normal thymic cortex; small foci of cells with squamoid features suggest abortive Hassall corpuscles. The perivascular spaces are narrow, and foci of medullary differentiation are not found or are inconspicuous.

Well-differentiated thymic carcinoma (WDTC) (type B3 thymoma) is a predominantly epithelial tumor in which epithelial cells are either similar to those in cortical thymoma (type B2 thymoma) (fig. 2-40), or squamoid in arrangement (figs. 2-31, 2-36, 2-54). A slight to moderate degree of cellular atypia and mitoses of up to 10 per 10 high-power fields are noted. The palisading of epithelial cells around the perivascular spaces is a characteristic feature (figs. 2-31, 2-36). WDTC generally shows invasive growth, but there may be a lobular growth pattern surrounded by fibrous tissue. According to Kirchner et al. (54), the diagnosis is established when typical features of WDTC occupy over 50 percent of the tumor areas, but according to Quintanilla-Martinez

et al. (114) any significant component of the tumor with features of WDTC is sufficient for a diagnosis. Combined thymomas exhibiting cortical thymoma and WDTC are common. They are classified as combined type B2/B3 thymoma by the WHO classification, although no definition regarding the amount of each component has been given.

Pescarmona et al. (109) reviewed 15 WDTCs and justified their separation from thymoma because of histologic characteristics and aggressive biologic behavior. Later, they recognized histologic progression in 5 of 9 recurrent thymomas with cortical differentiation from predominantly cortical thymoma to cortical thymoma and/or WDTC, usually associated with more advanced clinical stages (107).

Kuo et al. (66) compared the Müller-Hermelink system with the traditional morphologic classification in the evaluation of 71 thymomas, and supported the former system for predicting the aggressive potential of thymomas. Studies in Singapore and Denmark showed significant correlation of this classification system with invasive behavior (stage) (35,148). Ho et al. (45) also supported the histogenetic classification for thymic epithelial tumors after evaluating 87 tumors from Chinese patients in Hong Kong. The reproducibility of the classification has been confirmed (31). Quintanilla-Martinez et al. (113), using the Marino-Müller-Hermelink-Kirchner system, concluded that histologic subclassification is an independent prognostic factor, predicting relapse and the risk of death from thymoma. Conversely, Pan et al. (104) concluded that "epithelial subtyping is not indispensable for diagnosis because long-term survival is not conspicuously influenced," although they recognized the merits of the Müller-Hermelink system.

Controversies Surrounding Histogenetic and WHO Histologic Subtypes

There are several controversies concerning histogenetic classification. These include the: 1) terminology used for the cell type (either based on cell morphology or based on histogenesis); 2) categorization of small oval or polygonal epithelial cells with hemangiopericytoma-like arrangement, rosette-like or glandular structures; and 3) separation of well-differentiated

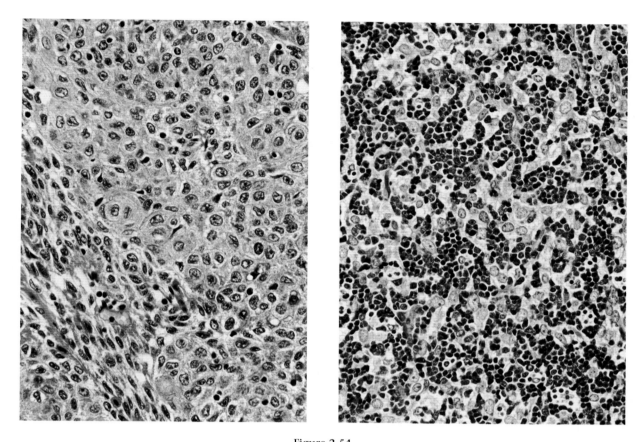

Figure 2-54

PREDOMINANTLY EPITHELIAL ATYPICAL (TYPE B3) THYMOMA (WELL-DIFFERENTIATED ORGANOTYPICAL LOW-GRADE THYMIC CARCINOMA BY HISTOGENETIC CLASSIFICATION)

Left: Metastasis in a lymph node consists of diffuse growth of moderately pleomorphic polygonal cells with hyperchromatic nuclei and a moderate amount of cytoplasm displaying an epidermoid arrangement.

Right: The primary tumor, removed together with a pulmonary lobe 6 years prior to death, reveals a mixture of lymphocytes and polygonal (cortical) epithelial cells with perivascular spaces (feature of type B1/B2 thymoma).

(organotypical low-grade) thymic carcinoma from cortical thymoma (61,61a,104,132,135). If the traditional morphologic system, which uses a subdivision into three types (predominantly lymphocytic, mixed lymphocytic and epithelial, and predominantly epithelial), is combined with a system using epithelial cell morphology (polygonal [round or oval] and spindle cell types graded by degree of atypia), and with tumor extension as circumscribed or invasive (Table 2-2), a system of subtyping similar to that of Müller-Hermelink and associates results. Since the cell of origin does not always determine the cell morphology, it is better not to use any term related to origin, but to stick to cell morphology for histologic classification. Thymoma with a hemangiopericytoma-like pat-

tern, rosette-like or glandular structures may metastasize to the lung, although growth is indolent (135) (see Factors Associated with Degree of Malignancy: Histologic Grading). Inclusion of such thymomas into the same category of medullary thymoma with spindle cells is not appropriate. WDTC can be classified as thymoma, predominantly epithelial polygonal cell type with atypia and increased proliferative activity, or simply as atypical thymoma (19,142). Table 2-5 presents the three representative classification systems for thymic epithelial tumors currently used: those of the WHO (121,151), Müller-Hermelink and associates (54,78), and Fascicle 21 of the Third Series (135), the last being a modification of that of Wick et al. (159) and Lewis et al. (75).

Although it is said that the histogenetic classification can be applied easily to most thymic epithelial tumors, we encountered some difficulty in deciding cell and histologic types using this system because of the presence of intermediate cell types (figs. 2-32, 2-33). When the tumor cells are small and oval, it is difficult to know to which cell type they belong. Within each cell type there seems to be at least two distinct cell morphologies, although there are cells with features transitional between the two types. That is, cortical cells include cells with round vesicular nuclei, prominent nucleoli, and indistinct cell borders (figs. 2-34, 2-35, 2-40) and cells with granular, occasionally folded nuclei, inconspicuous nucleoli, a moderate amount of cytoplasm, and distinct cell borders, which may show a squamoid arrangement (figs. 2-36, 2-54, left). In the medullary type, tumor cells may be spindle shaped and fibroblastic or small oval or polygonal epithelial with rosette-like or glandular structures. The absence of Hassall corpuscles in medullary thymoma and their presence in cortical thymoma is also difficult to understand, as is the presence of "cortical cells" within foci of medullary differentiation. From these observations, it is apparent that further studies on cell typing, cytogenesis, and appropriate terminology are required.

The same can be said for the new WHO classification. Rosai stated in the preface that the classification reflects the present state of knowledge, and modifications are almost certain to be needed as experience accumulates. Alphabetical letters and numbers will be replaced by proper terms, when the histogenetic, cytogenetic, and functional aspects of the thymus become clearly understood.

Suster and Moran (143a,143b) point out problem areas and inconsistencies in the WHO classification, mainly around the following issues: 1) histopathologic criteria for the diagnosis of various subtypes (types A, AB, B1, B2, and B3); 2) existence of rare and unusual types of thymoma (see the following section); 3) lack of interobserver reproducibility (117a); and 4) conflicting claims regarding the clinical significance and prognostic value of the various WHO diagnostic categories (25,117a). In 1999, Suster and Moran presented a novel conceptual approach to thymic epithelial neoplasms, which consisted of

three categories: thymoma (corresponding to the WHO types A, AB, B1, and B2 thymomas), atypical thymoma (type B3 thymoma), and thymic carcinoma (142). Recently, they proposed the following terminology: well-differentiated, moderately differentiated, and poorly differentiated thymic carcinoma for thymoma, atypical thymoma, and thymic carcinoma, respectively (139c,143b). An analogous trend is being adopted for neuroendocrine neoplasms in several organs (see chapter 4). For the surgical pathology report, the main diagnosis of thymoma or atypical thymoma is followed by a description of the invasiveness of the neoplasm and the morphology and histologic type as categorized by the traditional and/or WHO classification systems.

Variants and Uncommon Histologic Subtypes

Most thymomas can be classified into any of the WHO, histogenetic, and morphologic classification systems described already. There are uncommon or rare thymomas, however, with particular histologic features that should be added to the main diagnosis; some are already included in those classifications, but others are described as rare variants. They include thymomas with rosette-like structures, hemangiopericytoma-like patterns, papillary foci, glandular or mucus formation, clear cell features, marked squamous differentiation with Hassall corpuscles, and scattered myoid cells. These histologic features or patterns may be combined in a single tumor or may be present separately. Rare thymomas include micronodular thymoma, metaplastic thymoma, microscopic thymoma, and lipofibroadenoma.

Thymoma with Rosette-Like Structures (Type A Thymoma). In the second series Fascicle, rosettes were said to be identifiable in 20 percent of thymomas (120), but in our experience, thymomas with easily recognizable rosettes are less common. The rosettes are made up of epithelial cells with basal small nuclei, but do not form central lumens (124). The central portions of the rosettes are faintly eosinophilic and faintly fibrillar. A back-to-back arrangement of rosettes is the usual finding, with some lymphocytes rather than epithelial cells interspersed between them (fig. 2-44). There are tumors showing bundles of spindle-shaped epithelial cells intimately associated with rosettes (fig. 2-45). Many of the spaces between the rosettes are artifactual, produced by tissue processing. Rosette-forming cells are cytokeratin positive, without neuroendocrine markers or argyrophilia.

Thymoma with Hemangiopericytoma-Like Features (Type A Thymoma). Small nests and trabeculae of short spindle-shaped, oval to round epithelial cells may be closely associated with a fine vasculature, reminiscent of hemangiopericytoma (fig. 2-43). In these tumors, however, other features characteristic of thymoma are present and no smooth muscle actin is demonstrated in the hemangiopericytoma-like areas. True primary hemangiopericytoma in the thymus or mediastinum is extremely rare and only a single documented case was cited by Weiss and Goldblum (157). Tumors of the mediastinum with hemangiopericytoma-like areas should be examined carefully for features typical of thymoma.

Microcystic, Pseudoglandular Thymoma (Type A Thymoma). Microcysts or dilated spaces lined by cuboidal or flattened cells may be found in thymoma; the spaces either are empty, or contain amorphous eosinophilic material or cellular debris (figs. 2-47, 2-48). When these structures are seen in or near the capsule, the possibility of inclusion of mesothelial cells or preexistence of minute thymic cysts should be considered. A papillary arrangement of cuboidal epithelial cells is also seen, although infrequently. A glomeruloid body was noted in a single instance in our series (fig. 2-48, right).

Cystic Thymoma (Type A Thymoma). Microscopic foci of cystic spaces due to the liquefactive degeneration of thymoma are common. The spaces may be empty or contain cellular debris (fig. 2-49). Some cystic spaces become large enough to be recognized macroscopically, and are sometimes filled with proteinaceous material or foamy histiocytes. In rare cases, most or the entire lesion becomes cystic (145).

Glandular Thymoma (Type A Thymoma). True glandular spaces are found in thymoma. These are often small and lined by cuboidal or low columnar cells, with or without cytoplasmic snouts. They contain no visible material or periodic acid–Schiff (PAS)-positive eosinophilic secretion, and are surrounded by oval to short spindle-shaped epithelial cells (fig. 2-46). Rarely, the cytoplasm and glandular lumens contain epithelial mucin (fig. 2-49).

Clear Cell Thymoma (Type B2/B3 Thymoma). The polygonal cells of thymoma may possess abundant water-clear cytoplasm and centrally located, irregularly shaped or condensed small nuclei. A tumor composed predominantly of clear polygonal cells resembles renal cell carcinoma, but is distinguished from the latter by areas of polygonal cells with scanty cytoplasm, which are characteristic of type B3 thymoma, and the presence of perivascular spaces (fig. 2-55). If nuclear atypia is present, however, such a case could be interpreted as a developing clear cell carcinoma in a type B3 thymoma. In other cases, the epithelial cells of thymoma at times show ballooning type degenerative changes (fig. 2-56).

Thymoma with Marked Squamous Differentiation (Probably a Variant of Type B1/B2 Thymoma). Metaplastic squamous cell nests may be seen at the site of a degenerative process, although rarely (fig. 2-57). A thymoma with marked squamous differentiation and frequent Hassall corpuscles is rare, although a few Hassall corpuscles are seen in type AB (mixed) or type B1/B2 thymoma. The Hassall corpuscles may be so mature that it is difficult to exclude the possibility of inclusion of non-neoplastic thymic tissue, particularly when the Hassall corpuscles are near the capsule facing non-neoplastic thymic tissue (fig. 2-53). A thymoma with marked squamous differentiation is different from a thymoma with scattered Hassall corpuscles. It is largely composed of epithelial cell nests with a marked tendency for keratinization, surrounded by intimately associated lymphocytes. Individual cells possess bland nuclei, seldom showing mitotic activity, and the cellular arrangement is different than that of squamous cell carcinoma composed of solid tumor cell nests bordered by a stroma with lymphocytic infiltration (fig. 2-58).

Thymoma with Myoid Cells (Variant of Type A or Type AB Thymoma). Large myoid cells with abundant eosinophilic fibrillar cytoplasm may be scattered in the tumor; these cells are positive for desmin, actin, and myoglobin (fig. 2-59). Cross striations may be evident in these cells upon light and electron microscopic examination (fig. 2-60). The presence of myoid cells in normal thymic tissue, particularly in the medulla, supports the appearance of such cells

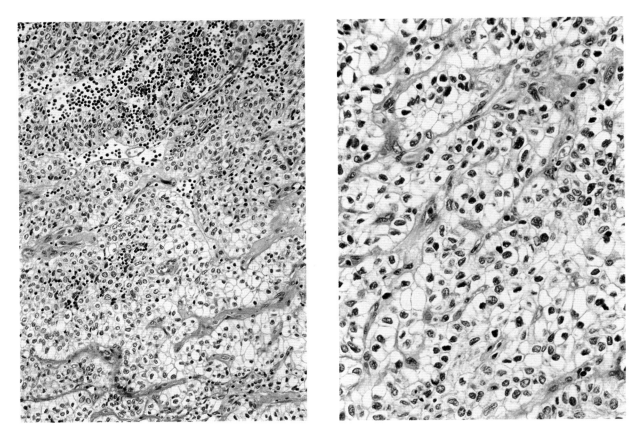

Figure 2-55

CLEAR CELL (TYPE B2/B3) THYMOMA

Left: The diffuse growth pattern of polygonal cells with slightly atypical nuclei and abundant water-clear cytoplasm resembles that of renal clear cell carcinoma, but features in the left lower corner are characteristic of thymoma (a mixture of lymphocytes and polygonal epithelial cells with perivascular spaces).

Right: Higher magnification of clear cell areas with nuclear atypia and hyperchromasia, which are due either to degeneration or neoplastic progression. (Courtesy of Dr. Tadaaki Eimoto, Nagoya, Japan.)

in neoplastic conditions (41,42). Myoid cells are considered to be transformed epithelial cells. Moran et al. (84) reported a rare case of thymoma containing numerous myoid cells, which they designated *rhabdomyomatous thymoma* (fig. 2-61). The presence of myoid cells is not associated with myasthenia gravis.

Micronodular Thymoma with Lymphoid Stroma (Possible Variant of Type A Thymoma). This rare entity is also termed *micronodular thymoma with lymphoid B-cell hyperplasia* (141,151). It is characterized by multiple, discrete epithelial nodules consisting of oval to spindle-shaped epithelial cells that are devoid of atypia or mitotic activity, and a few lymphocytes, similar to type A thymoma. The epithelial nodules are sepa-

rated by an abundant lymphoid stroma with prominent germinal centers (fig. 2-62). Rosette-like structures, glandular differentiation, and cystic changes may be seen (150). In addition to hyperplastic B cells and variable numbers of mature plasma cells, TdT-, CD1a-, and CD99-positive immature T cells are always present within and around the epithelial nodules. Over 90 percent of the tumors are encapsulated, but a few are minimally invasive; no cases with recurrence, metastasis, or death from tumor have been reported so far. Myasthenia gravis and other paraneoplastic syndromes have not been associated with these thymomas (141).

Recently, monoclonal B-cell populations were found in 6 of 18 micronodular thymomas,

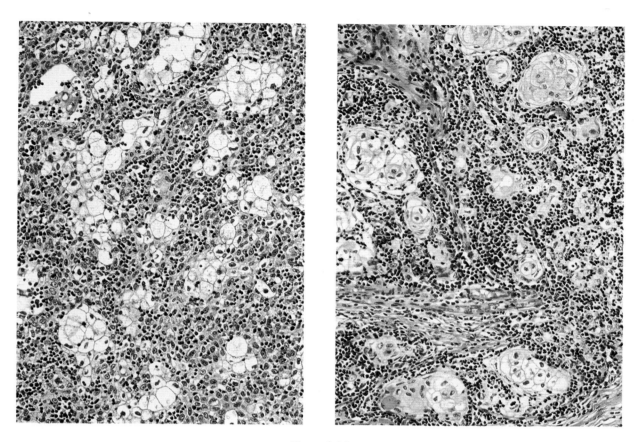

Figure 2-56

THYMOMA TYPE B1/B2 WITH BALLOONING DEGENERATION OF EPITHELIAL CELLS

Left: Within mixed lymphocytic and epithelial thymoma, there are multiple small aggregates of ballooned epithelial cells with a tendency to cytolysis.

Right: In a different case, ballooning is seen in epithelial cells showing squamous differentiation.

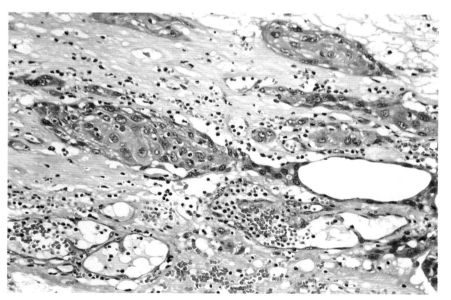

Figure 2-57

SQUAMOUS METAPLASIA IN THYMOMA

There are a few small nests of epithelial cells showing keratinization within a degenerating focus of thymoma. Keratinization of the nests is considered to be secondary to degeneration rather than residual Hassall corpuscles.

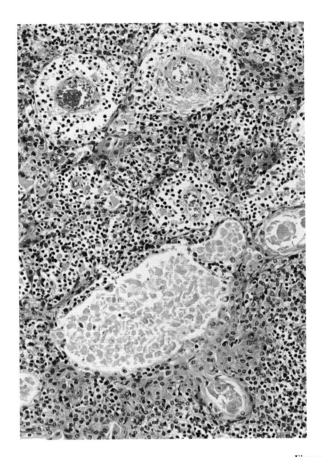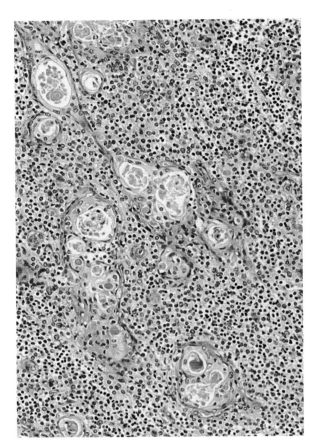

Figure 2-58

THYMOMA WITH MARKED SQUAMOUS DIFFERENTIATION

Left: This mixed lymphocytic and epithelial (type B1/B2) thymoma displays marked squamous differentiation, with abundant keratotic debris in some epithelial cell nests. A few perivascular spaces are lined by flattened epithelial cells.

Right: Hassall corpuscle–like cell nests interconnect. (Courtesy of Dr. Shojiro Morinaga, Tokyo, Japan.)

and intratumoral lymphoma was identified in 3 of 6 monoclonal micronodular thymomas (139b). The authors concluded that abnormal chemokine expression in micronodular thymoma can promote the formation of mucosa-associated lymphoid tissue (MALT), the emergence of monoclonal B cells, and eventually, the subsequent development of mediastinal lymphoma.

Tateyama et al. (149) divided micronodular thymic epithelial tumors into four groups based on the morphology of epithelial cells: group 1 tumors contained spindle cells (this is the typical micronodular thymoma with lymphoid stroma); group 2 contained an admixture of spindle and polygonal cells; group 3 had polygonal cells; and group 4 had features of lympho-epithelioma-like carcinoma. They considered

that each group may constitute a spectrum in the continuum of cytologic atypia.

A combination of micronodular thymoma and another type of thymoma, such as WHO B2 type, was reported (150). One patient with longstanding myasthenia gravis and lymphoid hyperplasia showed features of Castleman disease associated with thymic epithelial hyperplasia, the histology of which was suggestive of micronodular thymoma with lymphoid stroma in areas (see fig. 9-10).

Metaplastic Thymoma (Probably a Variant of Type A Thymoma). Thymomas are often circumscribed but may be invasive and composed of aggregates of polygonal epithelial cells and intervening bundles of spindle-shaped epithelial cells (fig. 2-63). These are metaplastic

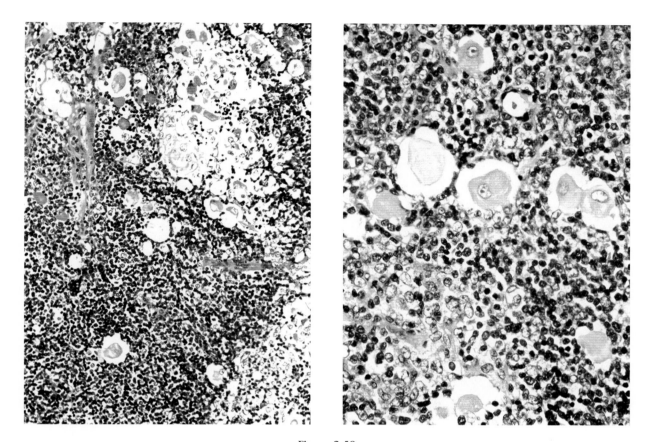

Figure 2-59

THYMOMA WITH MYOID CELLS

Left: Scattered within the tumor tissue are irregularly shaped large cells with vesicular nuclei, prominent nucleoli, and abundant eosinophilic fibrillar or homogenous cytoplasm.

Right: Higher magnification shows cellular detail. The cytoplasm of these cells was strongly positive for myoglobin (see fig. 2-95). (Figs. 2-59 and 2-95 are from the same patient.)

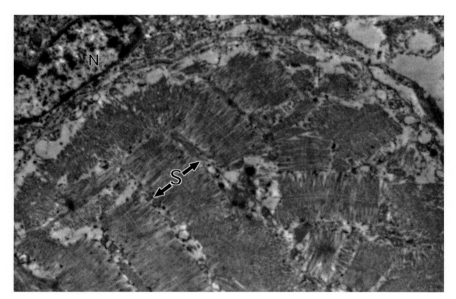

Figure 2-60

THYMOMA WITH MYOID CELLS

Electron micrograph shows that the cells contain numerous sarcomeres (S). The nucleus (N) belongs to a neighboring epithelial cell. (Fig. 3-72 from Fascicle 21, Third Series.)

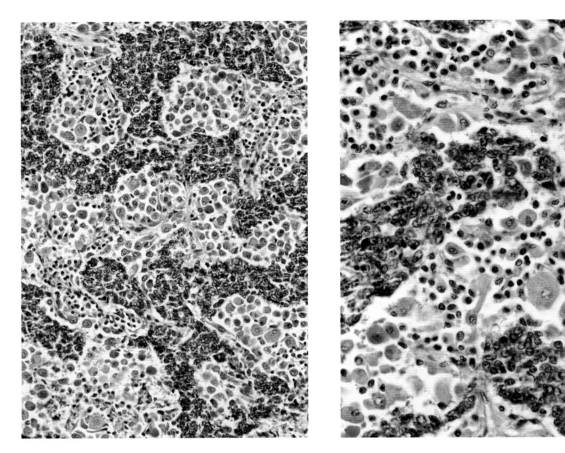

Figure 2-61

RHABDOMYOMATOUS THYMOMA

Left: Between the irregularly shaped nests of small epithelial cells of medullary type with vesicular nuclei and scanty cytoplasm, are numerous loosely arranged rhabdoid cells and some lymphoid cells.

Right: Higher magnification of the tumor reveals tadpole-shaped and round rhabdoid cells with a faintly fibrillar cytoplasm. (Courtesy of Dr. Cesar A. Moran, Houston, Texas.)

thymomas, also referred to as *thymoma with pseudosarcomatous stroma, biphasic thymoma of mixed polygonal and spindle cell type, biphasic metaplastic thymoma,* and *low-grade metaplastic carcinoma* (144,164). At a glance, these look like sarcomatoid carcinoma or malignant biphasic mesothelioma, but the nuclei are bland with little mitotic activity. The polygonal cells and occasional spindle cells are positive for cytokeratin. Lymphocytes are usually few in number. An association with myasthenia gravis and other paraneoplastic syndromes has not been reported.

Sclerosing Thymoma. Two cases of sclerosing thymoma, one each of predominantly epithelial and predominantly lymphocytic types, were re-

ported by Kuo (63), who considers sclerosis to be a phenomenon of spontaneous regression.

Plasma Cell–Rich Thymoma. A case of plasma cell–rich thymoma was reported by Moran et al. (87) in which a polyclonal hypergamma-globulinemia of unknown cause subsequently developed.

Pigmented Thymoma. A case of type A (spindle cell) thymoma with scattered melanin-containing, spindle or polygonal cells lying singly or forming small aggregates was encountered (fig. 2-64) (135). The cells were melanocytes, which may have originated from the neuroectodermal cells present in the thymic tissue. Neural features could not be demonstrated in the tumor, except for S-100 protein positivity in both polygonal and spindle

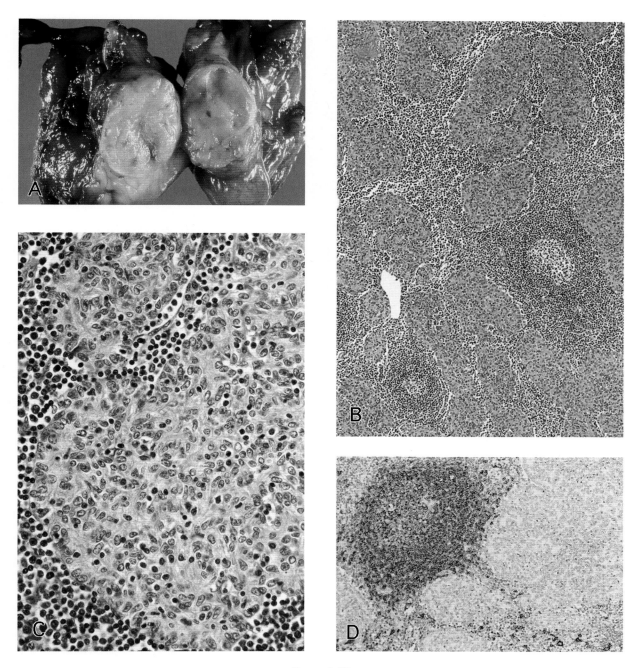

Figure 2-62

MICRONODULAR THYMOMA WITH LYMPHOID STROMA

An 80-year-old Japanese woman had a tumor in the anterior mediastinum, which was diagnosed as thymoma by needle biopsy and surgically resected.

A: The tumor, located in the lower pole of the right lobe of the thymus, is 3.5 x 2.5 cm and mostly encapsulated, and has a pale pinkish tan, rather homogeneous cut surface without lobulation.

B: Low-power view reveals multiple discrete epithelial cell nodules separated by lymphoid tissue with germinal centers.

C: High-power view shows epithelial cells forming nodules. These are polygonal and possess oval, small bland nuclei, inconspicuous nucleoli, and a moderate amount of cytoplasm. Epithelial nodules are scattered with a few lymphocytes.

D. Lymphocytes separating epithelial nodules stain for CD20, but those in the epithelial nodules are negative. (Courtesy of Dr. Tsunekazu Hishima, Tokyo, Japan.)

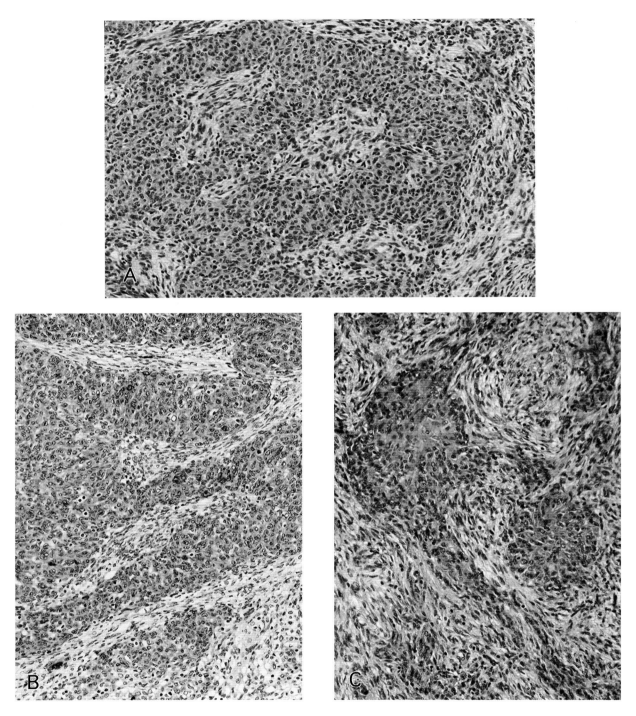

Figure 2-63

METAPLASTIC THYMOMA (BIPHASIC THYMOMA)

A: The tumor is composed of irregular anastomosing cords of polygonal cells and bundles of spindle cells somewhat resembling malignant mesothelioma of the biphasic epithelial and fibrous type.

B: Immunostaining for cytokeratin is positive in the epithelial tumor cells and weaker in the spindle tumor cells.

C: Another case of metaplastic thymoma has equal amounts of epithelial and spindle cell sarcomatoid elements. (Courtesy of Dr. Tadaaki Eimoto, Nagoya, Japan.)

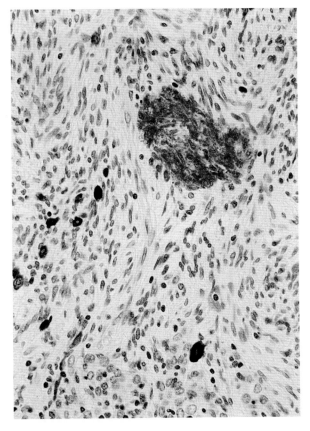

Figure 2-64

THYMOMA (TYPE A) WITH MELANOCYTES

Within the area of spindle cells are a few cell nests and scattered single cells with cytoplasmic brown (melanin) pigment (hematoxylin without eosin counterstain). Immunostaining for HMB45 was negative. (Figs. 2-64 and 2-85 are from the same patient.)

epithelial cells (see fig. 2-85). The presence of non-neoplastic melanocytes was also described in a thymic carcinoid tumor (46).

Microscopic Thymoma. These thymomas are invisible to the naked eye, but are found incidentally in routine sections of the thymus gland taken at the time of lung or cardiac surgery or at autopsy. They arise in the cortical and medullary compartments of the thymus. They may be multifocal and are found both in patients with or without myasthenia gravis but are said to be more frequent in the thymuses of patients with myasthenia gravis. The tumors are nonencapsulated and consist of bland-looking, pleomorphic, polygonal, or plump spindle cells, usually with few if any intraepithelial lympho-

cytes (figs. 2-65–2-67) (108,112,135). The tumor may be seen in a thymus with typical thymoma. There is no proof that microscopic thymoma is a precursor lesion of grossly recognizable thymoma, in spite of the fact that the histology is that of thymoma of various types.

Recently, Rosai (119) stated that a microscopic lesion such as that shown in figures 2-65 and 2-66 is probably nodular hyperplasia (or a thymic tumorlet) rather than microscopic thymoma. This interpretation has been supported by Cheuk et al. (29), who reported two small tumors of 5 mm and 7 mm that displayed histologic features of conventional type B1/B2 and type B2 thymoma, respectively. The tumors had perivascular spaces, a focus of medullary differentiation, and infiltration of TdT-positive immature T cells. They designated these tumors "microthymomas" to distinguish them from the microscopic thymoma described here. The microscopic lesion shown in figure 2-67 as a microscopic thymoma is considered by them to be microthymoma of type B2.

Lipofibroadenoma. This very rare entity has been listed in the new WHO classification (151). This tumor occurred adjacent to a type B1 thymoma in a patient with pure red cell aplasia (67). The tumor resembles fibroadenoma of the breast and shares morphologic features with thymolipoma. As with thymolipoma, it is unknown whether the lesion is neoplastic or hamartomatous.

Histologic Factors Associated with Degree of Malignancy

The problems related to the assessment of the prognosis of patients with thymoma were reviewed and described concisely by Wick in 1990 (158), who believed that staging procedures predicated on the degree of tumor invasion were the best prognosticators for thymoma. Studies at Memorial Sloan-Kettering Cancer Center also indicated that stage of the disease was the only independent prognostic factor affecting recurrence. Multivariate analysis showed that stage, tumor size, histology, and extent of surgical resection were independent predictors of long-term survival (22). Many reports support this concept (75,95,104).

Histology and Cell Types. Pathologists and clinicians agree that no histologic difference

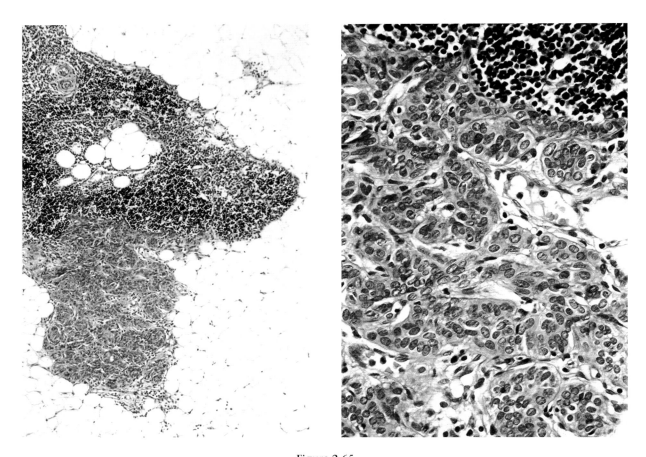

Figure 2-65

MICROSCOPIC THYMOMA

Left: In continuity with the cortex of the thymus is a microscopic lesion consisting of small, solid epithelial cell nests with scanty fibrous stroma.

Right: At higher magnification, the epithelial cells are polygonal with oval nuclei, indistinct nucleoli, and scanty cytoplasm. This lesion may be considered by some to be nodular hyperplasia. (Courtesy of Dr. Tetsuro Kodama, Matsudo City, Japan.) (Figs. 2-65 and 2-66 are from the same patient.)

exists between encapsulated, surgically curable thymoma and invasive thymoma with an unfavorable outcome. This appears to be generally true, but spindle cell (type A) thymoma is considered to be practically a benign tumor. Marino and Müller-Hermelink (78) include not only the medullary type (type A) but also mixed medullary and cortical type (type AB) thymomas in this category. The incidence of predominantly epithelial and polygonal cell type (type B3) thymoma in clinically advanced disease stage is high, and a majority of fatal cases are either predominantly epithelial polygonal cell type (type B3) or mixed lymphocytic and polygonal epithelial cell type (type B2); the prognosis of patients with the spindle cell type (type A) thymoma is much bet-

ter than those with other subtypes of thymoma (Tables 2-5, 2-6; fig. 2-68) (75). Therefore, thymoma of the polygonal cell type, particularly the predominantly epithelial cell type, can be said to be more aggressive biologically than other cell types or histologic subtypes.

The epithelial cells of thymomas that show nuclear atypia are almost always of the polygonal cell type. The nuclei are large, round, and vesicular, and often contain distinct nucleoli; mitotic figures are frequent in some cases (atypical thymoma) (fig. 2-40) (19,142). The epithelial cells may have epidermoid features, and such tumors are categorized by Marino and Müller-Hermelink (78) as well-differentiated (organotypical) carcinoma (type B3 thymoma),

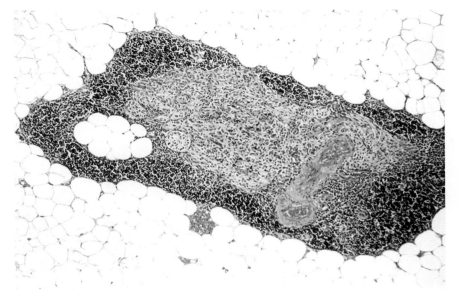

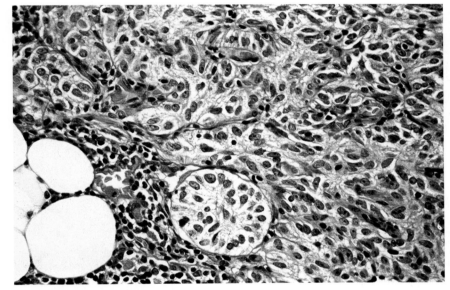

Figure 2-66

MICROSCOPIC THYMOMA

Top: A microscopic lesion occupies the central portion of a thymic lobule and is surrounded by the cortex. A small amount of medulla is seen in the lower right, adjacent to the lesion.

Bottom: Higher magnification reveals that the constituent cells are short spindled, with oval to elongated uniform nuclei and some small but distinct nucleoli. A single rosette-like structure is noted. Both microscopic lesions in figures 2-65 and 2-66 are considered to consist of medullary type epithelial cells (epithelial cells of type A thymoma of World Health Organization [WHO] classification). This lesion is also considered by some to be nodular hyperplasia rather than thymoma. (Courtesy of Dr. Tetsuro Kodama, Matsudo City, Japan.)

since they are more aggressive than thymomas of other subtypes (figs. 2-36, 2-54, left).

In a study by Kirchner et al. (54), all medullary (type A) thymomas (6 cases) and mixed medullary and cortical (type AB) thymomas (27 cases) were of either stage I or II of Masaoka's classification (81). Twelve percent of predominantly cortical (type B1) thymomas (9 cases) were stage III and none was stage IV. Thirty-eight percent and 9 percent of cortical (type B2) thymomas (57 cases) were stages III and IV, respectively. Fifty-seven percent and 26 percent of well-differentiated

thymic carcinomas (type B3 thymoma) (23 cases) were stage III and IV, respectively.

Quintanilla-Martinez et al. (113) studied 116 patients with thymic epithelial tumors classified according to the Müller-Hermelink histogenetic classification system (54,78). They concluded that "their histologic classification has prognostic significance independent of tumor stage; medullary and mixed (types A and AB) thymomas were benign tumors with no risk of recurrence; organoid (predominantly cortical, or type B1) and cortical (type B2) thymomas

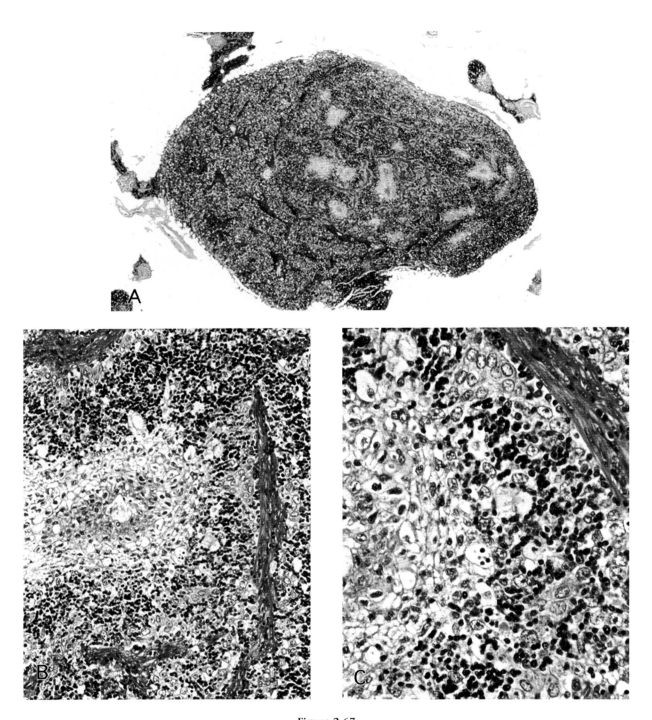

Figure 2-67

**INCIDENTALLY FOUND MICROSCOPIC
THYMOMA WITH EPIDERMOID FEATURES**

A: The 5-mm tumor is nonencapsulated. Several clear areas with epidermoid features are scattered within the tumor.

B: An area with epidermoid features is surrounded by a lymphocyte-rich zone with polygonal epithelial cells.

C: Higher magnification reveals cells transitional between those with epidermoid features and polygonal epithelial cells with vesicular nuclei and prominent nucleoli. This tumor is considered to correspond with "well-differentiated organotypical low-grade thymic carcinoma" (type B2/B3 thymoma of WHO classification).

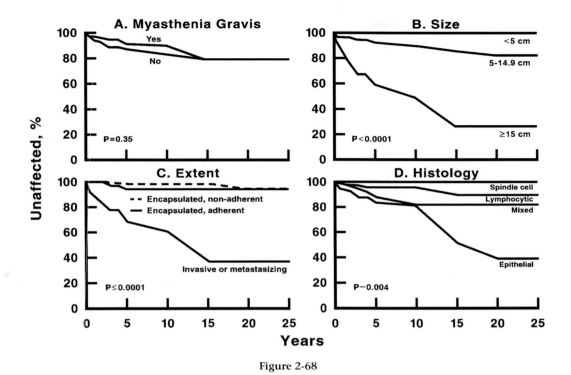

Figure 2-68

REPRESENTATIVE CURVES FOR SURVIVAL TO THYMOMA DEATH ACCORDING TO SELECTED VARIABLES

(Fig. 12 from Lewis JE, Wick MR, Scheithauer BW, Bernatz PE, Taylor WF. Thymoma: a clinicopathologic review. Cancer 1987;60:2737.)

showed intermediate invasiveness and a low but significant risk of late relapse. Well-differentiated thymic carcinomas (type B3 thymoma) were always invasive and had a significantly increased risk of relapse and death" (fig. 2-69).

Pan et al. (104) reported that further subclassification of cortical thymomas into organoid thymoma, conventional cortical thymoma, and well-differentiated thymic carcinoma did not provide more information about clinical behavior. By actuarial survival analyses, none of the epithelial subtypes displayed a statistically significant influence on prognosis; staging remains the most important factor affecting the patient's outcome.

According to the WHO classification system, types A, AB, B1, B2, and B3 thymoma are arranged in increasing order of malignancy (Table 2-5). Type A thymoma behaves like a benign tumor; types AB and B1 as low-grade malignant tumors (10-year survival rates of over 90 percent); type B2 has a greater degree of malignancy; and type B3 in the advanced stage shows a poor prognosis, just like thymic carcinoma and malignant

tumors of other organs (fig. 2-70) (100,151). Similar survival data, although with minor differences, were obtained by other studies (fig. 2-71) (95,139a). On the contrary, a study of 73 thymomas and 17 thymic carcinomas revealed that the prognosis for patients with types A/AB thymoma was not significantly different from that for patients with types B1/B2/B3 thymoma, but that a significant difference was noted between thymomas and thymic carcinoma (25).

In the pathology file of National Cancer Center Hospital in Tokyo, there were three patients with type A and AB thymomas with hematogenous metastases: multiple lung metastases in two cases and lung and liver metastases in one (135). The first case was a 10 cm thymoma in stage II. The tumor was partly predominantly lymphocytic and in part predominated by small polygonal to oval epithelial cells with frequent rosette-like structures (type AB) (fig. 2-44). Blood vessel invasion was frequently seen (fig. 2-72). Three years after surgery, the patient developed three metastatic nodules in the left lung, which were resected. Histologically, the epithelial

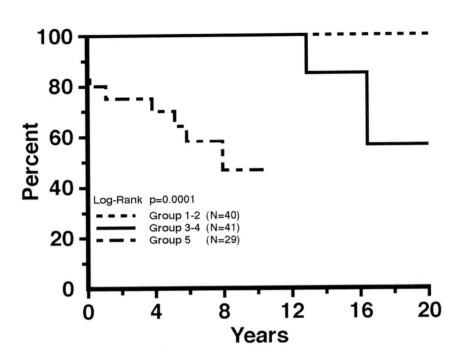

Figure 2-69

DISEASE-FREE SURVIVAL: FREEDOM FROM RELAPSE OF THYMIC EPITHELIAL TUMOR BY HISTOLOGIC SUBTYPE

Group 1: medullary; group 2: mixed; group 3: organoid; group 4: cortical; group 5; well-differentiated carcinoma (WDTC) (type B3 thymoma by WHO classification). Patients with WDTC relapsed more often and earlier than patients with other histologic subtypes. (Fig. 2 from Quintanilla-Martinez L, Wilkins EW Jr, Choi N, Efird J, Hug E, Harris NL. Thymoma. Histologic subclassification is an independent prognostic factor. Cancer 1994;74:613.)

component predominated (type A). The lung metastases were resected again 5 years later and the patient was alive with lung metastases 11 years after the first surgery.

In the second case, the mediastinal tumor projected into the lumen of the innominate vein, and invaded the lung and pericardium. The resected lobe of the lung contained three metastatic nodules. Both primary and metastatic tumors were similar, consisting of sheets of short spindle cells occasionally forming gland-like structures (type A thymoma) (fig. 2-73), Lung metastases were detected again 2 years after surgery, for which chemotherapy was given without effect. The patient was alive with multiple intrapulmonary metastases 5 years after surgery. In both cases no lymph node metastases were found (57,135). The third patient with lung and liver metastases had small round cell–predominant type A thymoma in the primary and spindle cell type A thymoma with pericytomatous areas in metastatic foci (fig. 2-74).

A case with lung and brain metastases was of predominantly small round epithelial cell type with round vesicular nuclei, inconspicuous nucleoli, and scanty cytoplasm forming questionable rosette-like structures (129). Scattered small aggregates of CD1a- and CD99-positive immature T cells (type AB) were seen (fig. 2-75). The patient

died of lung cancer with brain metastasis 12 years after detection of the mediastinal tumor.

The presence of such type A and type AB thymomas indicates that short spindle-shaped or small oval/round tumor cells showing rosette-like and glandular structures may behave in a malignant fashion at times, although growth is indolent. These tumors may be biologically different from type A thymoma with fibroblast-like spindle cells, although the case shown in figure 2-74 may indicate transformation of oval cells to long spindle cells.

By analyzing 81 type A (43 cases) and type AB (38 cases) thymomas, Pan et al. (102) concluded that all of type A and most type AB thymomas are detected at stages I and II; follow-up of the patients did not disclose relapse or tumor death. The outcome did not significantly differ from that of stage I and II thymomas of other types by a stage-matched survival analysis. They also divided these thymomas into short spindled (57 percent), long spindled (31 percent), and micronodular (12 percent) variants, but their staging and survival data did not support our hypothesis that the oval/short spindled variant is more aggressive than the long spindled form, although the patients with the long spindled variant were significantly younger. Further study of types A/AB thymoma is needed.

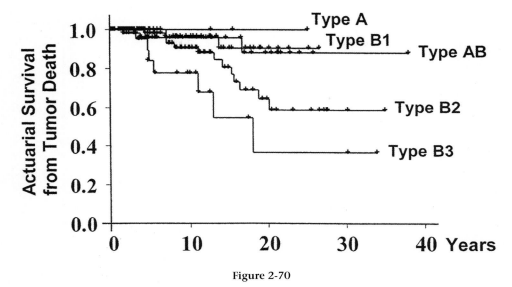

Figure 2-70

**SURVIVAL CURVES ACCORDING TO THE WHO HISTOLOGIC
CLASSIFICATION SYSTEM AMONG PATIENTS WITH THYMOMA**

Survival refers to freedom from tumor death. The curves reflect 17 patients with type A tumors, 66 with type AB tumors, 49 with type B1 tumors, 89 with type B2 tumors, and 22 with type B3 tumors. There was no significant difference in survival between patients with combinations of type A, type AB, and type B1 tumors. Conversely, there was a significant difference in survival between patients with type AB and type B3 tumors ($P = 0.004$), patients with type B1 and type B3 tumors ($P = 0.001$), and patients with type B2 and type B3 tumors ($P = 0.04$). Patients with type A tumors showed a tendency toward better survival compared with patients who had type B3 tumors ($P = 0.07$), and patients with type B1 tumors also showed a tendency toward better survival compared with patients who had type B2 tumors ($P = 0.06$). (Fig. 2 from Okumura M, Ohta M, Tateyama H, et al. The World Health Organization histologic classification system reflects the oncologic behavior of thymoma. A clinical study of 273 patients. Cancer 2002;94:628.)

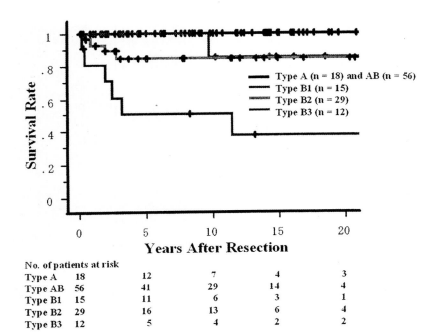

Figure 2-71

SURVIVAL CURVES ACCORDING TO THE HISTOLOGIC SUBTYPE OF THYMOMA

The 5- and 10-year survival rates according to the histologic subtype of thymoma are shown: 100% and 100% (type A and AB), 100% and 86% (type B1), 85% and 85% (type B2), and 51% and 38% (type B3), respectively. The difference in survival between patients with type B2 and type B3 is significant ($P = .000$). (Fig. 3 from Nakagawa K, Asamura H, Matsuno Y, et al. Thymoma: A clinicopathologic study based on the new World Health Organization classification. J Thorac Cardiovasc Surg 2003;126:1137.)

No. of patients at risk

Type A	18	12	7	4	3
Type AB	56	41	29	14	4
Type B1	15	11	6	3	1
Type B2	29	16	13	6	4
Type B3	12	5	4	2	2

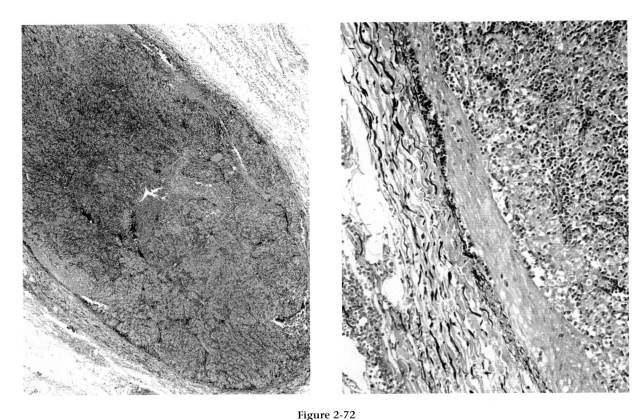

Figure 2-72

THYMOMA WITH BLOOD VESSEL INVASION

Left: Mixed lymphocytic and epithelial type thymoma forming frequent rosette-like structures occludes a medium-sized vein.

Right: Higher magnification (elastica stain).

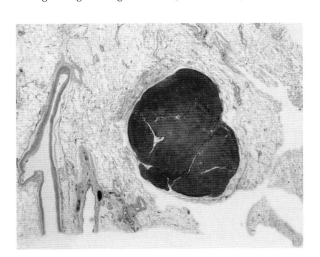
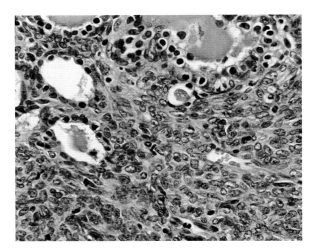

Figure 2-73

THYMOMA (TYPE A) WITH GLAND FORMATION METASTATIC TO THE LUNG

Left: A small, well-defined, nonencapsulated tumor metastatic to the lung.

Right: Higher magnification reveals glandular structures lined by cuboidal cells within an area of diffuse growth of oval to short spindle tumor cells.

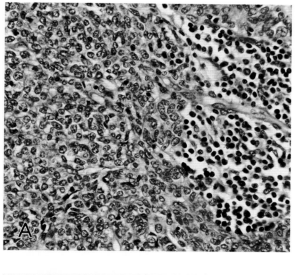

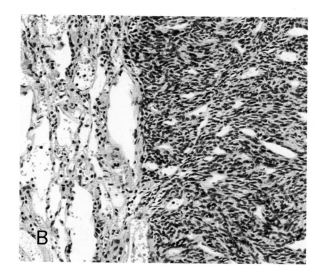

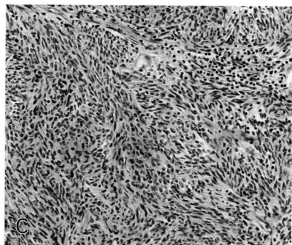

Figure 2-74

**THYMOMA (TYPE A OR AB) WITH
LUNG AND LIVER METASTASES**

A: The primary tumor is composed of areas with diffuse growth of small oval cells with vesicular nuclei, inconspicuous nucleoli, and scanty cytoplasm. Scattered, predominantly lymphocytic areas are suggestive of perivascular spaces filled with lymphocytes.

B: The lung metastasis is made up of long spindle cells arranged in a hemangiopericytomatous pattern.

C: Higher magnification of the lung metastasis shows moderately cellular, haphazardly arranged bundles of long spindle cells with a few lymphocytes.

D: Needle core biopsy of a liver metastasis discloses a similar but less vascular tumor than the lung metastasis.

E: Higher magnification of the liver metastasis shows features resembling the metastasis in the lung, and do not appear sarcomatous.

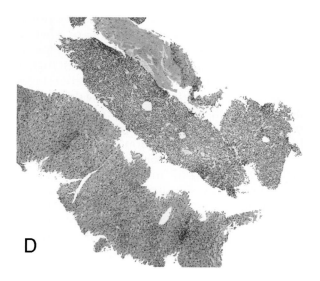

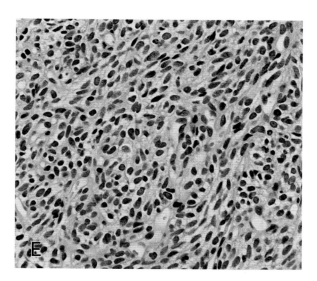

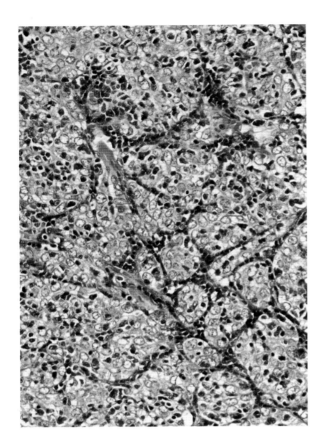 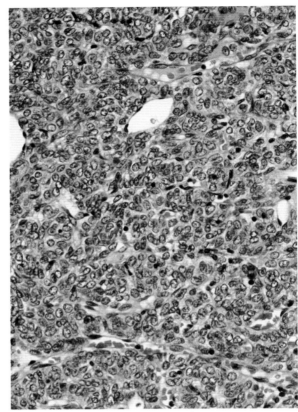

Figure 2-75

THYMOMA (TYPE AB) WITH LUNG AND BRAIN METASTASES

Left: In the primary tumor, small nests of small polygonal cells with vesicular nuclei, inconspicuous nucleoli, and scanty cytoplasm are often bordered by lymphocytes. (Figs. 2-75 and 2-92 are from the same patient.)

Right: The histology of the brain metastasis is similar to that of the primary tumor, although lymphocytes are reduced in number. (Courtesy of Dr. Minako Seki, Hiratsuka, Kanagawa, Japan.)

Proliferative Activity. The relationship between the frequency of mitotic figures in the epithelial cells and the degree of malignancy of the thymoma has not yet been studied in detail. Since the proliferative activity of tumor cells is considered to be one of several malignancy-associated factors in many tumors, such a study should be conducted for thymic epithelial tumors as well. Proliferative activity is determined not only by counting mitotic figures but also by the immunostaining of proliferating cell nuclear antigen (PCNA) or proliferation-associated nuclear antigen (Ki-67), and probably by investigating genetic abnormalities in growth-related oncogenes and tumor suppressor genes. However, no clinically applicable results have been obtained by immunohistochemical cell kinetic studies of

PCNA and Ki-67 in thymic epithelial tumors, although well-differentiated thymic carcinoma (type B3 thymoma) showed higher Ki-67 labeling indices compared with the medullary (type A) thymoma ($P<0.05$). Stage IV cases showed higher PCNA labeling indices than those of other stages ($P<0.05$). The results indicate that the differences in biologic behavior of the different histologic types may be, in part, explained by differences in the tumor growth fraction (163).

Similar results were obtained by Pan et al. (103) by using Ki-67 immunostaining; there were statistically significant differences in the labeling indices between stage I and stage III and between stage I and stage IV. Also, histologically, statistically significant differences were identified between predominantly epithelial thymoma and other subtypes of the conventional morphologic classification and between well-differentiated thymic carcinoma (type B3 thymoma) and medullary (type A) or mixed (type AB) thymomas. Regarding the prognostic implication of Ki-67 labeling indices, although there appeared to be a trend toward worse survival for patients with tumors with higher labeling indices, the difference was not statistically significant. Pan et al. concluded that the clinical usefulness of Ki-67 is limited because the indices of various stages and histologic types overlap and therefore this marker lacks prognostic significance (see chapter 3).

The argyrophilic proteins associated with the nuclear organizer regions (AgNORs) are related to cell proliferative activity. Pich et al. (110) found that the 10-year survival rate was 88 percent for patients with thymomas with 5.75 AgNORs or fewer per cell but only 34 percent for patients with thymomas with more than 5.75 AgNORs per cell (statistically significant), and that AgNOR counts as well as tumor stage retained independent prognostic significance on multivariate survival analysis.

Frozen Section Findings

A variety of mediastinal tumors show similar features on chest X ray, CT, and magnetic resonance imaging (MRI). Most of these cases can be diagnosed histologically or cytologically either by CT-guided percutaneous needle biopsy, biopsy through a mediastinoscope or thoracoscope, and rarely, by a fiberoptic bronchoscope. In the few cases without a preoperative histologic diagnosis, needle or incisional biopsy for frozen section evaluation during surgery is necessary to determine the histologic type of the tumor. Tumors that should be distinguished from thymoma include thymic carcinoma, carcinoid tumor, malignant lymphoma, germ cell tumors (mature and immature teratomas and malignant germ cell tumors), metastatic carcinoma, and a variety of other tumors that may occur in the mediastinum.

Subtyping of thymomas can be done on frozen section specimens in most instances; however, a different subtype may be present in the residual portion of the tumor. If the tissue is small in amount, imprint smears can be of help. Pleural and pulmonary lesions and enlarged lymph nodes, if present, can be sampled for frozen section analysis as well.

Cytologic Findings

Advances in imaging techniques make it much easier to approach and obtain material from mediastinal tumors, and thus needle biopsy or aspiration cytology under CT guidance is being increasingly performed (130,138,156). Needle core biopsy is more often performed than aspiration cytology just because of the preference of surgeons and pathologists, but it is obvious that pathologists should be well acquainted with the cytologic findings of various mediastinal tumors. Cytologic materials are obtained by needle aspiration through a mediastinoscope, bronchoscope, or thoracoscope, or by direct percutaneous harvesting. Pleural or pericardial fluids may be aspirated to prove implantation metastasis of the tumor. Touch imprints of the lesion can be used for diagnosis of anterior mediastinal neoplasms during surgery (62).

Smears prepared from the aspiration of thymoma frequently consist of a mixture of epithelial cells and lymphocytes. Tissue fragments composed of epithelial cell aggregates intimately associated with lymphocytes are called lymphoepithelial complexes, and their presence is generally diagnostic of thymoma (fig. 2-76) (34,117). Lymphoepithelial complexes are quite large at times. The cellular detail of the central portion of the complex can be difficult to analyze because of piling up of the cells and the resulting crushing effects. Cellular detail is clearly observed at the periphery, however. These complexes are seen in cases of mixed lymphocytic and epithelial (mixed, predominantly cortical, and cortical or types AB, B1, and B2) thymomas. The epithelial cells may be seen singly, in small aggregates, or in sheets. Cells arranged in sheets and aggregates with a few lymphocytes are seen in spindle/oval cell–predominant (type A or AB) thymoma, polygonal cell–predominant (type B3) thymoma, or thymic cancer. Dispersed single epithelial cells are seen in all types of thymomas.

Cytologically, there are two epithelial cell types in thymomas (155a), although identification of these two cell types is difficult at times because of the presence of a probable intermediate cell type. One is the spindle/oval cell type, which possesses oval or fusiform, normochromatic nuclei of up to 7 μm in the shortest dimension, with dispersed or unevenly distributed

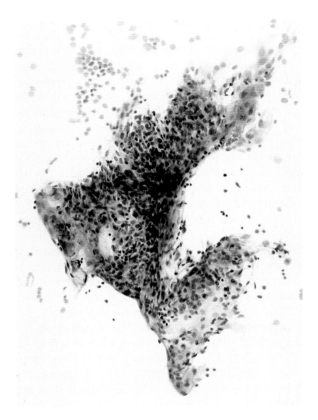

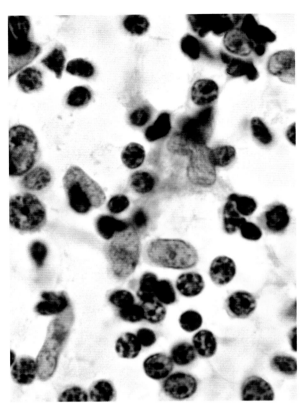

Figure 2-76

NEEDLE ASPIRATION CYTOLOGY OF THYMOMA: "LYMPHOEPITHELIAL COMPLEX"

Fragments of piled up epithelial cells are mixed with lymphocytes. Type A thymoma with medullary type epithelial cells. (Figs. 2-76 and 2-78 are from the same patient.)

Figure 2-77

NEEDLE ASPIRATION CYTOLOGY OF TYPE AB THYMOMA WITH MEDULLARY TYPE (SPINDLE) EPITHELIAL CELLS

There is a mixture of small lymphocytes and epithelial cells with oval or fusiform nuclei, unevenly distributed chromatin, inconspicuous nucleoli, and scanty or indistinct cytoplasm. (Fig. 1b from Ebihara Y, Dilnur P. Cytology of the mediastinal tumors. Byori to Rinsho 2002;20:609.)

chromatin, indistinct or small nucleoli, and lightly stained scanty or indistinct cytoplasm (fig. 2-77). These cells correspond to cells of spindle (type A) and mixed (type AB) thymoma, or the medullary epithelial cells of Müller-Hermelink et al. (figs. 2-78, 2-79). Figure 2-80 is from a rare case of pigmented thymoma, which was encapsulated and consisted predominantly of epithelial cells of short spindle to oval cell type, some containing brown granular pigment in the cytoplasm. Pigmented cells are negative for S-100 protein and HMB45, but some are positive for synaptophysin, indicating that the pigment could well be neuromelanin.

The other cytologic cell type is the polygonal/round cell. These cells possess round, normochromatic, and often clear nuclei, larger than the

nuclei of spindle cell type (8 to 11 μm), conspicuous round nucleoli, and variable amounts of light green-stained cytoplasm (figs. 2-81, 2-82). These epithelial cells correspond to the cells of polygonal/round cell (type B) thymoma or the cortical type epithelial cells of Müller-Hermelink et al. Although we are not familiar with the cytology of predominantly epithelial, atypical (type B3) thymoma with epidermoid features, the epidermoid cells are probably mixed with type B cells in smears and are expected to show round or irregular grooved nuclei, inconspicuous nucleoli, moderate amounts of cytoplasm, and well-defined cell borders.

Lymphocytes accompanying the epithelial cells of thymoma also consist of two cell types. One is a small mature lymphocyte with small

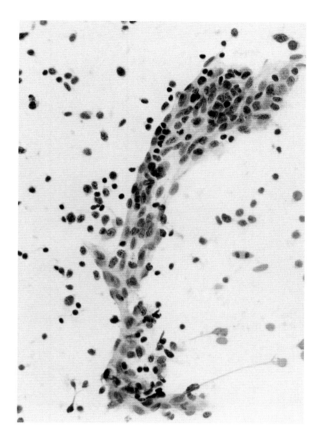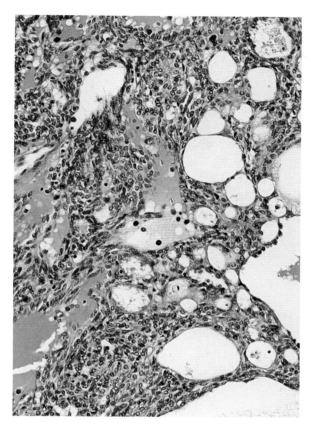

Figure 2-78

**NEEDLE ASPIRATION CYTOLOGY OF TYPE A THYMOMA WITH
MEDULLARY TYPE (SPINDLE) EPITHELIAL CELLS**

Left: An aggregate of spindle cells is mixed with some lymphocytes. The spindle cells have fusiform nuclei with evenly distributed fine chromatin and lightly stained cytoplasm.

Right: The histology of the resected tumor reveals features characteristic of cystic (type A) thymoma composed predominantly of short spindle epithelial cells.

dark-stained round nuclei without discernible internal structures and almost invisible cytoplasm (fig. 2-77). The other is a medium-sized lymphocyte with active-appearing, lighter-stained round nuclei with a recognizable chromatin pattern and cytoplasmic rim (figs. 2-81, 2-82). Mitotic figures may be seen. These lymphocytes correspond to immature (cortical) lymphocytes. Because of the morphology of such lymphocytes and the presence of epithelial cells misinterpreted as thyroid follicular cells, ectopic cervical thymoma mimicking a thyroid mass may lead to a misdiagnosis of malignant lymphoma when needle aspiration cytology is used (97,111).

Mature small lymphocytes predominate in spindle cell/medullary (type A) thymoma. Lym-

phocytes of both mature and immature forms are seen in thymomas of types AB and B. Lymphocytes in thymic cancer are of mature form.

The histologic subtype of the thymoma can be suspected from the cytologic findings in many cases, although the histologic features may vary from area to area of the thymoma. Rarely, necrotic material is present in thymoma smears, but its presence does not mean aggressiveness or a malignant nature.

The following is an instructive case kindly supplied by Dr. Tamiko Takemura. The patient was 53-year-old man who had an abnormal density in the left pulmonary hilar region on chest X-ray examination. Bronchial brushing cytology obtained from a polypoid tumor projecting into the left B6 bronchus revealed a mixture

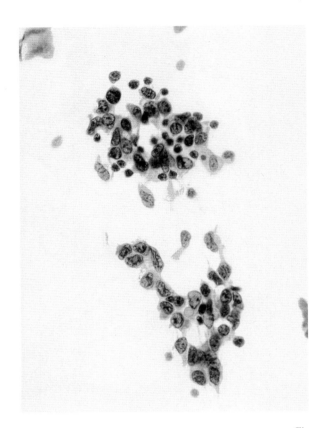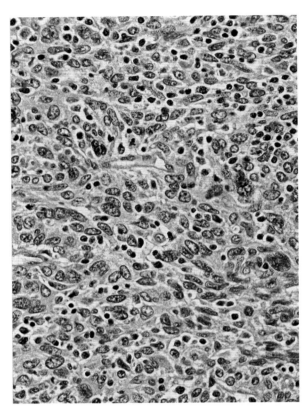

Figure 2-79

NEEDLE ASPIRATION CYTOLOGY OF TYPE AB THYMOMA WITH
MIXED MEDULLARY AND CORTICAL TYPE EPITHELIAL CELLS

Left: The smear shows a mixture of lymphocytes and larger epithelial cells. The latter possess either vesicular, oval to irregular nuclei and some small nucleoli, or irregular but bland nuclei and inconspicuous nucleoli, consistent with type AB (mixed) thymoma.

Right: The thymoma is composed predominantly of epithelial cells with varying sized short spindle cells having granular to vesicular nuclei and some small nucleoli. Small lymphocytes are scattered. This histologic picture is consistent with a diagnosis of type AB (mixed medullary and cortical) thymoma.

of lymphoid cells and scattered epithelial cells with round to oval, finely granular, bland nuclei; inconspicuous nucleoli; and a moderate amount of faintly stained cytoplasm. It was categorized as class III (suggestive of but inconclusive for malignancy) (fig. 2-83A). Since the tumor invaded the pericardium, left upper lobectomy with resection of the pericardium was performed. The tumor was diagnosed as mixed lymphocytic and epithelial (type B2-like) thymoma (fig. 2-83B), ectopic either in the lung or in the middle mediastinum. Imprint smears at the time of surgery revealed frequent active-appearing lymphocytes and scattered epithelial cells. The latter varied from small cells with oval to reniform nuclei, inconspicuous nucleoli, and a moderate amount of faintly

stained cytoplasm to large cells with vesicular nuclei and distinct nucleoli (fig. 2-83C). It was difficult to classify the small epithelial cells, which might well have been medullary type epithelial cells. Together with the presence of a few cortical type epithelial cells and frequent active lymphocytes, the tumor could be subtyped as a mixed medullary and cortical type thymoma. Retrospectively, bronchial smears were also consistent with the cytology of the thymoma, although the lymphocytes could be subclassified as either mature or immature.

Cytologic Differential Diagnosis. A needle aspiration cytology specimen of type A spindle cell type thymoma may pose significant diagnostic challenges (138). There are a variety of

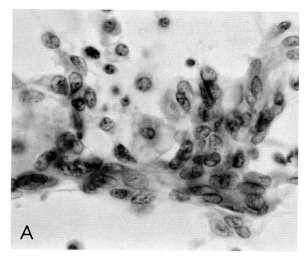

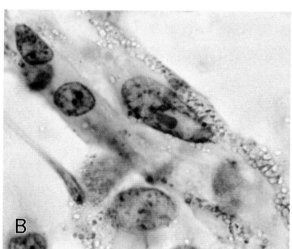

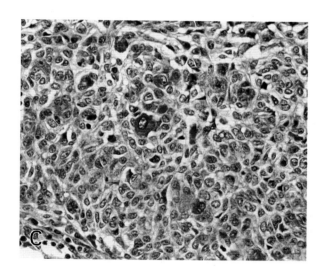

Figure 2-80

NEEDLE ASPIRATION CYTOLOGY OF TYPE A (SPINDLE CELL) THYMOMA WITH PIGMENTED CELLS

A: There is an aggregate of elongated cells with oval to fusiform, rather uniform nuclei and lightly stained cytoplasm.

B: Higher magnification of a different area reveals pigment granules in the cytoplasm.

C: Histologically, the tumor is composed of oval to short spindle cells with bland nuclei and scanty cytoplasm. Some cells have brown granular pigments in the cytoplasm. (Fig. 4A–C from Ebihara Y, Dilnur P. Cytology of mediastinal tumors. Byori to Rinsho 2002;20:610.)

Figure 2-81

NEEDLE ASPIRATION CYTOLOGY OF THYMOMA WITH CORTICAL EPITHELIAL CELLS

The two large epithelial cells have a large round clear nucleus, a single distinct nucleolus, and abundant cytoplasm. They are surrounded by lymphocytes with active nuclei. (Fig. 3 from Ebihara Y, Dilnur P. Cytology of the mediastinal tumors. Byori to Rinsho 2002;20:609.)

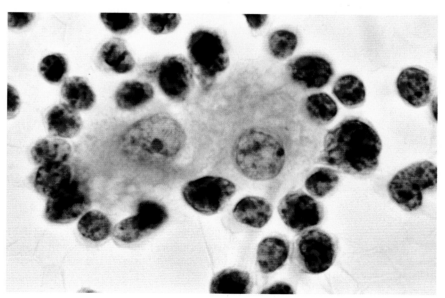

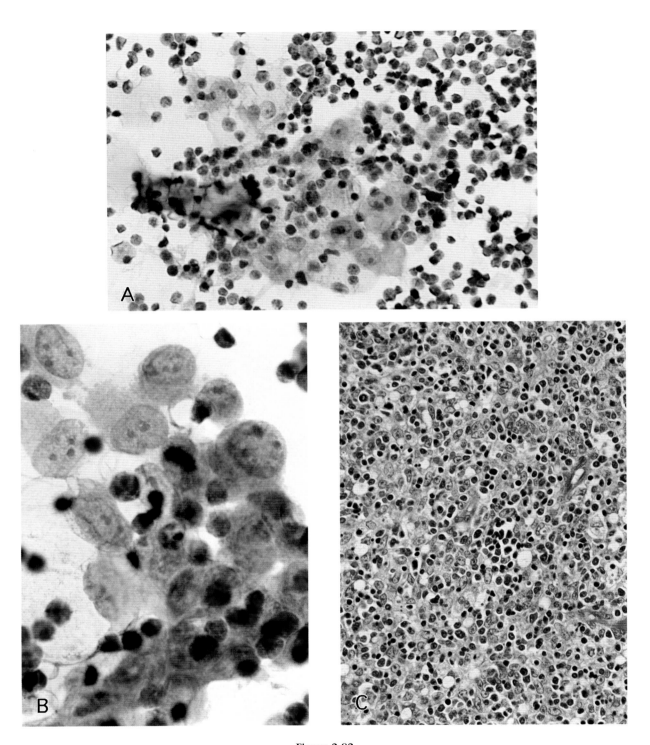

Figure 2-82

NEEDLE ASPIRATION CYTOLOGY OF TYPE B2 THYMOMA

A,B: Medium- and high-power views show a clump of epithelial cells with moderate to abundant cytoplasm and oval nuclei having a fine chromatin pattern and prominent nucleoli. The epithelial cells are surrounded by lymphoid cells, indicating cortical thymoma.

C: The histologic features are characteristic of type B2 (cortical) thymoma.

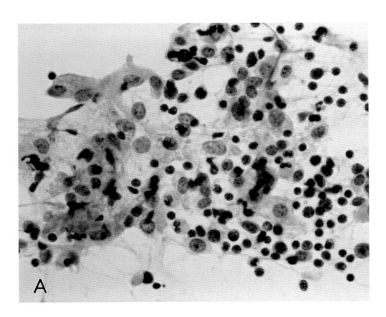

Figure 2-83

CYTOLOGY OF ECTOPIC THYMOMA

A: Cytologically, a bronchial scraping from a polypoid tumor projecting in left B6 bronchus shows a mixture of lymphocytes and scattered medium-sized epithelial cells with oval to round bland nuclei, inconspicuous nucleoli, and abundant faintly stained cytoplasm. This tumor was classified as class III, suggestive of, but inconclusive for, malignancy.

B: The resected tumor revealed a mixture of lymphocytes and small epithelial cells with bland oval nuclei and scanty cytoplasm. A diagnosis of type B2-like thymoma was made.

C: Imprint smears of a resected tumor shows a mixture of lymphocytes and scattered epithelial cells. The lymphocytes possess granular chromatin and appear active. Some epithelial cells are small, with oval to reniform bland nuclei and inconspicuous nucleoli, suggesting either medullary or small cortical type epithelial cells. Other tumor cells are large with vesicular nuclei and prominent nucleoli having features of cortical type epithelial cells. The cytologic findings are consistent with type B2 thymoma. (Courtesy of Dr. Tamiko Takemura, Tokyo, Japan.)

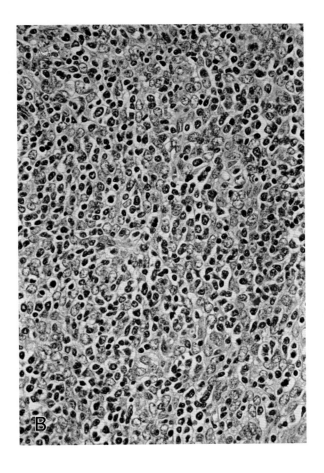

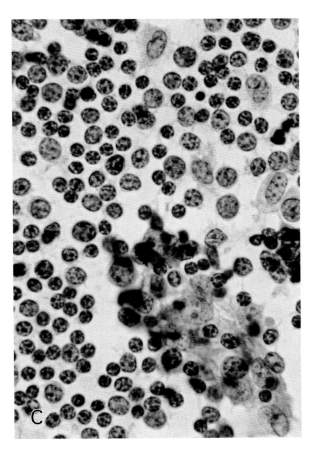

spindle cell lesions in the mediastinum and spindle cell thymoma may contain only a few lymphocytes, a large majority of which are mature T cells.

Thymic carcinoma of any type shows increased atypia (nuclear) of the epithelial cells (see chapter 3). Tumor cells with moderate atypia that mimic carcinoma cells may be seen in some invasive thymomas (117), but the presence of immature T cells with a TdT-, CD1a-, or CD99-positive profile is diagnostic of thymoma. The presence of plasma cells and eosinophils in smears often excludes the possibility of thymoma. Smears of carcinoid tumors contain monotonous medium-sized tumor cells with a peppered chromatin pattern and finely granular cytoplasm, and lymphocytes are mature, small, and few in number.

Singh et al. (137) reviewed 189 fine needle aspiration biopsies (FNAB) of the mediastinum and found 12 diagnostically discordant cases (6 percent) among the satisfactory FNAB specimens with histologic correlation. According to them, these errors primarily involved subclassification of small cell malignancies, such as small cell carcinoma and malignant lymphoma. In two cases, the classification of germ cell tumors and their distinction from metastatic carcinoma were problems. They concluded that FNAB of the mediastinum is an accurate diagnostic procedure.

Regarding malignant lymphoma (see chapter 6), recognition of Reed-Sternberg cells, lacunar cells, or Hodgkin cells leads to a diagnosis of Hodgkin lymphoma. Atypical large lymphoid cells with vesicular nuclei, distinct nucleoli, and frequent mitoses suggest diffuse large B-cell lymphoma with sclerosis. Predominant medium-sized lymphoid cells with round or indented granular nuclei, small nucleoli, and faintly granular cytoplasm suggest low-grade marginal zone B-cell lymphoma of MALT, in which epithelial cells derived from involuted Hassall corpuscles may be seen. Lymphoblastic lymphoma is composed of medium-sized mononuclear atypical lymphoid cells with convoluted or nonconvoluted nuclei (TdT positive), finely dispersed chromatin, inconspicuous nucleoli, and scanty cytoplasm. These cells resemble the cortical or immature T cells present in thymomas (37). The hyaline vascular type of

Castleman disease reveals many small mature B lymphocytes. Among germ cell tumors (see chapter 5), germinoma (seminoma) shows a mixture of lymphocytes, plasma cells, and tumor cells which possess much larger atypical nuclei and larger conspicuous nucleoli than those of thymoma .

The presence of benign-appearing epithelial cells and immature (cortical) lymphocytes points to a diagnosis of thymoma, unless contaminated with normal thymic tissue. The diagnostic accuracy of needle aspiration cytology is high, and when the cytologic diagnosis agrees with the clinical and radiographic findings, a definitive diagnosis can be generally rendered without open biopsy (136). If additional unstained smears are available, immunostaining for CD1a, CD99, or TdT helps to detect the presence of immature (cortical) T cells (131), which are present in thymoma but absent in thymic carcinoma and other thymic tumors, excluding lymphoblastic lymphoma of T-cell type.

Immunohistochemistry and Functional Correlation

The utilization of immunohistochemistry for the differential diagnosis of thymic tumors and tumors of other organs has been described briefly in the previous sections. Here, the immunohistochemical features of thymoma are summarized in comparison with those of other thymic tumors. An immunohistochemical approach is necessary for the characterization of both epithelial cells and lymphocytes. For the preservation of antigens and morphology, cold acetone (or methanol) fixation followed by paraffin embedding is recommended in addition to routine formalin fixation (126).

Epithelial cells of the normal thymus can be divided into subcapsular, cortical, and medullary epithelial cells. Müller-Hermelink et al. (91,92) reported that thymomas can be differentiated into those showing a cortical or medullary phenotype by using monoclonal antibodies such as 35β-H11 (against nonsquamous type keratin) and 34βE12, IV/82 (against squamous type keratin), respectively. Although van der Kwast et al. (155) divided thymomas into those composed mainly of cortical epithelial cells and those composed of medullary epithelial cells using the monoclonal antibodies antihuman

Table 2-7

**SUMMARY OF CYTOKERATIN PROFILE AND EXPRESSION OF
INVOLUCRIN IN DIFFERENT HISTOLOGIC TYPES OF THYMOMA[a]**

Thymoma Type	CK7[b]	CK8	CK10	CK13	CK14	CK18	CK19	CK20	IVL
Spindle cell	+[c]	+	–	–	+	+	+	–	–
Small polygonal cell	–	–	–	–	+	–	+	–	–
Mixed	+	+	–	–	+	+	+	–	–
Organoid	+	+	+	+	+	+	+	–	+
Large polygonal cell	+	–	–	–	–	–	+	–	–
Squamoid	+	–	+	–	–	–	+	–	–

[a]Table 6 from Kuo TT. Cytokeratin profiles of the thymus and thymomas: histogenetic correlations and proposal for a histological classification of thymomas. Histopathology 2000;36:410.
[b]CK = cytokeratin; IVL = involucrin.
[c]+ = majority of cases are focally and/or diffusely stained; – = negative or minority of cases are focally and/or diffusely stained.

leukocyte antigen (HLA)-DR and ER-TR5, and Chilosi et al. (30) found that variable numbers of spindle cells in most mixed thymomas, i.e., medullary type epithelial cells, were positive for the B-cell marker CD20/L26, there are no known antibodies available at present that are specific for either cortical or medullary epithelial cells. According to Pan et al. (102), 70 and 90 percent of spindle epithelial cells of type A and type AB thymomas, respectively, were positive for CD20, a B-cell marker, whereas the short-spindle epithelial cells in all micronodular thymomas were negative.

Recently, the expression of cytokeratins of different molecular weights and involucrin in epithelial cells of thymuses (Tables 1-3, 1-4) and thymomas (Table 2-7) was studied by Kuo (64). Small polygonal cells, spindle cells, and large polygonal cells of thymomas appeared to be related to subcapsular, medullary, and cortical cells of the thymus, respectively, while squamoid (type B3) thymoma acquired additional squamous type cytokeratin (Table 2-7). These findings support both the histogenetic and WHO histologic classifications, except for a group of small polygonal cell thymomas expressing only CK14 and CK19. At present, the authors are not aware of any antibodies that can identify the non-neoplastic thymic epithelial cells occasionally present within thymoma as inclusions.

In practice, the most important thymic epithelial cell antigen is cytokeratin. As already mentioned, recognition of a few epithelial cells in a lymphocyte-predominant thymoma can easily be done by using antibodies recognizing both high and low molecular weight cytokeratins (fig. 2-84). The presence of cytokeratin-positive cells in a spindle cell tumor indicates the epithelial nature of the tumor (figs. 2-39, 2-85, 2-86). Cytokeratin immunoreactivity is also useful for differentiating thymic epithelial tumors from other thymic neoplasms. Examples of tumors negative for cytokeratins include nodular sclerosing type Hodgkin lymphoma and primary mediastinal large B-cell lymphoma, which may resemble undifferentiated carcinoma or atypical germinoma (seminoma).

CD57 (leu-7), which is present in the subcapsular cortical cells of the thymus, is often immunohistochemically positive in the epithelial cells of thymoma (figs. 2-87, 2-88) (56). It has not been detected thus far in thymic squamous cell carcinoma, and therefore, may be used to distinguish thymoma from thymic squamous cell carcinoma. In the lung, however, CD57 has been shown to be positive in small cell carcinoma and differentiated adenocarcinoma, and so there is a possibility that some thymic carcinomas may show such immunoreactivity as well. Both CD5 and CD70 are expressed in many thymic squamous cell carcinomas (see fig. 3-35) and a few atypical (type B3) thymomas, but in no ordinary thymoma or carcinoma of nonthymic origin (43,44).

Recently, Nonaka et al. (96a) reported that Foxn1, a novel thymic epithelial marker and a transcription factor related to thymic organogenesis, is a specific marker for thymoma and thymic carcinoma and appears superior to CD5 and CD117. They also found that CD205

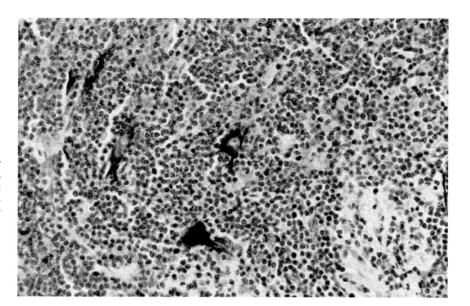

Figure 2-84

LYMPHOCYTE-PREDOMINANT THYMOMA (TYPE B1): CYTOKERATIN IMMUNOSTAINING

Scattered among the densely packed lymphocytes are cells with vesicular nuclei, prominent nucleoli, and cytoplasmic processes. These cells stain strongly for cytokeratin.

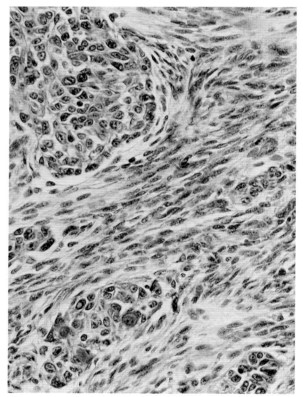
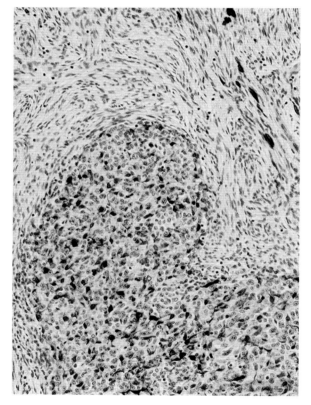

Figure 2-85

MIXED POLYGONAL/OVAL AND SPINDLE CELL THYMOMA (TYPE A): IMMUNOSTAINING FOR CYTOKERATIN AND S-100 PROTEIN

Left: Both the polygonal and spindle cells contain immunoreactive cytokeratin; the reaction is somewhat stronger in the former. This tumor may be called metaplastic (or biphasic) thymoma (cytokeratin immunostain).

Right: Many S-100 protein–positive cells are present in a polygonal/oval epithelial cell nest, but pigmented cells appear negative (S-100 protein immunostain).

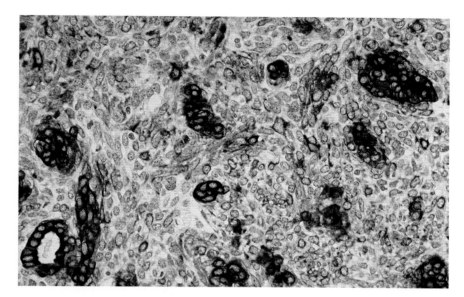

Figure 2-86

THYMOMA (TYPE A), WITH GLANDS: CYTOKERATIN IMMUNOSTAINING

The cuboidal and oval cells form tubules and small nests that are strongly reactive for cytokeratin. Oval to short spindle cells between the cell nests stain less intensely.

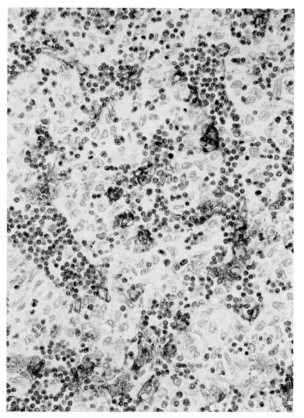

Figure 2-87

MIXED LYMPHOCYTIC AND EPITHELIAL TYPE THYMOMA (TYPE B2): CD57 IMMUNOSTAINING

CD57-positive epithelial cells are scattered, but many are nonreactive.

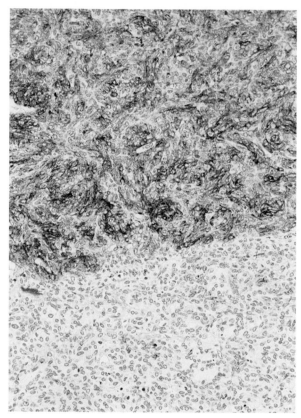

Figure 2-88

SHORT SPINDLE CELL THYMOMA (TYPE A): CD57 IMMUNOSTAINING

Although the constituent cells are morphologically similar, half of the figure contains strongly CD57-immunoreactive cells and the other half weakly or nonreactive cells.

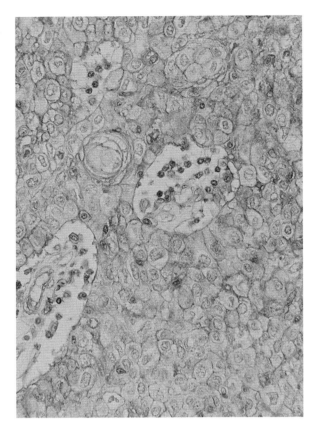

Figure 2-89

PREDOMINANTLY EPITHELIAL, POLYGONAL CELL THYMOMA (TYPE B3): IMMUNOSTAINING FOR β2-MICROGLOBULIN

Immunoreaction products are present in the cytoplasmic membrane of polygonal epithelial cells of a pleural implant and small round cells in the perivascular spaces.

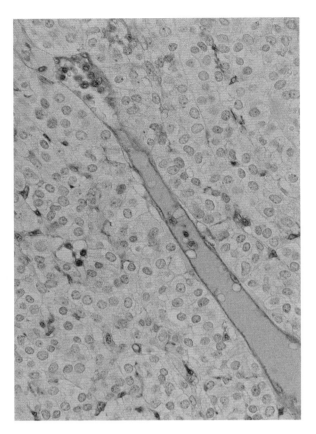

Figure 2-90

SHORT SPINDLE CELL THYMOMA (TYPE A): IMMUNOSTAINING FOR β2- MICROGLOBULIN

No or very weak reaction for β2-microglobulin is noted in the short spindle epithelial cells.

(DEC205), which is linked to the positive selection process for thymocytes, is a sensitive and specific marker for thymoma, but its sensitivity to thymic carcinoma is lower than CD5 and CD117 (see chapter 3, Thymic Carcinoma).

Changes in the expression of HLAs have been shown to occur at the time of neoplastic transformation. Matsuno et al. (unpublished data, National Cancer Center Hospital, Tokyo, 1990) investigated the expression patterns of β2-microglobulin, the light chain of HLA class 1 antigen, and the alpha chain of HLA-DR class 2 antigen on 17 thymomas and 16 thymic carcinomas. Only the 2 thymomas with metastasis showed diffuse immunostaining for β2-microglobulin on the cytoplasmic membrane, whereas the remaining 15 cases without

metastasis were negative or showed only focal immunostaining (figs. 2-89, 2-90). In contrast, 7 thymic carcinomas showed diffuse staining and only 3 were negative. A similar result was obtained for the alpha chain of HLA-DR class 2 antigen: none of the thymomas showed diffuse staining, whereas 8 thymic carcinomas stained diffusely and the remaining 8 stained focally; there were no unreactive cases. These results indicate that expression of β2-microglobulin and the alpha chain of HLA-DR is seen in thymoma with metastasis and in many cases of thymic carcinoma.

In a study (31a), the Ki-67 labeling index was higher in type B3 thymoma and thymic carcinoma than in types A, AB, and B2 thymoma. The Ki-67 labeling index correlated with prognosis, but multivariate analysis was not performed, so it is not clear whether the Ki-67 labeling index is an independent prognostic indicator. Cell cycle regulator proteins p21 and p27, together with p53, were studied immunohistochemically in thymomas (18b,82a). It was shown that low or negative expression of p21 and p27 and high expression of p53 correlated with a poor prognosis in cases of thymoma. Multivariate analysis suggests that low or negative p27 expression is the most significant variable for a poor prognosis.

Thymic lymphocytes (thymocytes) can be divided into medium-sized cortical (or immature) lymphocytes and small medullary (or mature) lymphocytes. The cortical lymphocytes are characterized by a CD1a-, CD3-, CD4-, and CD8-positive phenotype (double-positive thymocytes). Mitotic figures are observed. Mature lymphocytes are characterized by a CD1a-negative, CD3-positive, and CD4- or CD8-positive phenotype (single-positive thymocytes). Both types of lymphocytes can be identified in almost all thymomas, unless the tumors consist almost entirely of epithelial cells. A good example is shown in figure 2-91, which demonstrates double-positive thymocytes surrounding areas of medullary differentiation containing single-positive thymocytes. CD1a-positive lymphocytes are numerous in lymphocyte-predominant (types B1 and B2) and mixed lymphocytic and epithelial (type B2) thymomas, decrease in epithelial cell–predominant (type B3) thymoma, and cannot be detected in thymic carcinoma (127,135). Müller-Hermelink et al. (53,92) stated that well-differentiated, organotypic thymic carcinoma (type B3 thymoma) contained immature (cortical) thymocytes. In other words, thymoma retains the function of the thymus to attract immature T cells from the bone marrow to make them mature (127,128), whereas thymic carcinoma has lost this function. As a result, T lymphocytes infiltrating thymic carcinoma are mature T cells, as seen in cancer of other organs.

CD1a-positive immature (cortical) lymphocytes can be stained with the MIC2 antibody 013 (CD99) after formalin fixation (fig. 2-92). This antibody has been used for diagnosing Ewing sarcoma and peripheral primitive neuroectodermal tumors. It can be used to confirm a diagnosis of thymoma in small biopsy specimens, to distinguish invasive thymoma and thymic carcinoma, and to classify thymic epithelial tumors (27,33). Anti-TdT antibody also can be applied to formalin-fixed paraffin-embedded sections.

In addition to T cells, areas of medullary differentiation contain CD20-positive B lymphocytes, thus mimicking the medulla of the normal thymus. CD1a-negative and S-100 beta-positive interdigitating reticulum cells (Langerhans cells) are scattered in the parenchyma of thymoma and in nests of thymic carcinoma, but also appear as clusters in areas of thymoma showing medullary differentiation, as in the normal thymus (figs. 2-93, 2-94) (58).

Myoid cells, which are found in the fetal thymus of mammals including humans, and in a few thymomas, possess centrally located small nuclei and abundant cytoplasm containing eosinophilic fibrillar structures. Their cytoplasm is immunoreactive with antibodies recognizing desmin, myoglobin, and muscle-specific actin (fig. 2-95). No myoid cells have been found in thymic cancers examined thus far except for sarcomatoid carcinoma with rhabdomyoblastic differentiation, an example of which was reported by Snover et al. (139).

Ultrastructural Findings

The ultrastructural architecture of the normal thymus, consisting of reticular epithelial cells with elongated cytoplasmic processes and lymphoid cells, is retained to various degrees in thymoma (51,73,74). The epithelial cells, characterized by bundles of tonofilaments in their cytoplasm and the presence of a large number of desmosomes, extend their fine cellular reticula within and around the parenchyma. The outer surface of the epithelial cells is covered by a basement membrane (figs. 2-96, 2-97). In areas with epithelial cell predominance, solid cords and nests are formed instead of extensions of slender epithelial reticula. Keratinization is seen in areas corresponding to Hassall corpuscles by light microscopy. Spindle cells can also be identified as epithelial in nature from the presence of desmosomes and intracytoplasmic tonofilaments (72). Other cytoplasmic organelles include a moderate number of mitochondria, a well-developed Golgi apparatus, a scanty rough endoplasmic reticulum, lysosomes, and occasional lipid droplets. The nuclei of the epithelial cells of thymoma are oval or irregularly

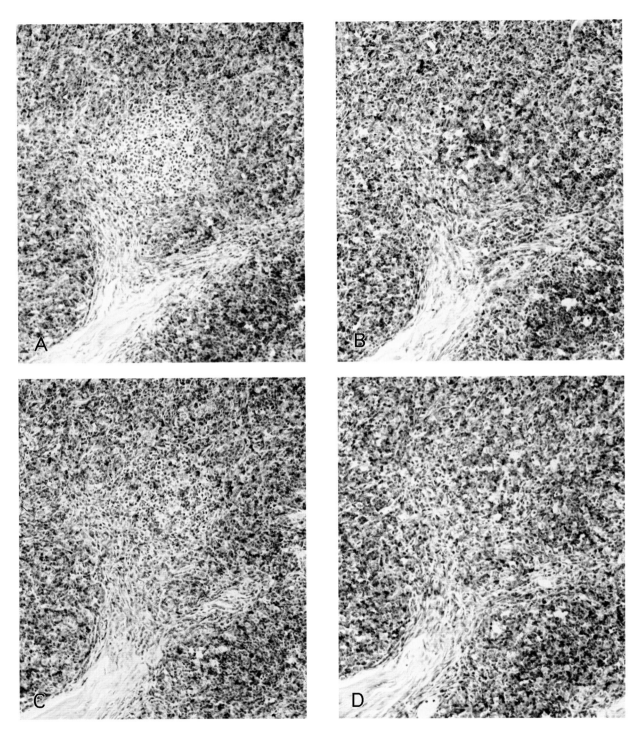

Figure 2-91

THYMOMA (TYPE B1) WITH MEDULLARY DIFFERENTIATION: IMMUNOSTAINING FOR LYMPHOCYTE MARKERS

Serial sections are immunostained for surface markers of lymphocytes. The area of medullary differentiation in the center of each photograph is composed of: cells nonreactive for CD1a (A); cells entirely immunoreactive for CD3 (B); cells partly reactive and partly nonreactive for CD4 (C); and cells partly reactive and partly nonreactive for CD8 (D). Areas surrounding a focus of medullary differentiation consist of lymphocytes with a CD1a-, CD3-, CD4-, and CD8-positive phenotype.

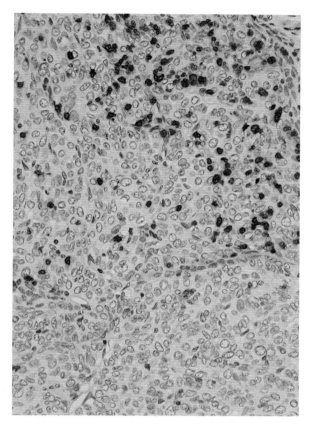

Figure 2-92

**TYPE "B2-LIKE" AREA IN TYPE AB THYMOMA
(MIXED LYMPHOCYTIC AND SMALL POLYGONAL
EPITHELIAL CELL TYPE): IMMUNOSTAINING
FOR MIC2 ANTIBODY 013 (CD99)**

Most lymphocytes are positive for MIC2 antibody.
(Courtesy of Dr. Minako Seki, Hiratsuka, Japan.)

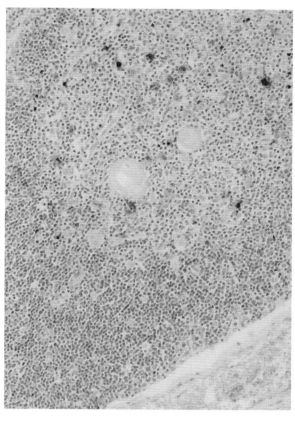

Figure 2-93

**NORMAL THYMUS WITH INTERDIGITATING
RETICULUM CELLS: IMMUNOSTAINING FOR S-100β**

Interdigitating reticulum cells positive for S-100β protein
are almost entirely confined to the medulla.

Figure 2-94

**LYMPHOCYTE-PREDOMINANT
THYMOMA (TYPE B1)
INTERDIGITATING
RETICULUM CELLS:
IMMUNOSTAINING
FOR S-100β**

An area of medullary differentiation is studded with interdigitating reticulum cells showing
an irregular outline and some
cytoplasmic processes that stain
for S-100β.

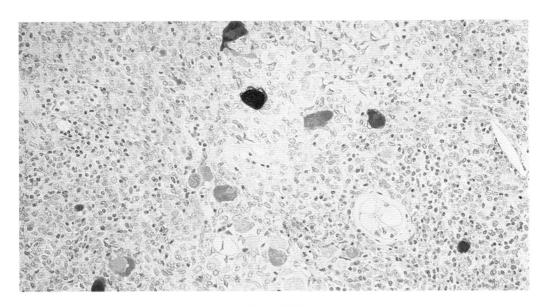

Figure 2-95

THYMOMA WITH MYOID CELLS: IMMUNOSTAINING FOR MYOGLOBIN

Scattered in this mixed lymphocytic and epithelial (type AB) thymoma are large cells with abundant cytoplasm that stain intensely for myoglobin.

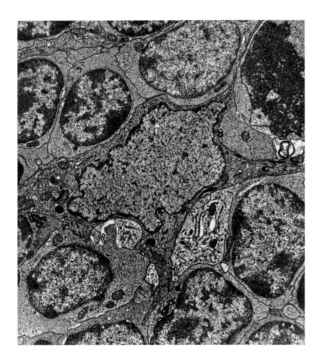

Figure 2-96

ULTRASTRUCTURE OF THYMOMA

The epithelial cells in the center have elongated cell processes and tonofilaments. A lymphocyte mitosis is seen at the upper right, close to an epithelial cell process. (Fig. 3-87 from Fascicle 21, Third Series.)

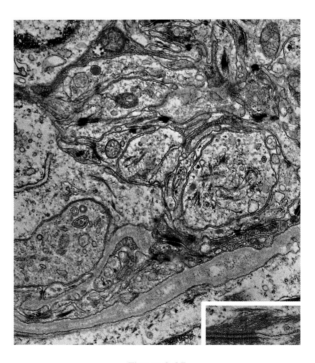

Figure 2-97

ULTRASTRUCTURE OF THYMOMA

Complex cellular interdigitations, many desmosomes, and a basal lamina characterize this area of thymoma. Inset: Tonofilaments are inserted into a typical desmosome. (Fig. 3-88 from Fascicle 21, Third Series.)

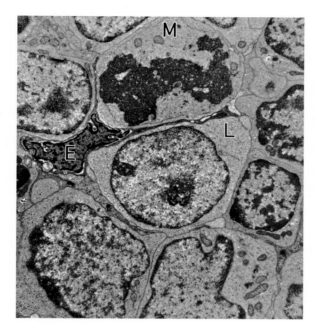

Figure 2-98

ULTRASTRUCTURE OF THYMOMA

Seen is an epithelial cell (E) with an attenuated process, an electron-dense nucleus, and cytoplasm. Lymphocyte activation is manifested by the presence of scant heterochromatin and nucleolar prominence (L). One of the lymphocytes is undergoing mitosis (M). Mature and inactive lymphocytes are also present. (Fig. 3-89 from Fascicle 21, Third Series.)

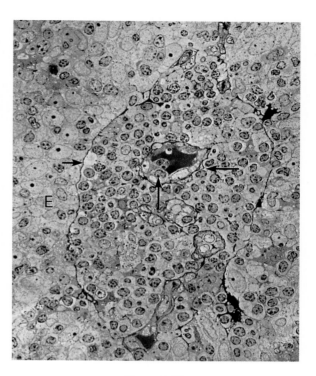

Figure 2-99

ULTRASTRUCTURE OF THYMOMA

A typical perivascular space has a central vessel and branches, endothelial lamina (horizontal arrow), a lymphocyte-packed space, epithelial lamina (short arrow), and palisading epithelial cells (E). The upward arrow indicates a lymphocyte within an endothelial cell. (Fig. 3-90 from Fascicle 21, Third Series.)

indented, with condensed heterochromatin beneath the nuclear membrane and various-sized nucleoli. Basement membranes are irregularly interspersed between tumor cells, although there is a tendency for the basement membrane to surround clusters of tumor cells (fig. 2-97).

Thymic lymphocytes (thymocytes) are characterized by smooth cytoplasmic borders, oval dark nuclei, and a paucity of cytoplasmic organelles. Mature (or medullary) lymphocytes in the resting phase are small, with nuclei containing abundant heterochromatin, whereas immature (cortical) lymphocytes are larger and have nuclei showing scanty heterochromatin, nucleolar prominence, and an increased number of cytoplasmic polyribosomes. Mitotic figures can be observed (fig. 2-98).

The perivascular spaces are frequently dilated. They contain amorphous material, lymphocytes, mast cells, macrophages, and collagen. Both vascular and epithelial basement membranes are observed (figs. 2-99, 2-100).

Gland-like spaces are lined by epithelial cells with tonofibrils and microvilli at the free cell surface. Junctional complexes are observed at the cell borders near the free cell surface.

Levine et al. (74) described a form of emperipolesis in thymoma, that is, the presence of degenerating lymphocytes in a space encompassed by epithelial cytoplasm. The epithelial cells, however, have no signs of degeneration. In the end-stage of this process, spaces in the epithelial cells contain myelin figures and other cellular debris.

Myoid cells, which may be present in thymoma, are characterized by numerous sarcomeres and Z-bands (fig. 2-60). Epithelial cells filled with mucus granules may be found, as well as spaces containing amorphous material. The spaces are lined by epithelial cells equipped with microvilli.

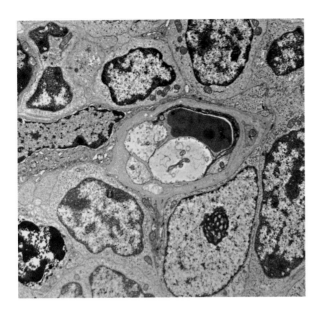

Figure 2-100

ULTRASTRUCTURE OF THYMOMA

The central vessel of a thymoma is completely surrounded by epithelial processes. The basal laminae of both the vessel and epithelial cells are well defined. A well-developed nucleolonema is present in the epithelial cells bellow the vessel. (Fig. 3-91 from Fascicle 21, Third Series.)

Although thymoma is ultrastructurally characteristic, electron microscopic studies are not common in routine practice since diagnosis by immunohistochemical methods is much easier.

Molecular and Other Special Techniques

Genetic Abnormalities. Thymomas have been attracting the interest of scientists for their histogenesis and functional differentiation. The morphologic classification proposed by the WHO has become a standard worldwide, and its correlation with malignant potential and functional status has been extensively studied. The functional/histogenetic classification used in Europe attempts to classify thymomas based on their morphologic or immunohistochemical resemblance to normal counterparts (93). It is expected that genetic abnormalities will shed light on the tumorigenesis, progression, and functional aspects of thymic epithelial tumors. However, it is difficult to genetically study abnormalities of neoplastic cells because of the abundance of accompanying lymphocytes.

Most thymomas previously studied genetically are those without a significant lymphocyte population, namely, type A and type B3 thymomas and thymic squamous cell carcinoma. Recent studies on the genetic aberrations in thymomas, including type B2 thymoma with a dense lymphocytic infiltration, used microdissection methods to increase the concentration of neoplastic epithelial cells.

Loss of heterozygosity (LOH) is frequently found on chromosomes 3p, 6, 13q, and 16q, and especially on 6q (165). Other LOHs are detected at 5q21-22, which includes the *APC* locus, and at 17p13.1, the site for *p53* locus. Comparing the allelotypes of the thymomas, the group at the University of Würzburg identified two pathways that lead to the development of thymoma: LOH of 6q23.3-25.3 and 5q21 (166).

Another important finding is the frequent and multiple aberrations of chromosome 6 (48). Genetic aberrations of chromosome 6 were found in 77.5 percent of thymic epithelial tumors (36 thymomas and 4 thymic carcinomas) (48). There are five hotspots indicating that several tumor suppressor genes on chromosome 6 are involved in the development of thymic epithelial tumors.

Type A thymomas show the least chromosomal abnormalities with consistent loss on chromosome 6p. In contrast, other types of thymic epithelial tumors show diverse genetic abnormalities (49). Types B2 and B3 thymomas and thymic carcinomas usually show genetic aberrations on multiple chromosomes. Type A thymomas almost never show multiple aberrations and type AB thymomas are intermediate between type A and type B thymomas. Type B3 thymomas often show gains on chromosome 1q and losses on chromosomes 6 and 13q. Type B2 thymomas are genetically related to type B3 thymomas. Thymic squamous cell carcinomas show gains on chromosomes 1q, 17q, and 18 and losses on chromosomes 3p, 6, 16q, and 17p. Similarity in genetic abnormalities indicates a close relationship between type B3 thymomas and thymic squamous cell carcinomas (151).

Multiple accumulations of genetic aberrations seem to contribute to the progression of thymomas. Chromosome alterations reported for the different WHO histologic thymoma subtypes are summarized in the WHO classification monograph (Table 2-8) (151).

Table 2-8

GENETIC ALTERATIONS REPORTED FOR THE DIFFERENT WORLD HEALTH ORGANIZATION (WHO) HISTOLOGIC THYMOMA SUBTYPES[a]

WHO Type	Chromoso-mal Gains	Chromosomal Losses
Type A	none	-6p
Type AB	none	-5q21-22, -6q, -12p, -16q
Type B3	+1q	-6, -13q
Thymic squamous cell carcinoma	+1q, +17q, +18	-3p, -6, -13q, -16q, -17p

[a]Section from Table 3.05 of Travis WD, Brambilla E, Müller-Hermelink HK, Harris CC, eds. World Health Organization Classification of Tumours. Pathology and genetics of tumours of the lung, pleura, thymus and heart. Lyon: IARC Press; 2004:153.

Point mutations of the *p53* gene has been demonstrated across the entire spectrum of thymic epithelial neoplasms (143). *p53* gene mutations may be an early event in thymic tumorigenesis (148a). Some immunohistochemical studies have shown that the number of p53-positive tumor cells increases with the progression of the neoplasm; others, however, have not found this correlation (42a,42b,148a) (see chapter 3, Molecular and Other Special Techniques). In one study, patients with thymomas immunoreactive with a polyclonal antibody CM-1 against p53 protein showed substantially lower survival rates than those with nonreactive thymomas (155b). Immunostaining of p53 with a monoclonal antibody D0-1 was negative in thymomas and positive in 4 of 9 thymic carcinomas. Although primary carcinoma is different from metastatic carcinoma in the lung by the *p53* gene mutation pattern, no genetic study on multiple thymomas has been reported as yet (95a).

Other genes that may be involved in the development or progression of thymic neoplasms are *APC*, *RB1*, *bcl-2*, *RAS*, and *EGF* (143). Since the number of cases studied are still small and only a few groups have published genetic data on thymomas, further accumulation of cases and more extensive analysis are necessary to further define the genetic background of thymic epithelial tumors.

Nuclear Areas and Nuclear DNA Contents. The nuclear areas of the epithelial cells of the normal thymus, hyperplastic thymus, and thy-

momas were measured by Nomori et al. (96). They found that the nuclei of epithelial cells in thymoma were significantly larger than those of both normal and hyperplastic thymus, and that the nuclei of epithelial cells of invasive thymoma (clinical stages III and IV) were even larger (47.4 ± 6.7 μm^2) than those of noninvasive thymoma (clinical stages I and II; 36.5 ± 7.5 μm^2). A similar study was carried out by Asamura et al. (18), who showed that the mean nuclear area increased significantly in increasing order from noninvasive thymoma to invasive thymoma to thymic carcinoma (49.27 ± 7.88 μm^2, 62.44 ± 5.10 μm^2, and 76.79 ± 10.27 μm^2, respectively [fig. 2-101]). The sizable overlap in the results of the above two studies shows that measurement of nuclear area is not satisfactory for predicting the behavior of individual cases of noninvasive and invasive thymoma.

Asamura et al. (18) also investigated the nuclear DNA content of noninvasive thymomas, invasive thymomas, and thymic carcinomas by cytofluorometry. They found that the mean nuclear DNA content of thymic carcinoma was significantly higher than that of both invasive and noninvasive thymomas ($3.82 \pm 0.98C$, $2.63 \pm 0.28C$, and $2.46 \pm 0.18C$, respectively). There was no significant difference between noninvasive and invasive thymoma (fig. 2-102). The aneuploid stem cell line appeared in 92.3 percent of thymic carcinomas, in only one invasive thymoma (7.7 percent), and in no noninvasive thymomas. Abnormal DNA histogram patterns were seen in about half of all thymic carcinomas but in none of the thymomas. As with nuclear area, the overlap between noninvasive and invasive thymomas and between invasive thymoma and thymic carcinoma precludes using mean nuclear DNA content as a predictor of behavior in individual cases of thymoma. The three parameters (the mean nuclear DNA content, the occurrence of an aneuploid stem cell line, and an abnormal DNA histogram pattern), are helpful, however, for distinguishing invasive thymoma from thymic carcinoma.

Gschwendtner et al. (39) determined the ploidy values of the epithelial component of various subtypes of thymoma using image cytometry. They found that the percentage of aneuploid tumors increased from medullary type (WHO type A thymoma), at 0 percent, through mixed type

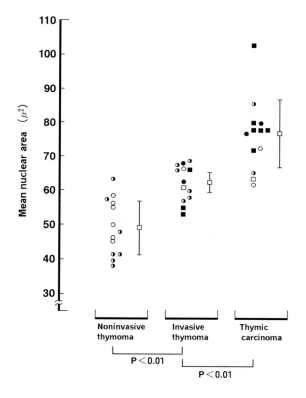

Figure 2-101

MEAN NUCLEAR AREAS OF NONINVASIVE THYMOMA, INVASIVE THYMOMA, AND THYMIC CARCINOMA

(Fig. 4 from Asamura H, Nakajima T, Mukai K, Noguchi M, Shimosato Y. Degree of malignancy of thymic epithelial tumors in terms of nuclear DNA content and nuclear area. An analysis of 39 cases. Am J Pathol 1988;133:620.)

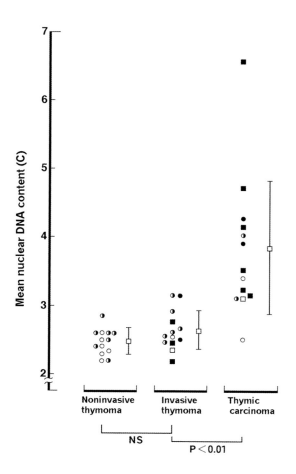

Figure 2-102

MEAN NUCLEAR DNA CONTENT OF NONINVASIVE THYMOMA, INVASIVE THYMOMA, AND THYMIC CARCINOMA

(Fig. 2 from Asamura H, Nakajima T, Mukai K, Noguchi M, Shimosato Y. Degree of malignancy of thymic epithelial tumors in terms of nuclear DNA content and nuclear area. An analysis of 39 cases. Am J Pathol 1988;133:618.)

(type AB thymoma), 44.4 percent; predominantly cortical (type B1 thymoma), 75 percent; cortical (type B2 thymoma), 83.3 percent; to well-differentiated thymic carcinoma (type B3 thymoma), 100 percent. The results correlate with the concept of the histogenetic and WHO classifications regarding the degree of malignancy of each histologic type.

Davies et al. (32) used flow cytometry to show that aneuploidy correlated with a more advanced stage of thymoma and occurred more frequently in epithelial-predominant (type B3) thymoma. Aneuploidy was predictive of tumor recurrence, independent of the effects of stage. Kuo et al. (65), also using flow cytometry, reported that the DNA indices of grossly invasive thymoma and thymic carcinoma were significantly higher than those of noninvasive

and microinvasive thymomas, and that the proportion of aneuploidy as well as the S-phase fraction in grossly invasive thymomas were significantly higher than in noninvasive and microinvasive thymomas. According to Pich et al. (110), the 10-year survival rate for patients with thymoma was 73 percent for those with diploid tumors, but only 38 percent for those with aneuploid tumors, a statistically significant difference. Although there is an opinion that flow cytometry is not a useful guide for predicting the malignant potential of thymic tumors or the prognosis of patients, the general consensus is that nuclear morphometry and nuclear DNA content analysis help in assessing the degree of malignancy and predicting the prognosis of patients with thymic epithelial tumors.

Differential Diagnosis

Differentiating thymoma from other thymic tumors is based not only on the histology but on other diagnostic approaches as well, such as immunohistochemistry, and in the future, genetic methods. In this section emphasis is placed mainly on the histologic and cytologic features of the tumors.

An important consideration in routine practice is distinguishing invasive thymoma from thymic carcinoma, which also includes carcinoma developing in thymoma. In particular, type B3 thymoma with epidermoid features must be distinguished from thymic squamous cell carcinoma. In the former, the general features of thymoma, such as partial encapsulation, lobulation, and perivascular spaces, as well as cytologic features including a wrinkled or folded nuclear membrane, are maintained. In addition, other histologic features of thymoma, such as those of type B2 thymoma, are found almost always in other portions of the tumor. Carcinoma very often shows infiltrative invasive growth at the advancing borders of the tumor, whereas invasive thymoma frequently shows encapsulation or at least well-defined borders in some parts, and at times even in the advancing border, such as in the lung. Also, sclerosis, particularly in the center of the tumor, is seen more frequently in thymic squamous cell carcinoma. Although liquefactive necrosis that forms various-sized cystic spaces is common in thymoma, coagulation necrosis is less frequent than in thymic carcinoma. Infarcted thymoma with extensive coagulation necrosis, however, may cause diagnostic difficulties (fig. 2-103). The cells of thymic carcinoma are atypical and can be easily distinguished from those of invasive thymoma, which frequently possess bland nuclei (133,152). Some thymomas, however, have atypical nuclei with some growth activity, like those in the well-differentiated thymic carcinoma of Müller-Hermelink et al. (type B3 thymoma) (54). The number of mitotic figures is not a useful distinguishing feature, unless it is very high. Atypical mitotic figures are almost nonexistent in thymoma, however, and their presence strongly suggests carcinoma. Inflamma-

tory cells are seen most frequently in the stroma of carcinoma rather than in the parenchyma. Plasma cells and eosinophils are seen occasionally in carcinoma, but rarely in thymoma.

It is on the basis of these general features that thymoma with frequent Hassall corpuscles is distinguished from keratinizing squamous cell carcinoma. Perivascular spaces, which were once considered to be peculiar to thymoma, may be seen in some carcinomas (e.g., basaloid carcinoma). In addition, basaloid carcinoma is frequently encapsulated, and encapsulation together with perivascular spaces suggest borderline malignancy. The cytologic atypia, however, defines basaloid carcinoma as carcinoma, and it has been categorized into the low-grade malignancy group by Suster and Rosai (146).

Features that allow differentiation from lymphoepithelioma-like carcinoma are marked atypia and anaplasia, together with increased mitotic activity in the individual carcinoma cells (see fig. 3-26). In addition, the phenotypes of the infiltrating lymphocytes are different. Immature (or cortical) T cells are almost always found in thymoma, but the infiltrating lymphocytes in carcinoma are mature T cells as well as B cells and plasma cells.

Clear cell carcinoma cells, which possess small nuclei like those seen in renal cell carcinoma, should be differentiated from the clear cells of epithelial cell–predominant (type B3) thymoma. In the latter, the tumor is at least partly encapsulated and shows typical features of thymoma in some parts, such as oval cells with distinct cell membranes and perivascular spaces (fig. 2-55).

Mucoepidermoid carcinoma, which is classified as low-grade carcinoma by Suster and Rosai (146), has normochromic, round and uniform nuclei with little pleomorphism. When encapsulated and containing perivascular spaces, the histologic classification is problematic, and the tumor could well be thymoma with bidirectional differentiation. As with mucoepidermoid tumors of other organs, some mucoepidermoid tumors behave as benign thymic tumors.

Besides morphology, the presence of a paraneoplastic syndrome, particularly myasthenia gravis, is important for distinguishing thymoma and thymic carcinoma. Myasthenia gravis has never been noted in patients with thymic

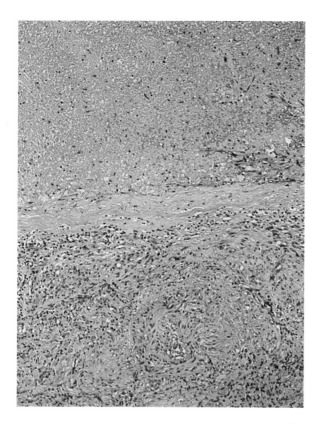 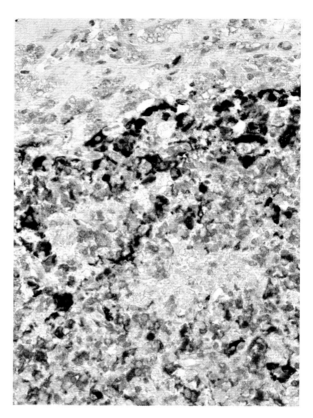

Figure 2-103

INFARCTED THYMOMA

This encapsulated tumor was filled with necrotic tissue. Scattered viable tumor tissue a few millimeters in size was attached to the capsule.

Left: Encapsulated tumor (left of image) is almost completely necrotic. Degenerating tumor tissue with a small occluded vessel is noted outside the capsule on the right.

Right: Necrotic epithelial cells are positive for cytokeratin using AE1/AE3. The diagnosis of thymoma was made from the histology of the degenerating tumor (left of image) and the cytokeratin-positive epithelial cell ghosts (right of image).

carcinoma, except when it coincidentally developed from typical thymoma. The high incidence of myasthenia gravis in the well-differentiated thymic carcinoma of Müller–Hermelink et al. (54) is an additional reason why that neoplasm is now classified as type B3 thymoma.

Other tumors to be differentiated from thymoma include Hodgkin disease, precursor T-lymphoblastic lymphoma, diffuse small cell lymphoma, marginal zone low-grade B-cell lymphoma of MALT, and atypical carcinoid tumor. Lymphocyte-predominant thymoma should not be misinterpreted as malignant lymphoma. The most important distinguishing feature is the presence of scattered, medium-sized to large cells with lightly stained nuclei in a diffuse lymphocytic background in the former. These cells pos-

sess features of polygonal (or cortical) epithelial cells with vesicular and round nuclei, distinct nucleoli, and often clear cytoplasm (fig. 2-6). For confirmation, immunostaining for cytokeratin makes the epithelial cells stand out among the nonstaining lymphocytes and histiocytes (fig. 2-84). Histiocytes scattered in thymoma may produce a starry sky appearance, which can be distinguished easily from epithelial cells by the presence of intracytoplasmic nuclear debris (fig. 2-51). This is never as prominent as that seen in Burkitt lymphoma and lymphoblastic lymphoma of the T-cell type.

Germ cell tumors and diffuse large B-cell lymphoma can be differentiated from thymoma with relative ease, but possibly with some difficulty from thymic carcinoma.

Although the nodular sclerosis type Hodgkin lymphoma was interpreted as granulomatous thymoma in the past (69), the presence of lacunar cells and a variety of inflammatory cells, and the absence of epithelial cells distinguish these two tumors. Non-Hodgkin lymphoma can also be diagnosed by the absence of epithelial cells and the presence of mitotic figures in the lymphoid cells, mitoses being particularly frequent in the lymphoblastic type.

Carcinoid tumors can be differentiated from thymoma with rosette-like features by the lack or paucity of lymphocytes and the presence of monotonous tumor cells with diffusely stippled nuclear chromatin and very finely granular cytoplasm. These features contrast with the medullary type epithelial cells in this type of thymoma.

Spindle cell thymoma and benign solitary fibrous tumor of the pleura can be differentiated histologically in most cases. If difficulty persists, immunohistochemistry for cytokeratin and CD34 should be performed (see figs. 11-8, 11-9). Demonstration of TdT, CD1a, and/or CD99 (phenotypes of immature or cortical T cells) in lymphocytes helps distinguish thymoma from other thymic or mediastinal tumors, excluding precursor T-lymphoblastic lymphoma.

Conditions and Diseases Associated with Thymoma

The most common paraneoplastic phenomenon associated with thymoma is myasthenia gravis, which affects one third to half of all thymoma patients. According to Lewis et al. (75), of 283 patients with thymoma treated at Mayo Clinic during a 40-year period, 130 (46 percent) had myasthenia gravis. Nonmyasthenic paraneoplastic phenomena were present in 28 patients (10 percent), 10 of whom also had myasthenia gravis. Eleven patients had hematologic disorders: hypogammaglobulinemia (5 patients), pure red cell aplasia (2 patients), and aplastic anemia (4 patients). Fifteen patients had possible autoimmune-related disorders: pernicious anemia (3 patients), a positive lupus erythematosus preparation (3 patients), and polymyositis (2 patients). One patient each had the following: keratoconjunctivitis sicca, alopecia areata, mixed collagen-vascular disease, Graves disease, Crohn disease, chronic ulcerative colitis, anhy-

drosis/orthostasis, and positivity for rheumatoid factor. Myocarditis and myopathy were seen in one patient each. Forty-eight patients (17 percent) had another primary tumor.

Myasthenia gravis is associated with predominantly lymphocytic thymoma (69,83), but several reports have shown a similar distribution of histologic subtypes in both myasthenic and nonmyasthenic patients (75,124). At the National Cancer Center Hospital in Tokyo, myasthenia gravis was a complication in 11 of 79 thymomas (13.9 percent), of which 9 were of the polygonal cell type (type B thymoma) and 2 were of the mixed polygonal and spindle cell type (type AB thymoma). None of the pure spindle cell type was complicated by myasthenia gravis (57). A recent study of 130 thymomas in the same institution revealed myasthenia gravis in 16 cases (12.3 percent) and no cases with pure red cell aplasia (95). The difference in incidence of a paraneoplastic syndrome in thymoma patients is evident between general hospitals and cancer hospitals.

According to Kirchner et al. (54), the association with myasthenia gravis was highest in well-differentiated thymic carcinoma (type B3 thymoma) (77 percent), followed by cortical (type B2) thymoma (66 percent) and other subtypes of thymoma (33 to 39 percent); no thymic carcinoma was associated with myasthenia gravis. About half of the patients with myasthenia gravis show lymph follicles with germinal centers in the residual thymus, whereas only a few nonmyasthenia patients do so (120). In those cases, lymph follicles with germinal centers are often seen within thymoma tissue (fig. 2-104).

Despite the frequent association of myasthenia gravis with thymoma, the causal relationship between the two conditions is not yet understood. It is known that myasthenia gravis is an autoimmune disease affecting the acetylcholine receptor at the neuromuscular junction; production of an autoantibody against the acetylcholine receptor alpha-subunit is assumed to be the cause of the disease (55,71). The source of acetylcholine receptors in the thymus is considered to be the myoid cells present in the medulla of the thymus. Unlike in adults, none of the patients with juvenile myasthenia gravis (15 years of age or less), had an associated autoimmune disease, and thymoma was

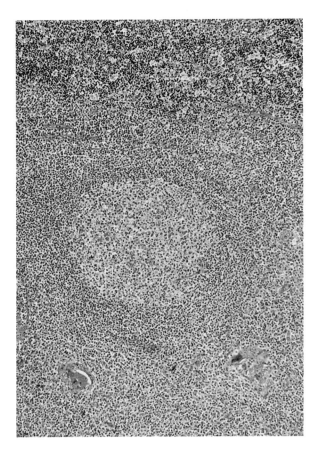

Figure 2-104

**THYMOMA CONTAINING LYMPH FOLLICLE
WITH GERMINAL CENTER IN A PATIENT
WITH MYASTHENIA GRAVIS**

A lymph follicle with a prominent germinal center is present within a lymphocyte-predominant (type B1) thymoma, which also contains Hassall-like bodies. The residual thymus also contained lymph follicles with germinal centers.

found in only 1 of 11 patients who underwent thymectomy (18a).

Kirchner et al. (53,55) found that the neoplastic epithelial cells in 15 of 17 thymic epithelial tumors associated with myasthenia gravis, but in only 2 of 8 tumors not so associated, showed cytoplasmic acetylcholine receptor-related antigenic determinants, but no epitopes of the extracellular main immunogenic region. Marx et al. (79) identified neurofilaments and titin-like epitope expressed aberrantly in many of the neoplastic epithelial cells of thymic epithelial tumors with cortical differentiation, including the cortical (type B2)

thymomas and well-differentiated thymic carcinoma (type B3 thymoma) of Kirchner et al. (54). They suggested that the abnormal expression of titin-like epitope in thymomas may trigger antititin autoimmunity for the pathogenesis of myasthenia gravis.

Many reports have described the presence of myasthenia gravis as an indicator of poor prognosis in patients with thymoma (20,70,124). Studies by Wilkins and Castleman (160), Maggi et al. (76), and Lewis et al. (75) have not supported this concept, and patients with myasthenia gravis have a survival rate equal to that of patients with nonmyasthenia-related thymoma. These authors attributed the equal prognosis to better postoperative respiratory support as well as improved long-term medical care of myasthenic patients. Monden et al. (83) found that thymoma was detected earlier, the recurrence rate was lower, and the survival curve better in patients with myasthenia gravis.

Spindle cell thymoma occurs more frequently in patients with hypogammaglobulinemia, pure red cell aplasia, and aplastic anemia (118). All of 17 cases of thymoma associated with pure red cell aplasia collected by Masaoka et al. (80) were of the spindle cell type, with a variable lymphocyte component; 2 were associated with myasthenia gravis and 3 with hypogammaglobulinemia. The Coombs and antinuclear antibody tests were positive in 5 cases. Thymic tissue attached to thymoma displayed epithelial clusters frequently (10 of 11 cases) but no germinal centers, and could well be a bud of another thymoma. In the series reported by Lewis et al. (75), only 3 of 11 patients with hematologic abnormalities had spindle cell thymomas. A study from Taiwan indicated that the five thymomas associated with pure red cell aplasia showed various histologic types. One was an unusual composite tumor of WHO type B1 thymoma and a so far unreported "lipofibroadenoma," and none was a spindle cell thymoma (67).

Hematologic disorders are associated less frequently with thymoma than myasthenia gravis, and are studied less. Pure red cell aplasia occurs in only 5 percent of thymoma patients, and thymomas are found in 50 percent of patients with pure red cell aplasia (122). Pure red cell aplasia is divided into that without any suspected cause or drug induction and that with some suspected cause. The aplasia associated with thymoma is chronic and of the latter category. This category is also associated with malignant lymphoma, chronic leukemia, systemic lupus erythematosus, and Sjögren syndrome. Pure red cell aplasia can be caused by any factors that inhibit the process of erythroid cell maturation from totipotent stem cells (colony forming unit-S [CFU-S]) to erythrocytes through the erythroid burst-forming unit (BFU-E) and erythroid colony-forming unit (CFU-E). In this process, various factors are known to be involved, such as interleukin 3 and erythropoietin. Not only autoantibodies against progenitor cells of the erythroid series and factors that enhance erythropoiesis, but also factors that inhibit erythropoiesis, such as suppressor T cells and gamma-interferon, can cause pure red cell aplasia (80). In Masaoka's cases (80), highly positive Coombs and antinuclear antibody tests, and a decrease of CD4/CD8 ratio were noted, suggesting involvement of other autoimmune diseases and activation of suppressor T cells.

Pure red cell aplasia occurs either concomitantly with thymoma or after treatment of thymoma, although the latter situation is rare. Thymectomy with resection of thymoma is effective treatment in 20 to 40 percent of cases of red cell aplasia. Steroid therapy is also administered in many cases, and sometimes immunosuppressive agents are given. The role of thymoma in the occurrence of pure red cell aplasia is unknown at present, but suggested explanations are: 1) thymoma shares an antigen in common with cells of the erythroid series; 2) thymoma overproduces suppressor T cells, at times resulting not only in pure red cell aplasia but also in hypogammaglobulinemia; and 3) both thymoma and pure red cell aplasia occur through the action of common causative agents (80). In a case of pure red cell aplasia with thymoma, the peripheral blood mononuclear cells were CD2 positive, CD3 positive, CD4 negative, and CD8 positive. A monoclonal rearrangement of the T-cell receptor–beta chain gene was found in the mononuclear cells of both the peripheral blood and the thymoma, indicating a T-cell clonal disorder in pure red cell aplasia (82).

Although the pathogenic agents causing thymoma are not known, and although it does not appear to be associated with Epstein-Barr virus (see chapter 3), a case of thymoma was reported in a patient with a pedigree of Li-Fraumeni syndrome (unpublished data, H. Sugimura, Hamamatsu, Japan, 1994). Tumors reported in this pedigree were carcinoma of the adrenal cortex, astrocytoma, hepatoblastoma, and carcinoma of the pancreas. The patient who developed the thymoma was a 19-year-old male student and a carrier of the *p53* germline mutation (exon 8). (The patient is family 2, III-5, in reference 125). The surgically resected tumor was 9.5 x 6.0 x 3.7 cm, weighed 100 g, and was predominantly lymphocytic, polygonal cell type thymoma with no cellular atypia (cortical [type B2] thymoma). Immunohistochemically, the p53 product accumulated in the nuclei of the epithelial cells, but loss of heterozygosity in the tumor cells was not detected. Occurrence of thymoma in a pedigree of Li-Fraumeni syndrome may be contingent, but a genetic approach not only determines etiology but is also important for evaluation of the degree of malignancy.

Spread and Metastases

According to the WHO classification system (121), thymomas are divided, irrespective of cytoarchitectural type, into six categories based on the invasive/metastasizing properties of the tumor (Table 2-9). This classification incorporates the criteria of a staging system.

The incidence of thymoma in these categories according to histologic subtypes varies among various institutions. Data collected from many reports by many participants in the histologic classification of thymic tumors are presented in the recent edition of the WHO classification (151). The following figures on incidence are transcribed from that publication. The majority of type A and AB thymomas are encapsulated (72 to 80 percent), followed by minimally invasive (17 to 22 percent), and rarely, widely invasive (3 to 6 percent). Type A and AB thymomas are, therefore, considered to be benign by many investigators. However, we encountered two cases with lung metastasis (57,135), one case of type A thymoma with lung and liver metastasis, and one case of type AB with brain metastasis, as already described. The patients are surviving over 10 years with metastasis, but none had lymph node metastases (see Histologic Factors Associated with Degree of Malignancy and figs. 2-72–2-75).

Table 2-9

WORLD HEALTH ORGANIZATION (WHO) CLASSIFICATION OF THYMOMA[a]

Encapsulated:	A thymoma completely surrounded by a fibrous capsule of varying thickness. (Thymic tumors infiltrating into, but not through the capsule still belong in this category.)
Minimally Invasive:	A thymoma surrounded by a capsule that is focally infiltrated by tumor growth or that invades the mediastinal fat. (The capsular invasion needs to be complete in order for the tumor to be placed in this category.)
Widely Invasive:	A thymoma spreading by direct extension into adjacent structures such as pericardium, large vessels, or lung.
With Implants:	A thymoma in which tumor nodules separated from the main mass are found on the pericardial or pleural surface.
With Lymph Node Metastases:	A thymoma that involves one or more lymph nodes anatomically separate from the main mass. (This excludes direct extension into the node by the tumor. The nodes most commonly involved by metastatic thymoma are the mediastinal and supraclavicular nodes.)
With Distant Metastases:	A thymoma accompanied by embolic metastases to a distant site. (This excludes metastases to lymph nodes and direct extension into any organ. The sites most commonly involved by embolic metastases are lung, liver, and skeletal system.)

[a]Data from reference 121.

Type B1 thymoma is considered to be a low-grade malignant tumor; a little more than half of the cases are encapsulated and about a quarter are minimally invasive and, less frequently, widely invasive. The incidence in relation to invasiveness of type B2 thymoma varies in different reports, but encapsulated, minimally invasive, and widely invasive tumors appear to occur with similar frequency and metastatic disease occurs less commonly (mean, 8.9 percent). Distant metastases are rare (less than 3 percent). In type B3 thymomas, encapsulated tumor is rare, widely invasive growth is noted in about half of the cases, and metastatic disease occurs in 6 to 26 percent of patients (mean, 15 percent). Distant metastases in lung, liver, bone, and soft tissue are noted in up to 7 percent.

Staging

Masaoka et al. (81) suggested criteria for the clinical staging of thymic epithelial tumors (Table 2-10), and later proposed the Tumor-Node-Metastasis (TNM) classification (Table 2-11) (162). Although the staging system has been used widely by many investigators, a minor modification in wording should be made: that is, "invasion into the capsule" in stage II should be "transcapsular invasion" and "invasion into the pleura and pericardium" (stage III) should be defined more precisely, as "adherent to, but not penetrating through, the pleura (or pericardium)" (stage II) and "invading and exposed at the pleural (or pericardial) surface" (stage III)

Table 2-10

MASAOKA CLINICAL STAGE[a]

Stage I:	Macroscopically completely encapsulated and microscopically no capsular invasion
Stage II:	1. Macroscopic invasion into surrounding fatty tissue or mediastinal pleura, or 2. Microscopic invasion into capsule
Stage III:	Macroscopic invasion into neighboring organs, i.e., pericardium, great vessels, or lung
Stage IVa:	Pleural or pericardial dissemination
Stage IVb:	Lymphogenous or hematogenous metastasis

[a]Modified from Table 1 from Masaoka A, Monden Y, Nakahara K, Tanioka T. Follow-up study of thymomas with special reference to their clinical stage. Cancer 1981;48:2485.

(Table 2-12). Similar modifications have been made in the WHO classification: "minimally invasive" corresponds to stage II and "widely invasive" to stage III.

The TNM classification and stage grouping has been applied to malignant tumors of many organs to group relatively homogeneous tumors in patients with similar prognoses in relation to stage and facilitate the treatment strategy (50). There is currently no authorized TNM system for thymic epithelial tumors, however. One of the reasons for this delay is the unique clinicopathological characteristics of these tumors, especially thymomas of benign and low-grade (borderline) malignancy, and thymic carcinoma and neuroendocrine carcinoma with high-grade malignancy. Not enough data have been reported

Table 2-11

YAMAKAWA-MASAOKA TNM CLASSIFICATION AND STAGING[a]

T Factor
T1: Macroscopically completely encapsulated and microscopically no capsular invasion
T2: Macroscopic adhesion or invasion into surrounding fatty tissue or mediastinal pleura, or microscopic invasion into capsule
T3: Invasion into neighboring organs, such as pericardium, great vessels, and lung
T4: Pleural or pericardial dissemination

N Factor
N0: No lymph node metastasis
N1: Metastasis to anterior mediastinal lymph nodes
N2: Metastasis to intrathoracic lymph nodes except anterior mediastinal lymph nodes
N3: Metastasis to extrathoracic lymph nodes

M Factor
M0: No hematogenous metastasis
M1: Hematogenous metastasis

Stage

Stage			
Stage I	T1	N0	M0
Stage II	T2	N0	M0
Stage III	T3	N0	M0
Stage IVa	T4	N0	M0
Stage IVb	any T	N1, 2, or 3	M0
	any T	any N	M1

[a]Modified from Table 5 from Yamakawa Y, Masaoka A, Hashimoto T, et al. A tentative tumor-node-metastasis classification of thymoma. Cancer 1991;68:1986.

to fully test the classification. In the TNM Supplement 3rd edition (154), a tentative classification of "malignant thymomas" is proposed (Table 2-13). This is mainly based on the Masaoka system and its revised versions (81,135,153). The following are our comments regarding TNM categories and stage groupings, which have also been included in the recent WHO publication (151).

Because of the presence of thymic tumors with a wide range of malignancy, there should be histologic confirmation of the tumors, and cases should be divided according to histologic type. Here, the discussion is restricted to thymoma. Crucial points in defining the T categories are invasion through the capsule and invasion into neighboring structures. Although invasive growth found at the time of thoracotomy has been repeatedly reported to have significant impact on the outcome (20,57), the prognostic significance of "encapsulation" remains controversial.

Many reports on thymoma have shown little or no difference in survival of patients with stage I and stage II thymomas (57,68,100,106, 116,161a). T1 (completely encapsulated) and T2 (with capsular invasion) may eventually be merged into a new T1 category, or at least made subsets of T1, e.g., T1a and T1b. Wilkins et al (161). reported that 2 out of 23 patients with stage II

Table 2-12

PROPOSED PATHOLOGIC TNM AND STAGING OF THYMIC EPITHELIAL TUMORS (National Cancer Center Hospital, Tokyo, 1994)[a]

pT
pT1: Completely encapsulated tumor
pT2: Tumor breaking through capsule, invading thymic tissue or fatty tissue (clinically may be adherent to mediastinal pleura or pericardium but not invading neighboring organs)
pT3: Tumor breaking through the mediastinal pleura or pericardium, or invading neighboring organs such as great vessels and lung
pT4: Tumor with pleural or pericardial implantation

pN
pN0: No lymph node metastasis
pN1: Metastasis in anterior mediastinal lymph nodes
pN2: Metastasis in intrathoracic lymph nodes excluding anterior mediastinal lymph nodes
pN3: Metastasis in extrathoracic lymph nodes

pM
M0: No distant organ metastasis
M1: With distant organ metastasis

Pathologic Stage Grouping

Stage I	T1, T2	N0	M0
Stage II	T1, T2	N1	M0
Stage III	T3	N0, N1	M0
Stage IVa	T4	N0, N1	M0
IVb	any T	N2, N3	M0
IVc	any T	any N	M1

[a]Table 2 from Tsuchiya R, Koga K, Matsuno Y, Mukai K, Shimosato Y. Thymic carcinoma: proposed pathological TNM and staging. Pathol Int 1994;44:506.

Table 2-13

TNM CLINICAL CLASSIFICATION (TENTATIVE FOR TESTING)[a]

T – Primary Tumor
TX: Primary tumor cannot be assessed
T0:   No evidence of primary tumor
T1:   Tumor completely encapsulated
T2:   Tumor invades pericapsular connective tissue
T3:   Tumor invades into neighboring structures, such as pericardium, mediastinal pleura, thoracic wall, great vessels and lung
T4:   Tumor with pleural or pericardial dissemination

N – Regional Lymph Nodes
NX: Regional lymph nodes cannot be assessed
N0:   No regional lymph node metastasis
N1:   Metastasis in anterior mediastinal lymph nodes
N2:   Metastasis in other intrathoracic lymph nodes excluding anterior mediastinal lymph nodes
N3:   Metastasis in scalene and/or supraclavicular lymph nodes

M – Distant Metastasis
MX: Distant metastasis cannot be assessed
M0:   No distant metastasis
M1:   Distant metastasis

Stage Grouping			
Stage I	T1	N0	M0
Stage II	T2	N0	M0
Stage III	T1	N1	M0
	T2	N1	M0
	T3	N0, N1	M0
Stage IV	T4	Any N	M0
	Any T	N2, N3	M0
	Any T	Any N	M1

[a]From Wittekind Ch, Greene FL, Henson DE, Hutter RV, Sobin LH, eds. TNM supplement. A commentary on uniform use, 3rd ed. New York: Wiley-Liss; 2003:118-119.

disease died from thymoma between 5 and 10 years after surgery, and recommended postoperative radiotherapy for all patients with stages II and III disease. Quintanilla-Martinez et al. (113) emphasized the importance of the microscopic assessment of invasion in stage II disease, since 1 of 16 stage IIa tumors (microscopic capsule invasion) recurred compared with 3 of 16 stage IIb tumors (invasion of mediastinal fat). The definition of "encapsulation" is meaningless, particularly in thymic carcinoma, since most thymic carcinomas are partially or entirely devoid of a capsule.

Although not referred to in the above-mentioned classification, tumor size has been used as an important parameter to define T categories: critical dimensions of 11 and 15 cm have been reported as a cut-off value for prognostication (22,75). In one report tumor size was stated to be one of the significant parameters of survival based on multivariate analysis (22).

Finally, the T3 denominator inevitably includes tumors with different characteristics: one extreme is an easily resectable tumor with minimal invasion of the pericardium and a good prognosis, and the other extreme is a nonresectable tumor with invasive growth into multiple neighboring organs. A further division of T3 tumors into potentially resectable and curable tumors (new T2) and nonresectable tumors with a poor prognosis (new T3) might be necessary, especially for planning treatment. According to Okumura et al. (99), involvement of the great vessels is an independent prognostic factor in patients with stage III disease: the 10-year and 20-year survival rates are 97 and 75 percent in the absence of involvement of the great vessels and 70 and 29 percent in the presence of it.

Regarding the N category, the anatomy of the lymphatic system in the anterior mediastinum is not yet fully understood. The appropriateness of the N1 to N3 nodal groupings requires further investigation. Depending on the tumor location in the anterior mediastinum, the lymphatic pathway by which tumor cells spread may vary. Consequently, the first lymph node into which tumor cells drain may not be located in the anterior mediastinum in some cases.

As proposed in the discussion for the T categories, the most important issue in staging is the therapeutic and prognostic appropriateness of the definitions of stages I and II. If the definition of T category remains unchanged, the present stages I and II should be merged into a new stage I. Stage III in the present tentative system, which is a heterogeneous group, is recommended to be divided into new stage II and III, i.e., a potentially resectable group with a favorable prognosis and an unresectable group with a poor prognosis, respectively. Furthermore, in the tentative classification, N1 is defined as stage III, but the prognostic equivalence of T3 and N1 has not yet been demonstrated.

Recently, a new staging system has been proposed that considers tumor size and number of involved organs/structures (17). Stage I was newly created by merging Masaoka stages I and II, and stage IV remains unchanged; stage II consists of tumors less than 10 cm in diameter and involving one neighboring organ/structure, and stage III consists of tumors of any size, involving two or more neighboring organs/structures, or tumors of 10 cm or more in diameter involving a single neighboring organ/structure. A well-balanced distribution of survival rates in each stage group has been obtained by this system.

Treatment

The primary curative treatment of thymoma is surgical removal (75–77). The extent of surgery is stage dependent. The therapeutic approach at the National Cancer Center Hospital in Tokyo is as follows. For encapsulated and minimally invasive thymomas (stages I and II), surgical resection is standard, usually thymothymomectomy via median sternotomy. Considering the multicentricity of thymoma and the possible postoperative development of myasthenia gravis, the complete removal of the thymus as well as the thymoma is recommended. Video-assisted thoracic surgery (VATS) for thymothymomectomy is considered for small (less than 5 cm in diameter), encapsulated or minimally invasive thymomas in institutions experienced in the VATS procedures. For larger thymomas of stage I or II, however, the intercostal space must be extended for removal of the resected tumors from the thoracic cavity in a VATS setting. This might compromise the less invasive nature of the procedure.

Systematic lymph node dissection is not usually indicated in thymothymomectomy for thymomas because of the rarity of lymph node metastases. The surgeons' approach is to remove the swollen nodes and submit them for frozen section diagnosis if they are present near the thymoma. Although postoperative radiotherapy may be indicated for minimally invasive thymoma on pathologic examination, its therapeutic significance is yet to be determined.

For potentially resectable stage III, widely invasive thymoma, complete resection by thymothymomectomy and combined resection of the invaded structures is still strongly recommended, and may be followed by radiotherapy or chemotherapy. A multimodal therapeutic approach is being adopted: induction systemic chemotherapy followed by definitive surgical resection is the representative example. For unresectable stage III and stage IV thymomas, a combination of radiation and systemic chemotherapy is indicated, although cure is less likely for these advanced tumors.

Recommendations for the management of thymoma by the Memorial Sloan-Kettering Cancer Center group are as follows (22): 1) small tumors (less than 5 cm) that appear encapsulated should be resected and if pathologically stage I, require no further treatment; 2) tumors 5 cm or more or those that appear invasive by CT scan have a high local recurrence rate and confer a low survival rate, therefore these patients should be considered for neoadjuvant therapy.

Prognosis

In the Lewis study (75) of 232 treated patients with thymoma who were discharged with no evidence of disease, 125 (44 percent) were alive after follow-up periods ranging from 1 to 30 years: 38 (14 percent) died of thymoma; 46 (16 percent) died of myasthenia gravis; 63 (22 percent) died due to unrelated causes. In 11 cases the cause of death was unknown. Recurrence occurred at or before 15 years of follow-up. Of 187 patients with circumscribed, noninvasive tumors, who underwent complete resection, 22 (12 percent) had thoracic recurrences. Fechner (36), after a review of the literature, stated that less than 2 percent of benign encapsulated thymomas recurred after resection, and that recurrent tumor took one of two forms, either pleural implants or localized mediastinal tumors. In one stage II case, type AB thymoma with rosette-like structures (fig. 2-44) showed vascular invasion histologically (fig. 2-72), and recurred with lung metastases 3 years after complete removal, but the patient was still alive with tumor 11 years after surgery for the primary tumor.

Analyses of death rates reveal that poor prognostic factors significant to overall survival ($P<0.05$) are an age exceeding 60 years, presence of mediastinal or constitutional symptoms, invasive or metastasizing thymoma at diagnosis, tumor size greater than or equal to 15 cm, and a predominantly epithelial histologic subtype. Slightly higher death rates in patients with myasthenia gravis are of marginal statistical significance. Illustrative survival curves with respect to tumor death are shown in figure 2-68. The importance of histologic subclassification by cell type has been stressed by Quintanilla-Martinez et al. (fig. 2-69) (113).

Rarely, extrathoracic spread of thymoma is seen. There were eight such cases in the series of Lewis et al. (75), involving the bone in five cases, extrathoracic lymph nodes in four, the liver in three, and central nervous system in two. Histologically, metastatic tumors maintain the characteristic features of thymoma in many cases, but may show a decrease in the number of lymphocytes as well as histologic progression (figs. 2-54, 2-73–2-75).

Although rare, carcinomatous transformation occurs in thymoma (see chapter 3) (140). There is a report describing an increased risk of a second malignancy in cases of thymoma, necessitating follow-up of patients with thymoma, even when benign, to enhance the early detection of another malignancy (101).

Most of the tumor deaths among our cases were observed within 3 years after the first surgery, regardless of the complete or incomplete removal of the tumor. If the tumor recurred more than 3 years after the first surgery, the prognosis was relatively good, despite the recurrence, indicating the slow growth of the thymoma in cases showing late recurrence. From these observations it can be extrapolated that the pathologic stage at the time of initial surgery may be regarded as a parameter of tumor aggressiveness, which influences the outcome of the disease; i.e., tumors at stages I and II frequently show slow growth in comparison with those at stages III and IV, which often proliferate faster. Therefore, the prognosis of patients with thymoma can be predicted on the basis of both disease stage and tumor aggressiveness. Tumor aggressiveness can be assessed by cell typing, as proposed by Müller-Hermelink et al. (54,78), or by cell typing and degree of cell atypia as proposed by Lewis et al. (75). The atypical thymomas based on cytologic atypia and organotypical features of differentiation described by Suster and Moran (142) are locally aggressive tumors with a high incidence of intrathoracic recurrence, but extrathoracic spread and death are uncommon (19). More accurate and objective methods for assessing the aggressiveness of tumors should be explored.

Three studies using the new WHO histologic classification system (121), evaluated by multivariate analysis, revealed that significant independent prognostic factors are staging and histologic classification (figs. 2-70, 2-105) (100); tumor size, completeness of resection, histologic subtype, and stage (figs. 2-71, 2-106) (95); and staging and completeness of resection (116a). The usefulness of the revised WHO histologic classification as a prognostic indicator in thymoma has been reported from other institutions (28,60). In contrast, one study reported that the prognoses for patients with types A and B thymoma did not significantly differ, and type A and B thymomas should be regarded as a morphologic continuum rather than as distinct histologic variants (25). Recently, Wright et al. (161a) concluded, from a prognostic viewpoint, that the Masaoka staging system could be collapsed into three groups by combining stage I and II; and the WHO histologic classification can be simplified for clinical use into A (A, AB), early B (B1, B2), advanced B (B3), and C; and a size of 8 cm or larger is an independent risk factor.

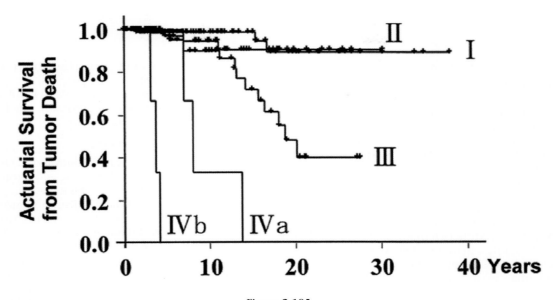

Figure 2-105

SURVIVAL CURVES ACCORDING TO THE MASAOKA STAGING SYSTEM AMONG PATIENTS WITH THYMOMA

Patients who died of myasthenia gravis, other diseases, or accidents were considered drop-outs at the time of the event. Survival refers to freedom from tumor death. There were 111 patients with stage I disease, 64 with stage II disease, 56 with stage III disease, 7 with stage IVa disease, and 5 with stage IVb disease. There were significant differences in actuarial survival between patients with stage I and stage III disease ($P = 0.0004$), patients with stage I and stage IVa disease ($P < 0.0001$), patients with stage I and stage IVb disease ($P < 0.0001$), patients with stage II and stage III disease ($P = 0.012$), patients with stage II and stage IVa disease ($P < 0.0001$), patients with stage II and stage IVb disease ($P < 0.0001$), patients with stage III and stage IVa disease ($P < 0.019$), patients with stage III and stage IVb disease ($P < 0.0001$), and patients with stage IVa and stage IVb disease ($P < 0.008$). There was no significant difference between patients with stage I and patients with stage II disease ($P = 0.56$). (Fig. 1 from Okumura M, Ohta M, Tateyama H, et al. The World Health Organization histologic classification system reflects the oncologic behavior of thymoma. A clinical study of 273 patients. Cancer 2002;94:628.)

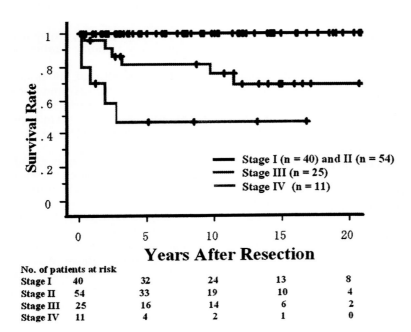

No. of patients at risk

Stage I	40	32	24	13	8
Stage II	54	33	19	10	4
Stage III	25	16	14	6	2
Stage IV	11	4	2	1	0

Figure 2-106

SURVIVAL ACCORDING TO TUMOR STAGE

The 5- and 10-year survival rates according to stage were 100% and 100% (stages I and II), 81% and 76% (stage III), and 47% and 47% (stage IV), respectively. The difference in survival between patients with stage III and stage IV is significant ($P = .000$). (Modified from fig. 4 from Nakagawa K, Asamura H, Matsuno Y, et al. Thymoma: A clinicopathologic study based on the new World Health Organization classification. J Thorac Cardiovasc Surg 2003;126:1138.)

REFERENCES

Classification

1. Kirchner T, Schalke B, Buchwald J, Ritter M, Marx A, Müller-Hermelink HK. Well-differentiated thymic carcinoma. An organotypical low-grade carcinoma with relationship to cortical thymoma. Am J Surg Pathol 1992;16:1153-69.
2. Levine GD, Rosai J. Thymic hyperplasia and neoplasia: a review of current concepts. Hum Pathol 1978;9:495-515.
3. Lewis JE, Wick MR, Scheithauer BW, Bernatz PE, Taylor WF. Thymoma. A clinicopathologic review. Cancer 1987;60:2727-43.
4. Marino M, Müller-Hermelink HK. Thymoma and thymic carcinoma. Relation of thymoma epithelial cells to the cortical and medullary differentiation of thymus. Virchow Arch A Pathol Anat Histopathol 1985;407:119-49.
5. Perrone T, Frizzera G, Rosai J. Mediastinal diffuse large-cell lymphoma with sclerosis. A clinicopathological study of 60 cases. Am J Surg Pathol 1986;10:176-91.
6. Quintanilla-Martinez L, Wilkins EW Jr, Choi N, Efird J, Hug E, Harris N. Thymoma. Histologic subclassification is an independent prognostic factor. Cancer 1994;74:606-17.
7. Rosai J, Levine GD. Tumors of the thymus. Atlas of Tumor Pathology, 2nd Series, Fascicle 13. Washington DC: Armed Forces Institute of Pathology; 1976.
8. Rosai J, Sobin LH. Histological typing of tumours of the thymus. World Health Organization, International histological classification of tumours, 2nd ed. New York: Springer; 1999.
9. Shimosato Y. Controversies surrounding the subclassification of thymoma. Cancer 1994;74:542-4.
10. Shimosato Y, Kameya T, Nagai K, Suemasu K. Squamous cell carcinoma of the thymus. An analysis of eight cases. Am J Surg Pathol 1977;1:109-21.
11. Shimosato Y, Mukai K. Tumors of the mediastinum. AFIP Atlas of Tumor Pathology, 3rd Series, Fascicle 21. Washington DC: American Registry of Pathology; 1997.
12. Snover DC, Levine GD, Rosai J. Thymic carcinoma. Five distinctive histological variants. Am J Surg Pathol 1982;6:451-70.
13. Suster S, Rosai J. Thymic carcinoma. A clinico-pathologic study of 60 cases. Cancer 1991;67:1025-32.
14. Travis WD, Brambilla E, Müller-Hermelink HK, Harris CC, eds. World Health Organization Classification of Tumours. Pathology and genetics of tumours of the lung, thymus and heart. Lyon: IARC Press; 2004.
15. Wick MR, Scheithauer BW, Weiland LH, Bernatz PE. Primary thymic carcinomas. Am J Surg Pathol 1982;6:613-30.

Thymoma

16. Asamura H, Morinaga S, Shimosato Y, Ono R, Naruke T. Thymoma displaying endobronchial polypoid growth. Chest 1988;94:647-9.
17. Asamura H, Nakagawa K, Matsuno Y, Suzuki K, Watanabe S, Tsuchiya R. Thymoma needs a new staging system. Interactive Cardiovasc Thorac Surg 2004;3:163-7.
18. Asamura H, Nakajima T, Mukai K, Noguchi M, Shimosato Y. Degree of malignancy of thymic epithelial tumors in terms of nuclear DNA content and nuclear area. An analysis of 39 cases. Am J Pathol 1988;133:615-22.
18a. Ashraf VV, Taly AB, Veerendrakumar M, Rao S. Myasthenia gravis in children: a longitudinal study. Acta Neurol Scand 2006;114:119-23.
18b. Baldi A, Ambrogi V, Mineo D, et al. Analysis of cell cycle regulator proteins in encapsulated thymomas. Clin Cancer Res 2005;11: 5078-83.
19. Baran JL, Magro CM, King MA, Williams TE Jr, Ross P Jr. Atypical thymoma: a report of seven patients. Ann Thorac Surg 2004;78:411-6.
20. Batata MA, Martini N, Huvos AG, Aguilar RI, Beattie EJ Jr. Thymomas: clinicopathological features, therapy, and prognosis. Cancer 1974;34:389-96.
21. Bernatz PE, Harrison EG, Clagett OT. Thymoma: a clinicopathologic study. J Thorac Cardiovasc Surg 1961;42:424-44.
22. Blumberg D, Port JL, Weksler B, et al. Thymoma: a multivariate analysis of factors predicting survival. Ann Thorac Surg 1995;60:908-14.
23. Ramon y Cajal SR, Suster S. Primary thymic epithelial neoplasms in children. Am J Surg Pathol 1991;15:466-74.
24. Castleman B. Tumors of the thymus gland. Atlas of Tumor Pathology, 1st Series, Fascicle 19. Washington, DC: Armed Forces Institute of Pathology; 1955.
25. Chalabreysse L, Roy P, Cordier JF, Loire R, Gamondes JP, Thivolet-Bejui F. Correlation of the WHO schema for classification of thymic epithelial neoplasms with prognosis. A retrospective study of 90 tumors. Am J Surg Pathol 2002;26:1605-11.

26. Chan JK, Rosai J. Tumors of the neck showing thymic or related branchial pouch differentiation: a unifying concept. Hum Pathol 1991;22:349-67.

27. Chan JK, Tsang WY, Seneviratne S, Pau MY. The MIC2 antibody 013. Practical application for the study of thymic epithelial tumors Am J Surg Pathol 1995;19:1115-23.

28. Chen G, Marx A, Wen-Hu C, et al. New WHO histologic classification predicts prognosis of thymic epithelial tumors: a clinicopathologic study of 280 thymoma cases from China. Cancer 2002;95:420-9.

29. Cheuk W, Tsang WY, Chan JK. Microthymoma: definition of the entity and distinction from nodular hyperplasia of the thymic epithelium (so-called microscopic thymoma). Am J Surg Pathol 2005;29:415-9.

30. Chilosi M, Castelli P, Martignoni G, et al. Neoplastic epithelial cells in a subset of human thymomas express the B cell-associated CD20 antigen. Am J Surg Pathol 1992;16:988-97.

31. Close PM, Kirchner T, Uys CJ, Müller-Hermelink HK. Reproducibility of a histogenetic classification of thymic epithelial tumours. Histopathology 1995;26:339-43.

31a. Comin CE, Messerini L, Novelli L, Boddi V, Dini S. Ki-67 antigen expression predicts survival and correlates with histologic subtype in the WHO classification of thymic epithelial tumors. Int J Surg Pathol 2004;12:395-400.

32. Davies SE, Macartney JC, Camplejohn RS, Morris RW, Ring NP, Corrin B. DNA flow cytometry of thymomas. Histopathology 1989;15:77-83.

33. Dorfman DM, Pinkus GS. CD99 (p30/32MIC2) immunoreactivity in the diagnosis of thymic neoplasms and mediastinal lymphoproliferative disorders. A study of paraffin sections using monoclonal antibody 013. Appl Immunohistochem 1996;4:34-42.

34. Ebihara Y, Dilnur P. Cytology of the mediastinal tumors. Byori to Rinsho 2002;20:608-13. [Japanese.]

35. Engel P, Marx A, Müller-Hermelink HK. Thymic tumours in Denmark. A retrospective study of 213 cases from 1970-1993. Pathol Res Pract 1999;195:565-70.

36. Fechner RE. Recurrence of noninvasive thymomas. Report of four cases and review of literature. Cancer 1969;23:1423-27.

37. Friedman HD, Hutchison RE, Kohman LJ, Powers CN. Thymoma mimicking lymphoblastic lymphoma: a pitfall in fine-needle aspiration biopsy interpretation. Diagn Cytopathol 1996;14:165-9.

38. Fukayama M, Maeda Y, Funata N, et al. Pulmonary and pleural thymomas. Diagnostic application of lymphocyte markers to the thymoma of unusual site. Am J Clin Pathol 1988;89:617-21.

39. Gschwendtner A, Fend F, Hoffmann Y, Krugmann J, Klingler PJ, Mairinger T. DNA-ploidy analysis correlates with the histogenetic classification of thymic epithelial tumours. J Pathol 1999;189:576-80.

40. Heitzman ER. The mediastinum: radiologic correlations with anatomy and pathology. St Louis: CV Mosby; 1977.

41. Henry K. Mucin secretion and striated muscle in the human thymus. Lancet 1966;1:183-5.

42. Henry K. An unusual thymic tumour with a striated muscle (myoid) component (with a brief review of the literature on myoid cells). Br J Dis Chest 1972;66:291-9.

42a. Hino N, Kondo K, Miyoshi T, Uyama T, Monden Y. High frequency of p53 protein expression in thymic carcinoma but not in thymoma. Br J Cancer 1997;76:1361-6.

42b. Hirabayashi H, Fujii Y, Sakaguchi M, et al. p16INK4, pRB, p53 and cyclin D1 expression and hypermethylation of CDKN2 gene in thymoma and thymic carcinoma. Int J Cancer 1997;73:639-44.

43. Hishima T, Fukayama M, Fujisawa M, et al. CD5 expression in thymic carcinoma. Am J Pathol 1994;145:268-75.

44. Hishima T, Fukayama M, Hayashi Y, et al. CD70 expression in thymic carcinoma. Am J Surg Pathol 2000;24:742-6.

45. Ho FC, Fu KH, Lam SY, Chin SW, Chan AC, Müller-Hermelink HK. Evaluation of histogenetic classification for thymic epithelial tumours. Histopathology 1994;25:21-9.

46. Ho FC, Ho JC. Pigmented carcinoid tumour of the thymus. Histopathology 1977;1:363-9.

47. Hofmann W, Moller P, Manke HG, Otto HF. Thymoma. A clinicopathologic study of 98 cases with special reference to three unusual cases. Pathol Res Pract 1985;179:337-53.

48. Inoue M, Marx A, Zettl A, Strobel P, Muller-Hermelink, HK, Starostik P. Chromosome 6 suffers frequent and multiple aberrations in thymoma. Am J Pathol 2002;161:1507-13.

49. Inoue M, Starostik P, Zettl A, et al. Correlating genetic aberrations with World Health Organization-defined histology and stage across the spectrum of thymomas. Cancer Res 2003;63:3708-15

50. International Union Against Cancer (UICC): TNM Classification of Malignant Tumours, 6th ed. Sobin LH, Wittekind CH, eds. New York: Wiley-Liss; 2002.

50a. Ishibashi H, Akamatsu H, Sunamori M. Multiple thymoma with myasthenia gravis: report of a case. Surg Today 2003;33:49-51.

51. Kameya T, Watanabe Y. Electron microscopic observations on human thymus and thymoma. Acta Pathol Jpn 1965;15:223-46.

52. Katzin WE, Fishleder AJ, Linden MD, Tubbs RR. Immunoglobulin and T-cell receptor genes in thymomas: genotypic evidence supporting the nonneoplastic nature of the lymphocyte component. Hum Pathol 1988;19:323-8.

53. Kirchner T, Müller-Hermelink HK. New approaches to the diagnosis of thymic epithelial tumors. Prog Surg Pathol 1989;10:167-89.

54. Kirchner T, Schalke B, Buchwald J, Ritter M, Marx A, Müller-Hermelink HK. Well-differentiated thymic carcinoma. An organotypical low-grade carcinoma with relationship to cortical thymoma. Am J Surg Pathol 1992;16:1153-69.

55. Kirchner T, Tzartos S, Hoppe F, Schalke B, Wekerle H, Müller-Hermelink HK. Pathogenesis of myasthenia gravis. Acetylcholine receptor-related antigenic determinants in tumor-free thymuses and thymic epithelial tumors. Am J Pathol 1988;130:268-80.

56. Kodama T, Watanabe S, Sato Y, Shimosato Y, Miyazawa N. An immunohistochemical study of thymic epithelial tumors. I. Epithelial component. Am J Surg Pathol 1986;10:26-33.

57. Koga K, Matsuno Y, Noguchi M, et al. A review of 79 thymomas: modification of staging system and reappraisal of conventional division into invasive and non-invasive thymoma. Pathol Int 1994;44:359-67.

58. Kondo K, Mukai K, Sato Y, Matsuno Y, Shimosato Y, Monden Y. An immunohistochemical study of thymic epithelial tumors. III. The distribution of interdigitating reticulum cells and S-100 beta-positive small lymphocytes. Am J Surg Pathol 1990;14:1139-47.

59. Kondo K, Sakiyama S, Takahashi K, Uyama T, Monden Y, Shimosato Y. Two cases of repeatedly recurrent atypical thymoma. Chest 1999; 115:282-5.

60. Kondo K, Yoshizawa K, Tsuyuguchi M, et al. WHO histologic classification is a prognostic indicator in thymoma. Ann Thorac Surg 2004;77:1183-8.

61. Kornstein MJ, Curran WJ Jr, Turrisi AT 3rd, Brooks JJ. Cortical versus medullary thymomas: a useful morphologic distinction? Hum Pathol 1988; 19:1335-9.

61a. Kornstein MJ. Controversies regarding the pathology of thymomas. Pathol Ann 1992;27:1-15.

62. Kornstein MJ, Max LD, Wakely PE Jr. Touch imprints in the intraoperative diagnosis of anterior mediastinal neoplasms. Arch Pathol Lab Med 1996;120:1116-22.

63. Kuo T. Sclerosing thymoma—a possible phenomenon of regression. Histopathology 1994;25:289-91.

64. Kuo T. Cytokeratin profiles of the thymus and thymomas: histogenetic correlation and proposal for a histological classification of thymomas. Histopathology 2000;36:403-14.

65. Kuo TT, Lo SK. DNA flow cytometric study of thymic epithelial tumors with evaluation of its usefulness in the pathologic classification. Hum Pathol 1993;24:746-9.

66. Kuo TT, Lo SK. Thymoma: a study of the pathologic classification of 71 cases with evaluation of the Müller-Hermelink system. Hum Pathol 1993;24:766-71.

67. Kuo T, Shih LY. Histologic types of thymoma associated with pure red cell aplasia: a study of five cases including a composite tumor of organoid thymoma associated with an unusual lipofibroadenoma. Int J Surg Pathol 2001;9:29-35.

68. Lardinois D, Rechsteiner R, Läng RH, et al. Prognostic relevance of Masaoka and Müller-Hermelink classification in patients with thymic tumors. Ann Thorac Surg 2000;69:1550-5.

69. Lattes R. Thymoma and other tumors of the thymus: an analysis of 107 cases. Cancer 1962;15:1224-60.

70. Legg MA, Brady WJ. Pathology and clinical behavior of thymomas. A survey of 51 cases. Cancer 1965;18:1131-44.

71. Lennon VA, Lambert EH, Leiby KR, Okarma TB, Talib S. Recombinant human acetylcholine receptor alpha-subunit induces chronic experimental autoimmune myasthenia gravis. J Immunol 1991;146:2245-8.

72. Levine GD, Bensch KG. Epithelial nature of spindle-cell thymoma. An ultrastructural study. Cancer 1972;30:500-11.

73. Levine GD, Rosai J. Thymic hyperplasia and neoplasia: a review of current concepts. Hum Pathol 1978;9:495-515.

74. Levine GD, Rosai J, Bearman RM, Polliack A. The fine structure of thymoma, with emphasis on its differential diagnosis. A study of ten cases. Am J Pathol 1975;81:49-86.

75. Lewis JE, Wick MR, Scheithauer BW, Bernatz PE, Taylor WF. Thymoma. A clinicopathologic review. Cancer 1987;60:2727-43.

76. Maggi G, Casadio C, Cavallo A, Cianci R, Molinatti M, Ruffini E. Thymoma: Results of 241 operated cases. Ann Thorac Surg 1991;51:152-6.

77. Maggi G, Giaccone G, Donadio M, et al. Thymomas. A review of 169 cases, with particular reference to results of surgical treatment. Cancer 1986;58:765-76.

78. Marino M, Müller-Hermelink HK. Thymoma and thymic carcinoma. Relation of thymoma epithelial cells to the cortical and medullary differentiation of thymus. Virchow Arch A Pathol Anat Histopathol 1985;407:119-49.

79. Marx A, Wilisch A, Schultz A, et al. Expression of neurofilaments and of a titin epitope in thymic epithelial tumors. Implications for the pathogenesis of myasthenia gravis. Am J Pathol 1996;148:1839-50.

80. Masaoka A, Hashimoto T, Shibata K, Yamakawa Y, Nakamae K, Iizuka M. Thymomas associated with pure red cell aplasia. Histologic and follow-up studies. Cancer 1989;64:1872-8.

81. Masaoka, A, Monden Y, Nakahara K, Tanioka T. Follow-up study of thymomas with special reference to their clinical stages. Cancer 1981;48:2485-92.

82. Masuda M, Arai Y, Okamura T, Mizoguchi H. Pure red cell aplasia with thymoma: evidence of T-cell clonal disorder Am J Hematol 1997;54:324-8.

82a. Mineo TC, Ambrogi V, Mineo D, Baldi A. Long-term disease-free survival of patients with radically resected thymomas: relevance of cell-cycle protein expression. Cancer 2005;104:2063-71.

83. Monden Y, Uyama T, Taniki T, et al. The characteristics of thymoma with myasthenia gravis: a 28-year experience. J Surg Oncol 1988;38:151-4.

84. Moran CA, Koss MN. Rhabdomyomatous thymoma. Am J Surg Pathol 1993;17:633-6.

85. Moran CA, Suster S. Thymoma with predominant cystic and hemorrhagic changes and areas of necrosis and infarction: a clinicopathologic study of 25 cases. Am J Surg Pathol 2001;25:1086-90.

86. Moran CA, Suster S, Fishback NF, Koss MN. Primary intrapulmonary thymoma. A clinicopathologic and immunohistochemical study of eight cases. Am J Surg Pathol 1995;19:304-12.

87. Moran CA, Suster S, Koss MN. Plasma cell-rich thymoma. Am J Clin Pathol 1994;102:199-201.

88. Moran CA, Travis WD, Rosado-de-Christenson M, Koss MN, Rosai J. Thymomas presenting as pleural tumors. Report of eight cases. Am J Surg Pathol 1992;16:138-44.

89. Morgenthaler TI, Brown LR, Colby TV, Harper CM Jr, Coles DT. Thymoma. Mayo Clin Proc 1993;68:1110-23.

90. Morinaga S, Sato Y, Shimosato Y, Shinkai T, Tsuchiya R. Multiple thymic squamous cell carcinoma associated with mixed type thymoma. Am J Surg Pathol 1987;11:982-8.

91. Müller-Hermelink HK, Marino M, Palestro G. Pathology of thymic epithelial tumors. In Müller-Hermelink HK, ed. The human thymus. Current topics in pathology, vol 75. Berlin: Springer-Verlag; 1986:208-68.

92. Müller-Hermelink HK, Marino M, Palestro G, Shumacher U. Kirchner T. Immunohistological evidence of cortical and medullary differentiation in thymoma. Virchow Arch A Pathol Anat Histopathol 1985;408:143-61.

93. Müller-Hermelink HK, Marx A. Towards a histogenetic classification of thymic epithelial tumours? Histopathology 2000;36:466-9.

94. Naidich DP, Zerhouni EA, Siegelman SS, eds. Computed tomography of the thorax. New York: Raven Press; 1984.

95. Nakagawa K, Asamura H, Matsuno Y, et al. Thymoma: a clinicopathological study based on the new World Health Organization classification. J Thoracic Cardiovasc Surg 2003;126:1134-40.

95a. Noguchi M, Maezawa N, Nakanishi Y, Matsuno Y, Shimosato Y, Hirohashi S. Application of the p53 gene mutation pattern for differential diagnosis of primary versus metastatic lung carcinomas. Diag Mol Pathol 1993;2:29-35.

96. Nomori H, Horinouchi H, Kaseda S, Ishihara T, Torikata C. Evaluation of the malignant grade of thymoma by morphometric analysis. Cancer 1988;61:982-8.

96a. Nonaka D, Henley JD, Chiriboga L, Yee H. Diagnostic utility of thymic epithelial markers CD205 (DEC205) and Foxn1 in thymic epithelial neoplasms. Am J Surg Pathol 2007;31:1038-44.

97. Oh YL, Ko YH, Ree HJ. Aspiration cytology of ectopic cervical thymoma mimicking a thyroid mass. A case report. Acta Cytol 1998;42:1167-71.

97a. Okada M, Tsubota N, Yoshimura M, Miyamoto Y, Sakamoto T. Two cases of synchronous multiple thymoma. Surg Today 1998;28:1323-25.

98. Okumura M, Miyoshi S, Fujii Y, et al. Clinical and functional significance of WHO classification on human thymic epithelial neoplasms: a study of 146 consecutive tumors. Am J Surg Pathol 2001;25:103:10.

99. Okumura M, Miyoshi S, Takeuchi Y, et al. Results of surgical treatment of thymomas with special reference to the involved organs. J Thorac Cardiovasc Surg 1999;117:605-13.

100. Okumura M, Ohta M, Tateyama H, et al. The World Health Organization histologic classification system reflects the oncologic behavior of thymoma: a clinical study of 273 patients. Cancer 2002;94:624-32.

101. Pan CC, Chen PC, Wang LS, Chi KH, Chiang H. Thymoma is associated with an increased risk of second malignancy. Cancer 2001;92:2406-11.

102. Pan CC, Chen WY, Chiang H. Spindle cell and mixed spindle/lymphocytic thymomas: an integrated clinicopathologic and immunohistochemical study of 81 cases. Am J Surg Pathol 2001;25:111-20.

103. Pan CC, Ho DM, Chen WY, Huang CW, Chiang H. Ki67 labeling index correlates with stage and histology but not significantly with prognosis in thymoma. Histopathology 1998;33:453-8.

104. Pan CC, Wu HP, Yang CF, Chen WY, Chiang H. The clinicopathological correlation of epithelial subtyping in thymoma: a study of 112 consecutive cases. Hum Pathol 1994;25:893-9.

105. Pescarmona E, Giardini R, Brisgotti M, Callea F, Pisacane A, Boroni CD. Thymoma in childhood: a clinicopathological study of five cases. Histopathology 1992;21:65-8.

106. Pescarmona E, Rendina EA, Venuta F, et al. Analysis of prognostic factors and clinicopathological staging of thymoma. Ann Thorac Surg 1990;50:534-8.

107. Pescarmona E, Rendina EA, Venuta F, Ricci C, Baroni CD. Recurrent thymoma: evidence for histological progression. Histopathology 1995;27:445-9.

108. Pescarmona E, Rosati S, Pisacane A, Rendina EA, Venuta F, Baroni CD. Microscopic thymoma: histological evidence of multifocal cortical and medullary origin. Histopathology 1992;20:263-6.

109. Pescarmona E, Rosati S, Rendina EA, Venuta F, Baroni CD. Well-differentiated thymic carcinoma: a clinicopathological study. Virchows Arch A Pathol Anat Histopathol 1992;420:179-88.

110. Pich A, Chiarle R, Chiusa L, et al. Long-term survival of thymoma patients by histologic pattern and proliferative activity. Am J Surg Pathol 1995;19:918-26.

111. Ponder TB, Collins BT, Bee CS, Silverberg AB, Grosso LE, Dunphy CH. Diagnosis of cervical thymoma by fine needle aspiration biopsy with flow cytometry. A case report. Acta Cytol 2002;46:1129-32.

112. Puglisi F, Finato N, Mariuzzi L, Marchini C, Floretti G, Beltrami CA. Microscopic thymoma and myasthenia gravis. J Clin Pathol 1995;48:682-3.

113. Quintanilla-Martinez L, Wilkins EW Jr, Choi N, Efird J, Hug E, Harris NL. Thymoma. Histologic subclassification is an independent prognostic factor. Cancer 1994;74:606-17.

114. Quintanilla-Martinez L, Wilkins EW Jr, Ferry JA, Harris NL. Thymoma— morphologic subclassification correlates with invasiveness and immunohistologic features: a study of 122 cases. Hum Pathol 1993;24:958-69.

115. Ramon y Cajal S, Suster S. Primary thymic epithelial neoplasms in children. Am J Surg Pathol 1991;15:466-74.

116. Regnard JF, Magdeleinat P, Dromer C, et al. Prognostic factors and long-term results after thymoma resection: a series of 307 patients. J Thorac Cardiovasc Surg 1996;112:376-84.

116a. Rena O, Papalia E, Maggi G, et al. World Health Organization histologic classification: an independent prognostic factor in resected thymomas. Lung Cancer 2005;50:59-66.

117. Riazmontazer N, Bedayat C, Izadi B. Epithelial cytologic atypia in a fine needle aspirate of an invasive thymoma. A case report. Acta Cytol 1992;36:387-90.

117a. Rieker RJ, Hoegel J, Morresi-Hauf A, et al. Histologic classification of thymic epithelial tumors: comparison of established classification schemes. Int J Cancer 2002;98:900-6.

118. Rogers BH, Manaligod JR, Blazek WV. Thymoma associated with pancytopenia and hypogammaglobulinemia. Report of a case and review of the literature. Am J Med 1968;44:154-64.

119. Rosai J. Rosai and Ackerman's Surgical Pathology, 9th ed. Edinburgh: Mosby; 2004:459-513.

120. Rosai J, Levine GD. Tumors of the thymus. Atlas of Tumor Pathology, 2nd Series, Fascicle 13. Washington, D.C.: Armed Forces Institute of Pathology; 1976.

121. Rosai J, Sobin LH. Histological typing of tumours of the thymus. World Health Organization international histological classification of tumours, 2nd ed. New York: Springer; 1999.

122. Rosenow EC 3rd, Hurley BT. Disorders of the thymus. A review. Arch Intern Med 1984;144:763-70.

123. Sagel SS, Glazer HS. Mediastinum. In Lee JK, Sagel SS, Stanley RJ, eds. Computed body tomography with MRI correlation, 2nd Ed. New York: Raven Press; 1989:245-94.

124. Salyer WR, Eggleston JC. Thymoma: a clinical and pathological study of 65 cases. Cancer 1976;37:229-49.

125. Sameshima Y, Tsunematsu Y, Watanabe S, et al. Detection of novel germ-line p53 mutations in diverse cancer prone families identified by selecting patients with childhood adrenocortical carcinoma. J Natl Cancer Inst 1992;84:703-7.

126. Sato Y, Mukai K, Watanabe S, Goto M, Shimosato Y. The AMeX method. A simplified technique of tissue processing and paraffin embedding with improved preservation of antigens for immunostaining. Am J Pathol 1986;125:431-5.

127. Sato Y, Watanabe S, Mukai K, et al. An immunohistochemical study of thymic epithelial tumors. II. Lymphoid component. Am J Surg Pathol 1986;10:862-70.

128. Scarpa A, Chilosi M, Capelli P, et al. Expression and gene rearrangement of the T-cell receptor in human thymomas. Virchows Arch B Cell Pathol Incl Mol Pathol 1990;58:235-9.

129. Seki M, Jinn Y, Du W. A case of type AB thymoma (World Health Organization) with brain metastasis. Haigan no Rinsho 2004;44:795-799. [In Japanese with English abstract.]

130. Shabb NS, Fahl M, Shabb B, Haswani P, Zaatari G. Fine-needle aspiration of the mediastinum: a clinical, radiologic, cytologic, and histologic study of 42 cases. Diagn Cytopathol 1998;19:428-36.

131. Sherman ME, Black-Schaffer S. Diagnosis of thymoma by needle biopsy. Acta Cytol 1990;34:63-8.

132. Shimosato Y. Controversies surrounding the subclassification of thymoma. Cancer 1994;74:542-4.

133. Shimosato Y, Kameya T, Nagai K, Suemasu K. Squamous cell carcinoma of the thymus. An analysis of eight cases. Am J Surg Pathol 1977;1:109-21.

134. Shimosato Y, Miller RR. Biopsy interpretation of the lung. New York: Raven Press; 1994.

135. Shimosato Y, Mukai K. Tumors of the mediastinum. AFIP Atlas of Tumor Pathology, 3rd Series, Fascicle 21. Washington, DC: American Registry of Pathology; 1997.

136. Shin HJ, Katz RL. Thymic neoplasia as represented by fine needle aspiration biopsy of anterior mediastinal masses. A practical approach to the differential diagnosis. Acta Cytol 1998;42:855-64.

137. Singh HK, Silverman JF, Powers CN, Geisinger KR, Frable WJ. Diagnostic pitfalls in fine-needle aspiration biopsy of the mediastinum. Diagn Cytopathol 1997;17:121-6.

138. Slagel DD, Powers CN, Melaragno MJ, Geisinger KR, Frable WJ, Silverman JF. Spindle-cell lesions of the mediastinum: diagnosis by fine-needle aspiration biopsy. Diagn Cytopathol 1997;17:167-76.

139. Snover DC, Levine GD, Rosai J. Thymic carcinoma. Five distinctive histological variants. Am J Surg Pathol 1982;6:451-70.

139a. Sonobe S, Miyamoto H, Izumi H, et al. Clinical usefulness of the WHO histological classification of thymoma. Ann Thorac Cardiovasc Surg 2005;11:367-73.

139b. Strobel P, Marino M, Feuchtenberger M, et al. Micronodular thymoma: an epithelial tumour with abnormal chemokine expression setting the stage for lymphoma development. J Pathol 2005;207:72-82.

139c. Suster S. Diagnosis of thymoma. J Clin Pathol 2006;59:1238-44.

140. Suster S, Moran CA. Primary thymic epithelial neoplasms showing combined features of thymoma and thymic carcinoma. A clinicopathologic study of 22 cases. Am J Surg Pathol 1996;20:1469-80.

141. Suster S, Moran CA Micronodular thymoma with lymphoid B-cell hyperplasia: clinicopathologic and immunohistochemical study of eighteen cases of a distinct morphologic variant of thymic epithelial neoplasm. Am J Surg Pathol 1999;23:955-62.

142. Suster S, Moran CA. Thymoma, atypical thymoma, and thymic carcinoma. A novel conceptual approach to the classification of thymic epithelial neoplasms. Am J Clin Pathol 1999;111:826-33.

143. Suster S, Moran CA. The mediastinum. In Weidner N, Cote RJ, Suster S, Weiss LM, eds. Modern surgical pathology. Philadelphia: Saunders; 2003:439-504.

143a. Suster S, Moran CA. Problem areas and inconsistencies in the WHO classification of thymoma. Semin Diagn Pathol 2005;22:188-97.

143b. Suster S, Moran CA. Thymoma classification: current status and future trends. Am J Clin Pathol 2006;125:542-54.

144. Suster S, Moran CA, Chan JK. Thymoma with pseudosarcomatous stroma: report of an unusual histologic variant of thymic epithelial neoplasm that may simulate carcinosarcoma. Am J Surg Pathol 1997;21:1316-23.

145. Suster S, Rosai J. Cystic thymomas. A clinicopathologic study of ten cases. Cancer 1992;69:92-7.

146. Suster S, Rosai J. Thymic carcinoma. A clinicopathologic study of 60 cases. Cancer 1991;67:1025-32.

147. Talerman A, Amigo A. Thymoma associated with a regenerative and aplastic anemia in a five-year-old child. Cancer 1968;21:1212-8.

148. Tan PH, Sng IT. Thymoma–a study of 60 cases in Singapore. Histopathology 1995;26:509-18.

148a. Tateyama H, Eimoto T, Tada T, et al. p53 protein expression and p53 gene mutation in thymic epithelial tumors. An immunohistochemical and DNA sequencing study. Am J Clin Pathol 1995;104:375-81.

149. Tateyama H, Saito Y, Fujii Y, et al. The spectrum of micronodular thymic epithelial tumours with lymphoid B-cell hyperplasia. Histopathology 2001;38:519-27.

150. Thomas De Montpreville V, Zemoura L, Dulmet E. [Thymoma with epithelial micronodules and lymphoid hyperplasia: six cases of a rare and equivocal subtype.] Ann Pathol 2002;22:177-82. [French.]

151. Travis WD, Brambilla E, Müller-Hermelink HK Harris CC, eds. World Health Organization Classification of Tumours. Pathology and genetics of tumours of the lung, thymus and heart. Lyon: IARC Press; 2004.

152. Truong LD, Mody DR, Cagle PT, Jackson-York GL, Schwartz MR, Wheeler TM. Thymic carcinoma. A clinicopathological study of 13 cases. Am J Surg Pathol 1990;14:151-66.

153. Tsuchiya R, Koga K, Matsuno Y, Mukai K, Shimosato Y. Thymic carcinoma: proposal for pathological TNM and staging. Pathol Int 1994;44:505-12.

154. Wittekind Ch, Greene FL, Henson DE, Hutter RV, Sobin LH, eds. TNM supplement. A commentary on uniform use, 3rd ed. New York: Wiley-Liss; 2003:118-119.

155. van der Kwast TH, van Vliet E, Cristen E, van Ewijk W, van der Heul RO. An immunohistologic study of the epithelial and lymphoid components of six thymomas. Hum Pathol 1985;16:1001-8.

155a. Wakely PE Jr. Cytopathology of thymic epithelial neoplasms. Semin Diagn Pathol 2005;22:213-22.

155b. Weirich G, Schneider P, Fellbaum C, et al. p53 alterations in thymic epithelial tumours. Virchows Arch 1997;431:17-23.

156. Weisbrod GL, Lyons DJ, Tao LC, Chamberlain DW. Percutaneous fine-needle aspiration biopsy of mediastinal lesions. AJR Am J Roentgenol 1984;143:525-9.

157. Weiss SW, Goldblum JR. Enzinger and Weiss's soft tissue tumors, 4th ed. St Louis: Mosby Inc; 2001.

158. Wick MR. Assessing the prognosis of thymomas. Ann Thorac Surg 1990:50:521-2.

159. Wick MR, Scheithauer BW, Weiland LH, Bernatz PE. Primary thymic carcinomas. Am J Surg Pathol 1982;6:613-30.

160. Wilkins EW Jr, Castleman B. Thymoma: a continuing survey at the Massachusetts General Hospital. Ann Thorac Surg 1979;28:252-6.

161. Wilkins EW Jr. Grillo HC, Scannell JG, Moncure AC, Mathisen DJ. J. Maxell Chamberlain Memorial Paper. Role of staging in prognosis and management of thymoma. Ann Thorac Surg 1991;51:888-92.

161a. Wright CD, Wain JC, Wong DR, et al. Predictors of recurrence in thymic tumors: importance of invasion, World Health Organization histology, and size. J Thorac Cardiovasc Surg 2005;130:1413-21

162. Yamakawa Y, Masaoka A, Hashimoto T, et al. A tentative tumor-node-metastasis classification of thymoma. Cancer 1991;68:1984-7.

163. Yang W, Efird JT, Quintanilla-Martinez L, Choi N, Harris NL. Cell kinetic study of thymic epithelial tumors using PCNA (PC10) and Ki-67 (MIB-1) antibodies. Hum Pathol 1996;27:70-6.

164. Yoneda S, Marx A, Heimann S, Shirakusa T, Kikuchi M, Müller-Hermelink HK. Low-grade metaplastic carcinoma of the thymus. Histopathology 1999,35:19-30.

164a. Yoneda S, Matsuzoe D, Kawakami T, et al. Synchronous multicentric thymoma: report of a case. Surg Today 2004;34:597-9.

164b. Yonemori K, Tsuta K, Tateishi U, et al. Diagnostic accuracy of CT-guided percutaneous cutting needle biopsy for thymic epithelial tumours. Clin Radiology 2006;61:771-5.

165. Zettl A, Strobel P, Wagner K, et al. Recurrent genetic aberrations in thymoma and thymic carcinoma. Am J Pathol 2000;157:257-66.

166. Zhou R, Zettl A, Strobel P, et al. Thymic epithelial tumors can develop along two different pathogenetic pathways. Am J Pathol 2001;159:1853-60.

3 THYMIC CARCINOMA

Thymic carcinoma is defined in the World Health Organization (WHO) Blue Book (75) as "a tumor exhibiting clear-cut cytologic atypia and a set of cytoarchitectural features no longer specific to the thymus, but rather analogous to those seen in carcinomas of other organs, and lacking immature lymphocytes." This same definition is used in the third series Fascicle on mediastinal tumors (79), and other publications (78,80,87,92,93,95)

In the second series Fascicle, Tumors of the Thymus, thymic carcinoma was included in the category of "thymoma" (74). Malignant thymoma included thymomas with local invasion, pleural implantation, or true lymphatic or hematogenous metastasis, and tumors with features characteristic of carcinoma as seen in other organs, with or without evidence of metastasis. These tumor types were designated later as malignant thymoma of types I and II, respectively (43). Levine and Rosai (43) used the terms "encapsulated thymoma," "true invasive thymoma," and "thymic carcinoma" for various stages in the spectrum of thymoma to carcinoma.

Synonyms and related terms for thymic carcinoma include *invasive thymoma, type II malignant thymoma, metastasizing thymoma*, and a variety of thymic carcinoma subtypes described separately.

Müller-Hermelink and coworkers followed the definition of thymic carcinoma by Levine and Rosai in their earlier publications in 1985 (45,57). Later, however, they proposed an entity of well-differentiated organotypical low-grade thymic carcinoma previously classified as cortical thymoma (30,31,69), which is now classified as type B3 thymoma by the WHO classification. The usefulness of their classification of thymic epithelial tumors has been questioned by some investigators (36,79)

GENERAL FEATURES

Because of the rarity of thymic carcinoma, the wide variation in histology, and the differences in diagnostic criteria among investigators, the exact incidence of this tumor in any given country as well as geographic differences in frequency are unknown. More than 300 cases have been reported in the literature (3). The largest series, by Suster and Rosai (87), is made up of consultation cases. The largest series from a single institution, reported by Wick et al. (95), comprised 20 cases collected over 75 years at the Mayo Clinic, during which more than 200 thymomas were assessed. The 13 cases reported by Truong et al. (92) were collected from two hospitals over a 22-year period. Of cases surgically resected at the National Cancer Center Hospital in Tokyo over a 40-year period, 64 were thymic carcinomas (46 squamous cell carcinomas and 18 cases of other histologic types including unclassifiable carcinomas), 138 were thymomas, and about 4,000 were lung cancers. The 1,320 cases of thymic epithelial tumors from 115 institutions in Japan collected by Kondo and Monden (33) by a questionnaire consisted of 1,093 thymomas (82.8 percent), 186 thymic carcinomas (14.1 percent), and 41 carcinoid tumors (3.1 percent). An analysis of thymic carcinoma subtypes in the literature shows a difference in geographic incidence: a higher frequency of well-differentiated squamous cell carcinoma and a much lower frequency of small cell carcinoma in the Orient than in the United States (39,78,87,92,95).

Most cases reported from various institutions occurred in cancer-age patients; only a few patients were below the age of 30 years, and the youngest was a 4-year-old boy. However, 25 of the 60 consultation cases of Suster and Rosai (87) occurred in patients under 40 years of age. This inconsistency cannot be explained at present. Thymic carcinoma occurs rarely in children: only 14 patients younger than 18 years of age are reported in the English language literature (99). The male to female ratio varies from almost equal to 2.3 to 1.0, contrasting with a tendency toward female predominance among patients

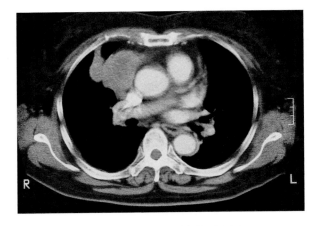

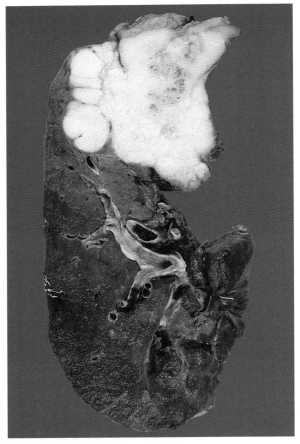

Figure 3-1

THYMIC CARCINOMA

Top: Computerized tomography (CT) shows an irregular but homogeneous density in the anterior mediastinum, which faces the density of the ascending aorta and invades S3 (anterior segment) of the right upper lobe of the lung.

Bottom: A horizontal slice of the tumor invading the lung roughly corresponds to the tumor shape depicted by CT. (Figs. 3-101B and C from Fascicle 21, Third Series.)

with thymoma. Kondo and Mondon (33) also stated that thymoma had a predisposition for females, but thymic carcinoma and thymic carcinoid affected more males than females.

Multiplicity has been reported (56), albeit rarely, although this has to be verified by excluding the possibility of intrathymic metastasis. Etiologic factors have not been clarified. A possible association between Epstein-Barr virus and lymphoepithelioma-like carcinoma is discussed separately.

CLINICAL FEATURES

The most frequent symptom in patients with thymic carcinoma is chest pain or dull ache. Coughing and general symptoms such as fatigue, fever, anorexia, and weight loss may also be present. Superior vena cava syndrome may be observed. In asymptomatic patients, the tumors are sometimes found by routine chest X-ray examination. There have been no reports of accompanying paraneoplastic syndromes, such as myasthenia gravis or pure red cell aplasia, although a few thymomas associated with myasthenic gravis have progressed to thymic carcinomas (87).

A tumor in the anterior mediastinum can be detected by imaging techniques in almost every instance, either by conventional chest X ray or with computerized tomography (CT) (fig. 3-1). Cystic changes and calcium deposits are rare. Frequently, the abnormal density involves the neighboring organs, such as the lungs, pericardium, and major vessels. Transbronchial biopsy or cytology via fiberoptic bronchoscopy, however, fails to reveal a tumor in most cases.

Imaging techniques are of no value for the determination of tumor type, and the diagnosis is made by either percutaneous needle biopsy (fig. 3-2) (249b), or aspiration cytology at the time of mediastinoscopy or thoracoscopy. If a biopsy yields only necrotic or crushed tissue (fig. 3-3), it should be repeated. Thymic carcinoma should be distinguished from predominantly epithelial thymoma, malignant germ cell tumors such as embryonal carcinoma, or diffuse large cell lymphoma with sclerosis. It may be difficult to determine whether the carcinoma is primary in the mediastinum or metastatic, unless clinical findings suggest a primary mediastinal tumor and biopsy specimens show features characteristic of thymic carcinoma.

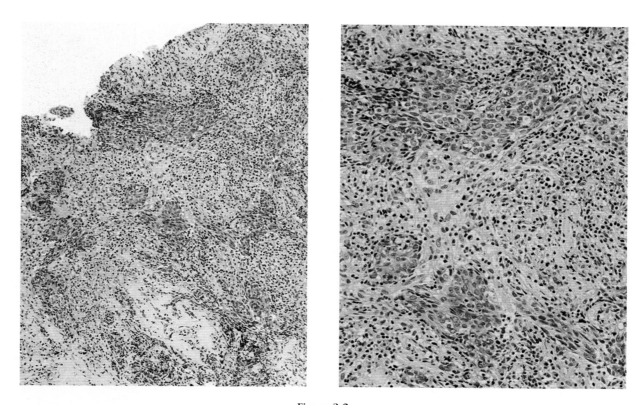

Figure 3-2

THYMIC CARCINOMA DIAGNOSED BY PERCUTANEOUS NEEDLE BIOPSY

Left: Irregular solid nests of infiltrating tumor are composed of polygonal to short spindle cells with hyperchromatic nuclei and distinct nucleoli. A partially sclerotic fibrous stroma is infiltrated by lymphocytes and plasma cells.

Right: Higher-power view of a poorly differentiated carcinoma nest.

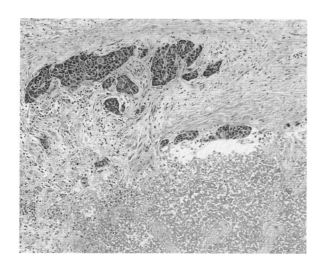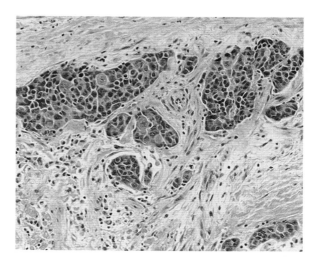

Figure 3-3

THYMIC CARCINOMA DIAGNOSED BY PERCUTANEOUS NEEDLE BIOPSY

Left: An extensively necrotic tumor is bordered by fibrous tissue. A few, apparently viable tumor cell nests are present at the periphery of the tumor.

Right: Higher-power view of the tumor suggests a squamous cell character.

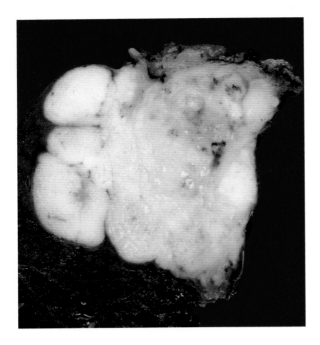

Figure 3-4

THYMIC CARCINOMA INVADING THE LUNG

Horizontal section of the tumor shown in figure 3-1 reveals that the main tumor in the anterior mediastinum has irregular invasive borders and a fibrotic central portion with small scattered foci of coagulation necrosis. Three nodules with a few anthracotic pigments on the left side of the tumor represent tumor invasion into the lung. The pseudoencapsulated border of the tumor on the right abutted the ascending aorta. Thymic tissue is attached to the tumor.

GROSS FINDINGS

The gross features of thymic carcinoma depend on tumor histology and size. In cases at the National Cancer Center Hospital, Tokyo, tumor diameter ranged from 3 to 5 cm or more. Squamous cell carcinoma with keratinization (low-grade histology by the Suster and Rosai classification [87]) is firm, with a rather homogeneous, ivory colored cut surface, a scalloped border, and often, a sclerotic center. Granularity may be noted, but lobulation is not evident or is inconspicuous, and there are small foci of necrosis and cystic changes (figs. 3-4–3-6). A false capsule is seen where the tumor reaches the capsule of the thymus, pleura, and pericardium. A true capsule is rare unless the carcinoma develops from a thymoma (fig. 3-7). A partially encapsulated basaloid carcinoma is shown in figure 3-8. Thymic carcinoma may arise in a multilocular

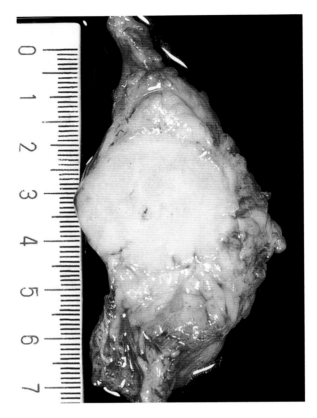

Figure 3-5

WELL-DIFFERENTIATED SQUAMOUS CELL CARCINOMA

A tumor about 3 cm in diameter is present within the thymus. It is ivory colored and homogeneous, with a sclerotic center and scalloped borders. No lobulation is noted.

thymic cyst, projecting into the cystic space as a nodular or papillary excrescence.

The degree of coagulation necrosis and the areas of hemorrhage tend to increase in less-differentiated tumors, or in tumors of high-grade histology. In some undifferentiated tumors, the surgical specimens consist of blood-stained fragments, probably because en bloc resection is impossible.

MICROSCOPIC FINDINGS AND HISTOLOGIC SUBTYPES

Microscopically, thymic carcinoma constitutes a heterogeneous group of tumors. The histologic subtypes employed by several investigators are listed in Table 2-2 (79,87,93,95) and in the WHO classification in Table 2-3 (75,91). In the United States, the most common type is

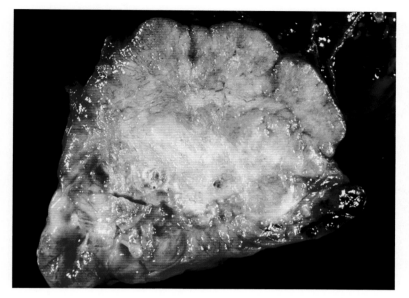

Figure 3-6

WELL-DIFFERENTIATED SQUAMOUS CELL CARCINOMA INVADING THE LUNG

The tumor is centrally sclerotic and peripherally granular. The granularity is reflected by solid tumor nests bordered by bands of fibrous connective tissue. Because of compressive growth, no anthracotic pigments are present within the tumor. The lung tissue is seen in the right upper corner, and swollen lymph nodes are located in the right lower corner.

Figure 3-7

THYMUS WITH MULTIPLE TUMORS

In this horizontal section, multiple tumors range from a few millimeters to 3.3 cm. The larger tumors are encapsulated, at least partially, and contain squamous cell carcinoma. This squamous cell carcinoma appears to have progressed from thymoma. A slice of the left upper lobe of the lung shows a few peribronchial and mediastinal lymph nodes containing metastases. (Fig. 3 from Morinaga S, Sato Y, Shimosato Y, Shinkai T, Tsuchiya R. Multiple thymic squamous cell carcinomas associated with mixed type thymoma. Am J Surg Pathol 1987;11:984.) (Figs. 3-7 and 3-17 are from the same patient.)

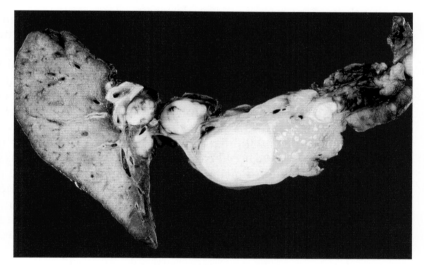

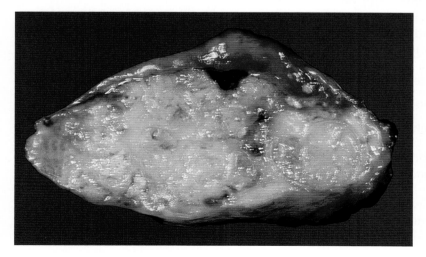

Figure 3-8

BASALOID CARCINOMA

The tumor is confined to within the thymic tissue and associated with a few cystic spaces. It is partly encapsulated and partly invasive. (Figs. 3-8 and 3-20 are from the same patient.)

119

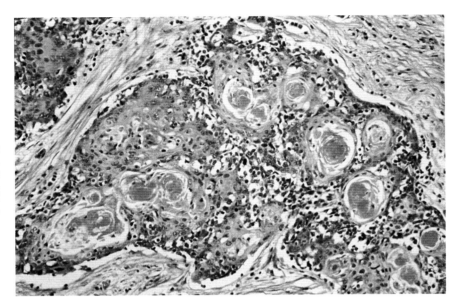

Figure 3-9

WELL-DIFFERENTIATED SQUAMOUS CELL CARCINOMA

Solid geographic nests are made up of polygonal cells with oval nuclei and moderately prominent nucleoli. Keratinization is present. The nests are separated by bands of fibrous tissue. (Figs. 3-9 and 3-14 are from the same patient.)

lymphoepithelioma-like carcinoma (poorly differentiated squamous cell carcinoma), followed by small cell/neuroendocrine carcinoma. At the National Cancer Center Hospital in Tokyo, as elsewhere in Japan, squamous cell carcinoma is by far the most common, followed by undifferentiated large cell carcinoma. Lymphoepithelioma-like carcinoma is infrequent, and small cell/neuroendocrine carcinoma, mucoepidermoid carcinoma, and clear cell carcinoma are rare. This may represent a racial difference in the histology of thymic carcinoma.

Although rare, thymic carcinoma can arise in any histologic type of thymoma. Of five cases of thymic carcinomas reported by Kuo and Chan (38), two arose from large polygonal cell thymomas, two from squamoid thymomas, and one from a spindle cell thymoma. The malignant components included two undifferentiated carcinomas and one each of spindle cell carcinoma, squamous cell carcinoma, and clear cell carcinoma with squamous differentiation.

Squamous Cell Carcinoma

Squamous cell carcinoma is defined as carcinoma showing keratinization or a keratotic tendency and/or intercellular bridges. *Well-differentiated squamous cell carcinoma of low-grade histology* (78,87) is characterized by solid nests of polygonal cells, often with vesicular nuclei, moderately prominent round nucleoli, a small to moderate amount of eosinophilic cytoplasm,

and well-defined cell borders showing keratinization and intercellular bridges in some areas (fig. 3-9). The keratinization may be abrupt, resembling Hassall corpuscles. Palisading or a radial arrangement of cells at the borders of nests, as is often seen in squamous cell carcinoma of the lung and esophagus, is not commonly observed (figs. 3-10, 3-11).

Tumor cell nests are surrounded by a broad zone of fibrous stroma, which is often hyalinized in the central portion of the tumor (fig. 3-11). Coagulation necrosis in the central tumor nests is either absent or minimal and rare in tumors of differentiated form or low-grade histology. Tumor cell nests in some areas have a lobular arrangement, with intermingled epithelial cells and lymphocytes, and closely associated fine blood vessels, simulating mixed epithelial and lymphocytic thymoma (fig. 3-12). The phenotypes of the lymphocytes here, however, do not resemble those seen in thymoma but rather those encountered in cancer of other organs (T lymphocytes that are CD1a negative, CD3 positive, and CD4 or CD8 positive [fig. 3-13], and B lymphocytes that are CD20 and CD79a positive). Plasma cells and eosinophils may also be found. The number of mitotic figures varies from area to area and from case to case.

In *less-differentiated squamous cell carcinoma*, keratotic foci are rare but intercellular bridges are identified in some areas. The general arrangement of the tumor cells, however, is similar

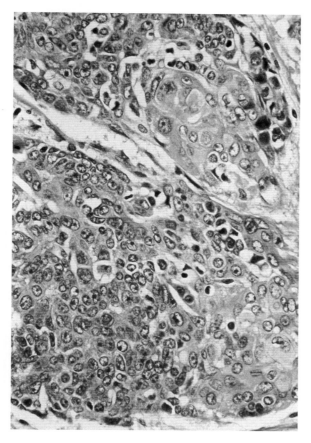

Figure 3-10

WELL-DIFFERENTIATED SQUAMOUS CELL CARCINOMA

The solid tumor nests are composed of polygonal cells with vesicular nuclei, prominent nucleoli, and a keratotic tendency. Palisading of tumor cells at the border of nests is not evident.

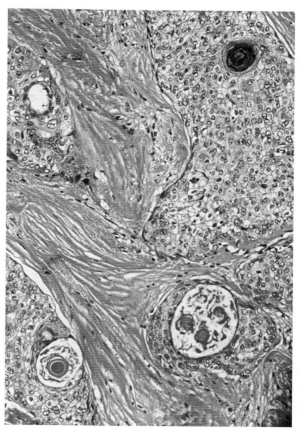

Figure 3-11

WELL-DIFFERENTIATED SQUAMOUS CELL CARCINOMA

Nests of squamous cell carcinoma showing Hassall corpuscle-like keratotic pearls with calcification or degeneration are bordered by broad bands of hyalinized stroma. Palisading of tumor cells is not seen at the periphery of nests.

to that of the differentiated form (78,87). The amount of coagulation necrosis increases in the less-differentiated form (fig. 3-14). Typical perivascular spaces seen in thymoma are rarely present in thymic carcinoma (figure 3-15 reveals probable organized perivascular spaces in a poorly differentiated squamous cell carcinoma).

A case of well-differentiated papillary squamous cell carcinoma arising in a preexisting thymic cyst was reported (42). There was also a case of well-differentiated basaloid squamous cell carcinoma arising in a multilocular thymic cyst (fig. 3-16A), which revealed malignant progression and invaded the sclerotic cyst wall. In this case (Shojiro Morinaga, Tokyo, unpublished case, 2004), features of basaloid carcinoma occurred

in a small part of the neoplasm and undifferentiated large cell carcinoma made up the rest (fig. 3-16B–E). This tumor was incidentally detected by a chest X-ray examination in a 52-year-old Japanese man, who already had pleural implantation metastases at the time of surgery. Immunohistochemically, the intracystic, papillary, well-differentiated basaloid squamous cell component was CD5 negative but the invasive basaloid and poorly differentiated large cell carcinoma was CD5 positive.

Squamous cell carcinoma coexisting with thymoma is uncommon (see chapter 4) (56). Truong et al. (92) reported two cases, and Kuo et al. (39) found a spindle cell thymoma and lymphoepithelioma-like carcinoma together;

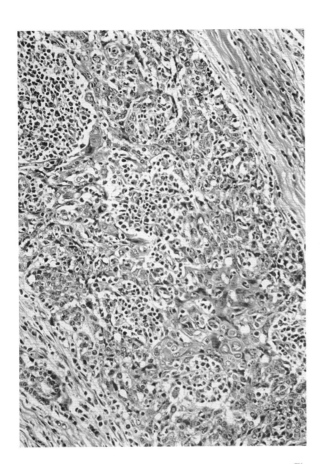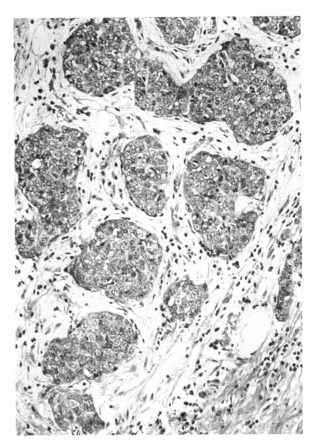

Figure 3-12

WELL-DIFFERENTIATED SQUAMOUS CELL CARCINOMA PARTLY SIMULATING THYMOMA

Left: Solid nests near the central portion of the tumor show foci of keratinization and are infiltrated by lymphocytes, reminiscent of thymoma. The stroma within the nest is loose, suggestive of an organized perivascular space, but the stroma surrounding the nest is sclerotic.

Right: Near the periphery and advancing border of the tumor, nests are composed of less differentiated and more atypical cells with coarsely granular or vesicular nuclei and prominent nucleoli. The loosely arranged stroma is infiltrated by lymphocytes, resembling carcinoma rather than thymoma.

the latter may be considered a variety of poorly differentiated squamous cell carcinoma. They also saw a cystic thymoma and a coexistent keratinizing squamous cell carcinoma. Wick et al. (95) described a thymoma together with lymphoepithelioma-like carcinoma. Suster and Moran (84) studied 22 thymic epithelial tumors characterized by the admixture of areas displaying features of thymoma and areas showing features of thymic carcinoma. Histologically, a combination of thymoma and well-differentiated squamous cell carcinoma was seen in 10 cases, thymoma and poorly differentiated squamous cell carcinoma in 7, and spindle cell thymoma with poorly differentiated squamous

cell carcinoma in 5. The features of clear cell carcinoma or lymphoepithelioma-like carcinoma were seen in some cases.

The authors have seen a patient with multiple tumors in the thymus, some of which were type B2 thymomas, while others showed features of keratinizing squamous cell carcinoma in some areas and poorly differentiated large cell carcinoma in others. Transition from thymoma to carcinoma was also observed (figs. 3-7, 3-17). Another patient with thymoma/carcinoma was a 36-year-old man in whom myasthenia gravis was diagnosed at the age of 21. Thymectomy was carried out at the age of 23. A locally recurrent tumor was removed and followed by

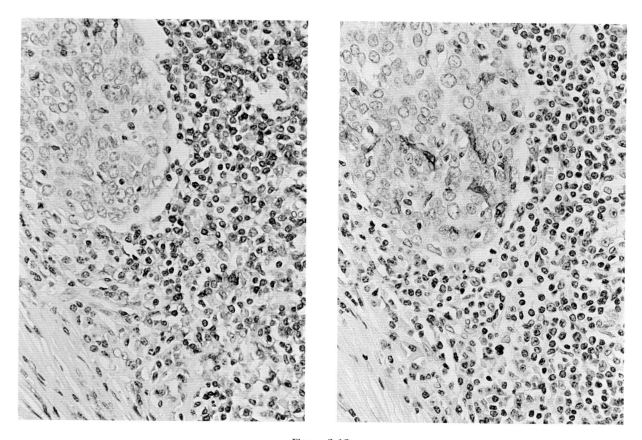

Figure 3-13

LYMPHOCYTE MARKERS IN SQUAMOUS CELL CARCINOMA

Left: The majority of infiltrating lymphocytes in the stroma are CD3-positive T lymphocytes.

Right: CD1a-positive lymphocytes are not evident. This indicates that the majority of CD3-positive cells are mature T cells, as is the case in carcinoma of other organs. The stained cells within a tumor nest are interdigitating reticulum cells.

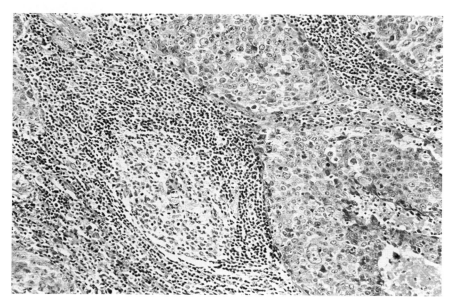

Figure 3-14

METASTATIC POORLY DIFFERENTIATED CARCINOMA IN A CERVICAL LYMPH NODE

Large solid nests consist of polygonal cells with vesicular nuclei and moderately prominent nucleoli. Coagulation necrosis is present at the left lower corner.

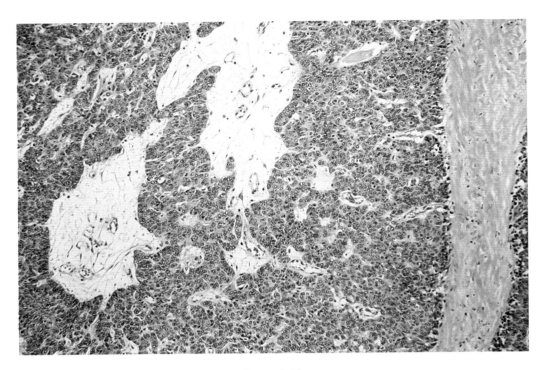

Figure 3-15

PROBABLE ORGANIZING PERIVASCULAR SPACE IN THYMIC CARCINOMA

In contrast to hyalinizing stroma around tumor nests, within solid nests, and in irregular anastomosing cords, there are fine thin-walled blood vessels in loose fibroblastic tissue bordered by palisading, poorly differentiated carcinoma cells. This finding suggests early organization of the perivascular spaces.

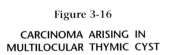

Figure 3-16

CARCINOMA ARISING IN MULTILOCULAR THYMIC CYST

A: The cut surface of a multilocular thymic cyst shows an intracystic papillary tumor invading a thickened, somewhat sclerotic wall and attached fatty tissue.

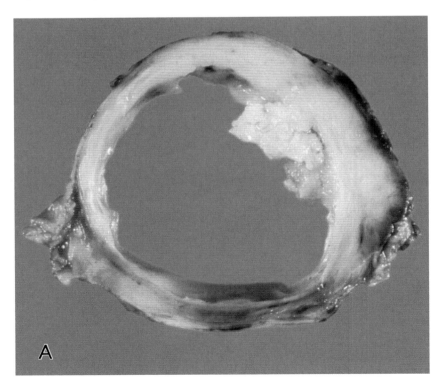

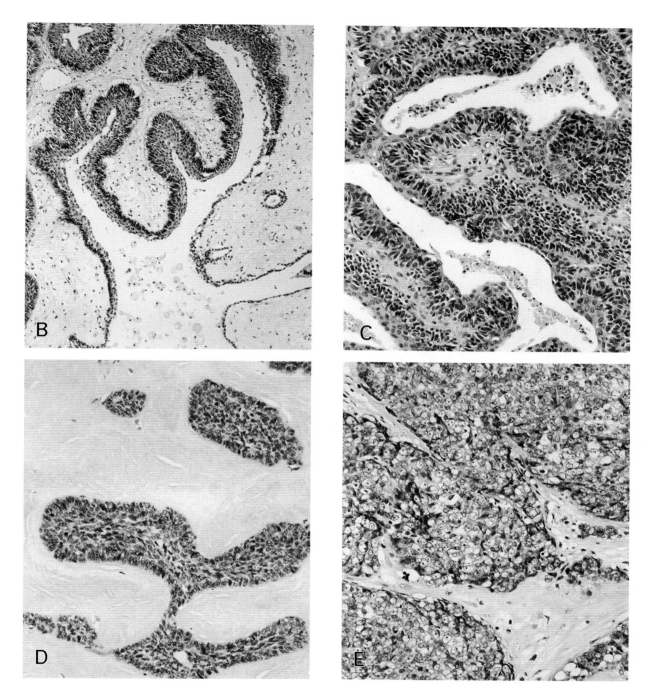

Figure 3-16 (Continued)

B: The papillary growth is basaloid squamous tumor with mild nuclear atypia growing beneath a single cell layer of cyst-lining epithelium, suggesting papilloma or low-grade carcinoma. The tumor cells were CD5 negative.

C: Higher-power view of other parts of the papillary tumor shows basaloid tumor cells beneath still recognizable, preexisting cyst-lining epithelium.

D: Carcinoma invading the sclerotic cyst wall has features of basaloid carcinoma. The tumor cells were positive for CD5. Basaloid squamous cell carcinoma was seen in other areas.

E: Malignant progression in and outside of the cyst wall resulted in a poorly differentiated large cell carcinoma with vesicular nuclei and distinct nucleoli. Pleural dissemination was evident at the time of surgery. (Courtesy of Dr. Shojiro Morinaga, Tokyo, Japan.)

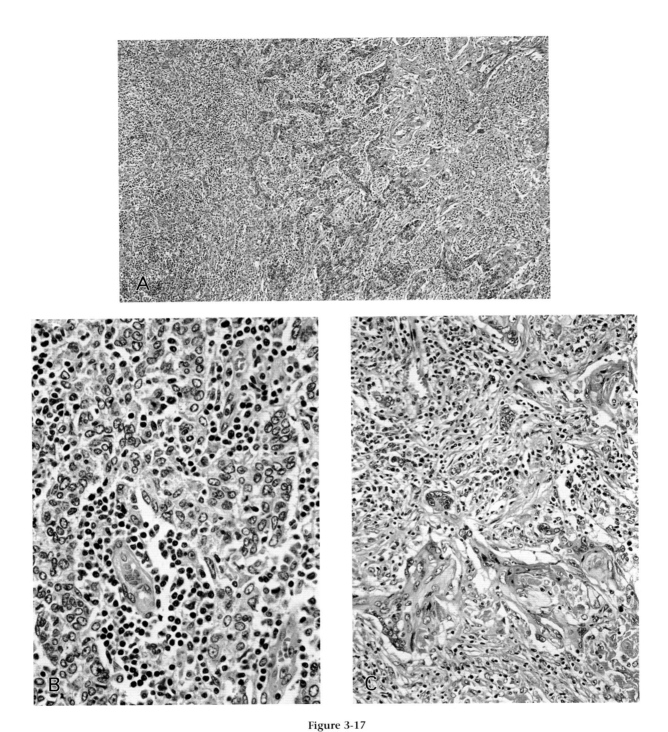

Figure 3-17

SQUAMOUS CELL CARCINOMA THAT APPEARS TO HAVE ORIGINATED IN THYMOMA

A: A low-power view of the tumor shows features of thymoma on the left and features of keratinizing squamous cell carcinoma on the right.

B: Higher magnification of a thymomatous area shows a mixture of lymphocytes and epithelial cells with bland nuclei (type B2 thymoma) and perivascular spaces with lymphocytes.

C: The same magnification of an area with keratinizing squamous cell carcinoma shows more evident individual cell atypia and marked keratinization.

radiotherapy at age 30. At age 36, a recurrent tumor involving the right upper lobe of the lung and a subcutaneous and intramuscular tumor of the epigastric region corresponding to the site of mediastinal drainage at the time of the previous surgical treatment were resected. All recurrent tumors were histologically similar, consisting of type B2/B3 thymoma with small areas of epidermoid features. At the tumor border, the epithelial cells showed increased nuclear atypia and eosinophilic cytoplasm with a tendency toward keratinization. The cells were arranged in irregular, solid infiltrating nests suggestive of poorly differentiated squamous cell carcinoma (fig. 3-18). Histologically, the tumor could be interpreted as type B2/B3 thymoma displaying malignant progression to squamous cell carcinoma. Two cases of thymic carcinoma involving the thyroid gland (52) can be classified as squamous cell carcinoma.

Basaloid Carcinoma

Basaloid carcinoma is a rare thymic carcinoma that frequently originates in multilocular thymic cysts. It is characterized by solid nests of small tumor cells with a high nuclear to cytoplasmic ratio and distinct peripheral palisading. There is only one case of basaloid carcinoma in the pathology file of National Cancer Center Hospital, Tokyo. Basaloid carcinoma is thought to be of low-grade malignancy, but hepatic metastasis was reported in one patient (50).

Grossly, the tumors are well circumscribed, often encapsulated and solid, with areas of hemorrhage and cyst formation, or are multilocular cystic (fig. 3-8). Microscopically, the tumors are composed predominantly of relatively small, uniform, spindled to polygonal cells with scanty cytoplasm and round to oval nuclei with inconspicuous nucleoli. The cells are arranged in solid nests, trabeculae, and anastomosing cords. The tumor cells at the periphery of the nests and trabeculae show a radial or palisading arrangement similar to the patterns seen in basal cell carcinoma of the skin (fig. 3-19) (80,87). Differentiation toward squamous cells may be seen in small areas, as well as gland-like or cystic spaces. Mitotic figures are frequent.

Although basaloid carcinomas often arise in thymic cysts (55,80), experience indicates that any histologic type of cancer, such as poorly differentiated squamous cell carcinoma and mucoepidermoid carcinoma, can arise from multilocular thymic cysts (fig. 3-16) (19,54). In one case, the cuboidal cells lining the cysts were replaced by carcinoma cells that resembled transitional cells or cells of urothelial carcinoma rather than typical basaloid cells (fig. 3-20). In this case, perivascular spaces were also noted. The tumor shown in figure 3-16 may also be considered basaloid carcinoma arising in multilocular thymic cysts, displaying squamous metaplasia and anaplasia.

Mucoepidermoid Carcinoma

Mucoepidermoid carcinoma is also a rare subtype, and only a small number of cases have been reported. Grossly, the tumor is solid or cystic and may be encapsulated. Its cut surface is nodular, with a granular or mucoid appearance (54,61,80)

Microscopically, tumor cell nests are separated by bands of fibrous stroma, and are composed of a mixture of three cell types (figs. 3-21, 3-22, left) (80). The most common cells are "intermediate cells," which are polygonal to short spindle cells, and have a moderate amount of eosinophilic cytoplasm, round to oval finely granular nuclei, and inconspicuous nucleoli. The second cell type is larger than the first and characterized by basophilic intracytoplasmic mucin that displaces the nuclei eccentrically to resemble signet ring cells or goblet cells. These cells occasionally form small glandular spaces. Cytoplasmic mucin, glandular spaces, and small cystic spaces within solid nests stain with Alcian blue–periodic acid Schiff (ABPAS) (fig. 3-22, right). The third cell type is squamous cells with a tendency to keratinize. Two or three cell types are often present within a single cell nest. Mitotic figures are hardly evident in any of these three cell types. The features described are consistent with the histology of mucoepidermoid carcinoma in other organs such as salivary glands and bronchi. The differential diagnosis includes epithelial cell–predominant thymoma with areas of mucin-producing cells (see fig. 2-49) and adenosquamous carcinoma (fig. 3-23).

At first, mucoepidermoid carcinoma of the thymus was included as a thymic carcinoma of low-grade malignancy (87). It has become apparent, however, that there is a wider histologic

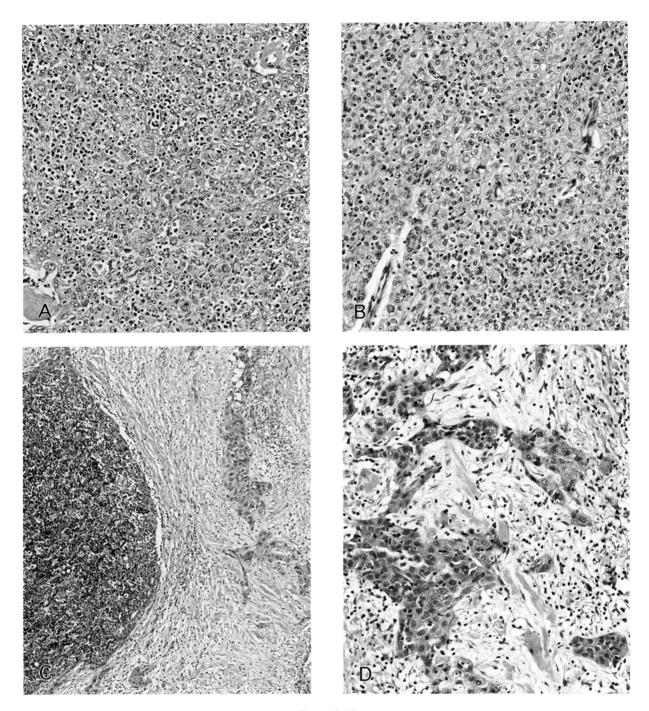

Figure 3-18

ATYPICAL (TYPE B2/B3) THYMOMA PROGRESSING TO POORLY DIFFERENTIATED SQUAMOUS CELL CARCINOMA

A: Polygonal epithelial cells have vesicular nuclei with prominent nucleoli, typical of B2 thymoma.

B: In small areas, the epithelial cells display epidermoid features (B3 thymoma).

C: At the border of the tumor (upper right) is a small focus of carcinoma consisting of irregular infiltrating nests of polygonal cells with vesicular nuclei, moderately prominent nucleoli, and eosinophilic cytoplasm showing a keratotic tendency. This carcinoma apparently arose from a lobule of thymoma (left side).

D: Higher magnification of the carcinoma. (Courtesy of Drs. Yasumasa Monden and Kazuya Kondo, Tokushima, Japan.)

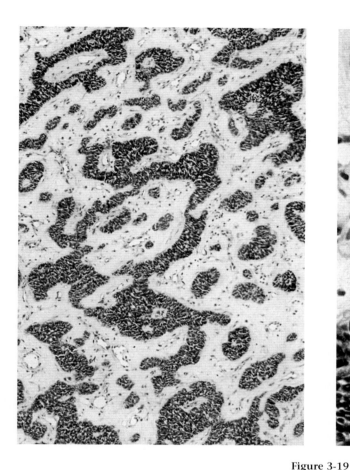 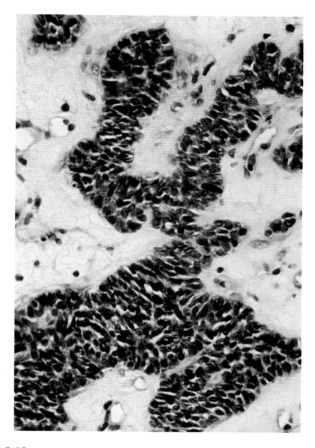

Figure 3-19

BASALOID CARCINOMA

Left: Palisading of cells at the periphery of tumor nests, trabeculae, and anastomosing cords are evident, resembling basal cell carcinoma of the skin.

Right: Higher-power view. (Courtesy of Dr. Juan Rosai, Milan, Italy.)

spectrum of differentiation, from well to poorly differentiated, and that the biologic behavior closely correlates with the degree of differentiation and cytologic atypia. In one study, two patients with intermediate- and high-grade tumors died within 2 and 7 years of initial diagnosis, four of six patients were between 17 and 26 years of age, and four tumors were closely associated with cystic structures having the features of acquired multilocular thymic cysts (54). In another study of eight low-grade tumors and two high-grade tumors, the two patients with the high-grade tumors died 1 year after diagnosis, whereas only 1 patient with a low-grade tumor (but high-stage disease) died after developing a local recurrence (61). Three of the tumors were associated with multilocular thymic cysts.

Adenosquamous Carcinoma

Carcinomas with combined squamous and glandular features uncharacteristic of mucoepidermoid carcinoma are placed in the category of *adenosquamous carcinoma* (fig. 3-23). Among squamous cell carcinomas of the thymus are cases with minor components of glandular differentiation in addition to the squamous component. In routine practice, glandular components may be so minor that their presence is merely added descriptively to the main diagnosis of squamous cell carcinoma.

The small cystic spaces within the squamous cell nests may contain mucinous material and cellular debris that stain with the ABPAS stain (fig. 3-23), although mucin-containing cells are rarely seen. The small cystic spaces result

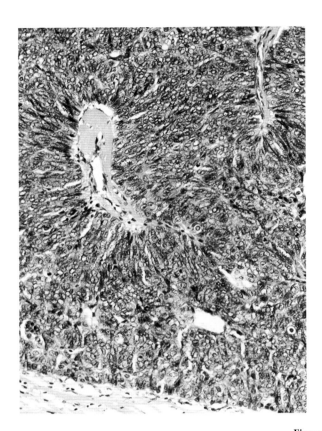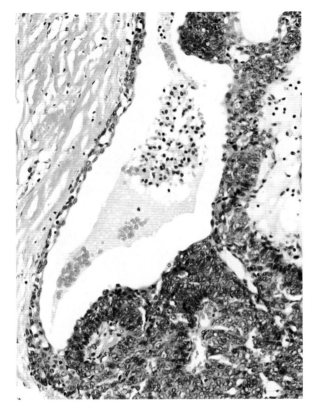

Figure 3-20

BASALOID CARCINOMA

Left: The tumor cells facing the perivascular space and the fibrous stroma surrounding the nest display pronounced palisading. The cellular arrangement and individual tumor cells with vesicular nuclei, however, simulate urothelial (transitional cell) carcinoma rather than basal cell carcinoma.

Right: Several cystic spaces were evident in the periphery of the tumor. They are lined by a few layers of less atypical, non-neoplastic cells, and are replaced in some areas by carcinoma cells.

Figure 3-21

MUCOEPIDERMOID CARCINOMA

Tumor nests are composed of polygonal cells with a tendency to squamous cell differentiation and mucus-producing cells. Small spaces filled with mucus are also present within the nests. (Courtesy of Dr. Juan Rosai, Milan, Italy.)

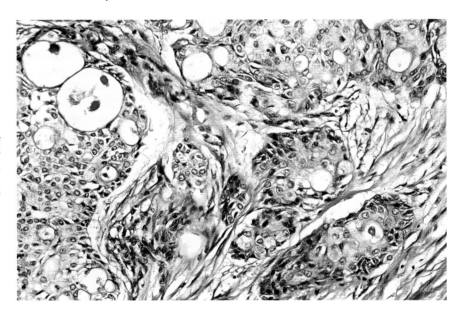

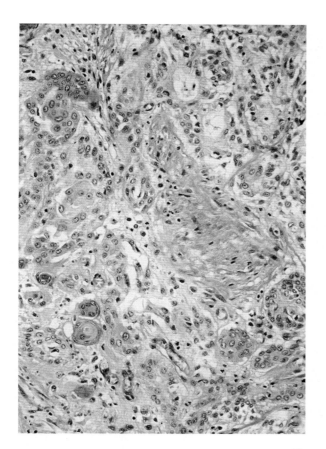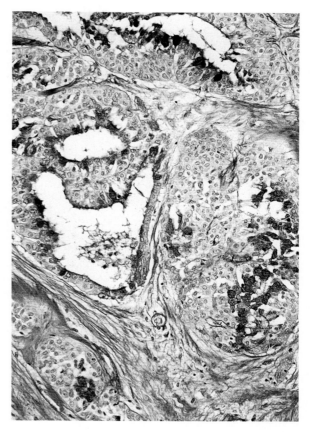

Figure 3-22

MUCOEPIDERMOID CARCINOMA

Left: This encapsulated, partly necrotic tumor consists largely of intermediate cells. The tumor cells are arranged in acini lined by low columnar cells with clear cytoplasm and basal nuclei. In some areas the cells show epidermoid features with a keratotic tendency.

Right: Alcian blue–periodic acid–Schiff (ABPAS) staining reveals abundant mucin in the cytoplasm of the tumor cells forming the acini. (Courtesy of Dr. Tadaaki Eimoto, Nagoya, Japan.)

from focal liquefactive degeneration of the tumor cells. However, immunostaining for a secretory component, which is considered to be a marker of glandular cells, reveals foci of aggregated, stained tumor cells, indicative of glandular cell characteristics (48). The presence of such structures alone, without definite glandular structures or mucin-containing cells, is not sufficient evidence for a diagnosis of adenosquamous carcinoma.

Preliminary studies indicate that patients with adenosquamous carcinoma have a better outcome than those with pure squamous cell carcinoma (48). The rarer *mucoepidermoid carcinoma* may be considered a variety of adenosquamous carcinoma of the thymus.

Adenocarcinoma

Adenocarcinoma is a carcinoma showing a papillary or glandular pattern. Papillae covered by a single layer of neoplastic epithelial cells are indicative of a glandular nature. It is not unreasonable to expect adenocarcinoma to occur in the thymus because of the presence of intracytoplasmic mucin in the thymic epithelial cells (21), the presence of glandular structures in a few thymomas, and the occurrence of mucoepidermoid and adenosquamous carcinomas in the thymus.

Thymic adenocarcinoma was first reported by Matsuno et al. (47) as papillary carcinoma. Two reported cases from the National Cancer Center Hospital in Tokyo were similar histologically

131

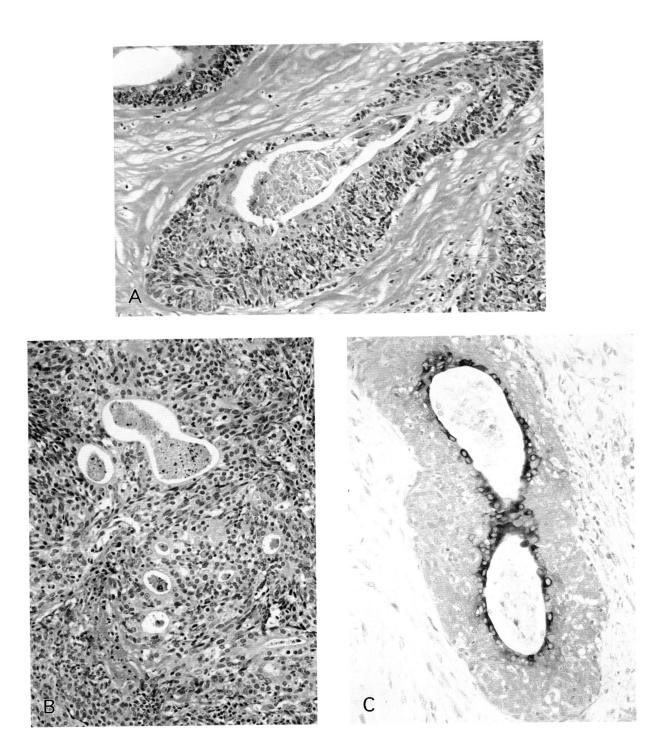

Figure 3-23

ADENOSQUAMOUS CARCINOMA

A: Histologically, the tumor has a variegated appearance. Solid nests of tumor cells are surrounded by hyaline stroma and show keratinization.

B: Within a tumor nest are several tubular structures lined by low columnar to cuboidal cells with basal nuclei.

C: The cytoplasm of the tumor cells facing a cystic space in a solid tumor nest stains for secretory component, a marker of glandular cells, even in the absence of demonstrable mucin-producing cells.

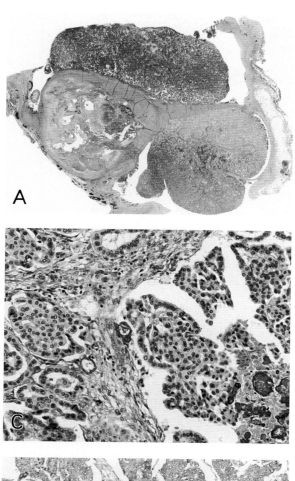

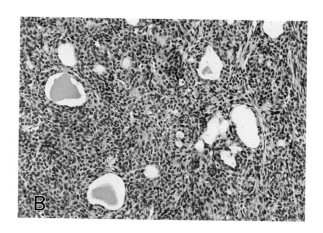

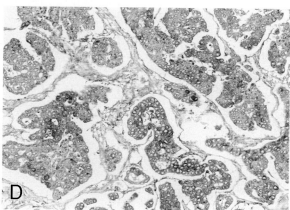

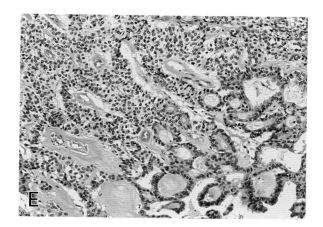

Figure 3-24

**PAPILLARY ADENOCARCINOMA
ARISING IN TYPE A THYMOMA**

A: A thickly encapsulated cystic thymoma is on the left and nodular, partly encapsulated tumors are in the upper portion and right lower corner.

B: The thymoma is partly cystic. There is diffuse growth of oval to short spindle cells with uniform nuclei.

C: A tubular and pseudopapillary arrangement with slight nuclear atypia and psammomatous bodies.

D: Positive immunostaining of carcinoma cells for carcinoembryonic antigen (CEA).

E: Collision of (or transition between) thymoma with a trabecular, hemangiopericytomatous pattern (left upper corner) and adenocarcinoma (right lower corner) within the thickly encapsulated nodule.

(figs. 3-24, 3-25) (79). In one case, a needle biopsy of an anterior mediastinal tumor, considered to be part of a teratoma, revealed adenocarcinoma. The resected tumor was composed of two parts: a thickly encapsulated cystic and predominantly short spindle cell (type A) thymoma and a papillotubular adenocarcinoma with occasional psammoma bodies that resembled ovarian serous papillary adenocarcinoma (fig. 3-24). Transitional features between the two parts were noted within a thickly encapsulated nodule of thymoma, strongly suggestive of adenocarcinoma arising in thymoma (fig. 3-24E). Although these two tumors were designated as papillary carcinoma originally, the term papillary adenocarcinoma is preferred.

133

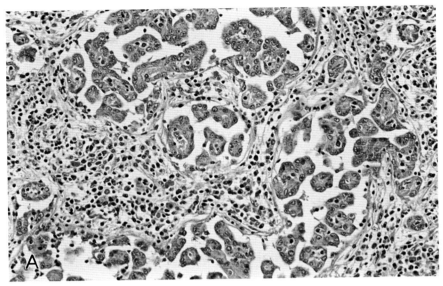

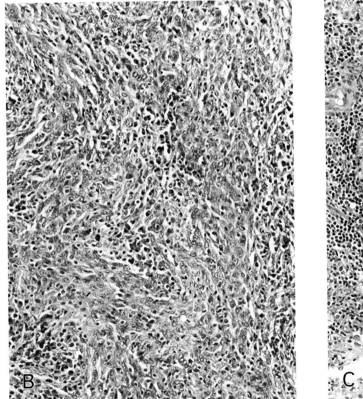
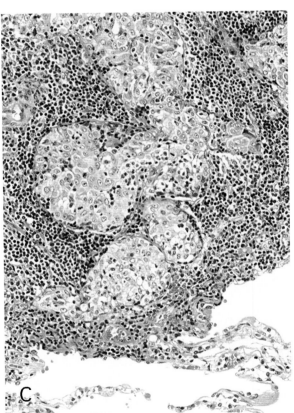

Figure 3-25

PAPILLARY ADENOCARCINOMA

A: An area of well-differentiated papillary adenocarcinoma with lymphoid stroma.

B: In another area, the tumor is poorly differentiated, with features of spindle cell carcinoma.

C: An advancing border invading the lung shows poorly differentiated solid carcinoma with a lymphoid stroma. (Courtesy of Dr. Hiroshi Fujita, Shimonoseki, Japan.)

A case of thymic carcinoma with glandular differentiation arose in a congenital thymic cyst (2). Choi et al. (7) described two cases of adenocarcinoma of the thymus: one with papillary carcinoma of high nuclear grade and the other with adenocarcinoma of mucinous subtype. They reviewed seven previously reported cases of adenocarcinoma as well and concluded that thymic adenocarcinomas usually arise from a thymic cyst or type A thymoma, and the clinical course varies. Recently, Takahashi et al. (88) reported another case of thymic mucinous adenocarcinoma unrelated to thymic cyst or thymoma, and Ra et al. (70) reported two more cases of mucinous adenocarcinoma of the thymus, one with numerous psammoma bodies and the other arising from a thymic cyst.

Carcinoma with Adenoid Cystic Carcinoma-Like Features

Recently, Di Tommaso et al. (10) reported four cases of *thymic epithelial tumor with adenoid cystic carcinoma-like features*. The tumors were multicystic and contained true glandular spaces filled with PAS-positive material. They presented as a continuum from benign looking and well circumscribed to overtly malignant and highly infiltrative. The authors interpreted the tumors as a histologic subtype of well-differentiated thymic carcinoma of low-grade malignancy. Isolated gain of chromosome 8 was noted in one case. The tumors somewhat resembled type A thymoma of oval cell type. Further study with accumulation of cases is needed.

Lymphoepithelioma-Like Carcinoma

Lymphoepithelioma-like carcinoma resembles undifferentiated (lymphoepithelioma-like) carcinoma of the nasopharynx. It is composed of large nests and diffuse growth of large polygonal cells with large vesicular nuclei, single prominent and round eosinophilic nucleoli, and scanty cytoplasm. The cells have ill-defined borders that often show syncytial features and are infiltrated to various degrees with lymphocytes and some plasma cells (fig. 3-26). When the lymphocytic infiltration is minimal, the histology is interpreted by some as poorly differentiated squamous cell carcinoma or large cell undifferentiated carcinoma (fig. 3-27).

Lymphoepithelioma-like carcinoma may be associated with areas of squamous cell carcinoma. One case was composed partly of ordinary epithelial thymoma (95) and another was composed partly of spindle cell thymoma (39). What looks like lymphoepithelioma-like carcinoma at the light microscopic level may reveal combined squamous and neuroendocrine differentiation at the ultrastructural level (95).

This subtype of thymic carcinoma appears to be rare among Japanese compared with the incidence among Caucasians, and is seen in younger patients. One of our few cases occurred in a 10-year-old boy, and the youngest patient reported was a 4-year-old boy. The prognosis of patients with this subtype is poor, and it is placed in the high-grade histology group by Suster and Rosai (87). An association with the Epstein-Barr virus is discussed separately.

Clear Cell Carcinoma

Clear cell carcinoma is a poorly differentiated carcinoma composed largely of clear cells. This is also a rare subtype, but more cases have been reported than for the mucoepidermoid and basaloid carcinomas.

Grossly, clear cell carcinoma is a solid tumor. Microscopically, there are lobules or sheets of polygonal cells with abundant clear cytoplasm, small nuclei with inconspicuous nucleoli or medium-sized vesicular nuclei with eosinophilic nucleoli, and a scanty fibrovascular stroma (fig. 3-28) (80). The clear cytoplasm contains abundant glycogen and some neutral fat but no mucin. It may be included in the category of large cell carcinoma. Several cases studied by electron microscopy and immunohistochemistry were believed to be a form of squamous cell carcinoma because of the presence of tonofibrils, desmosomes, and high molecular weight cytokeratin (92). Areas of necrosis and occasional mitotic figures (0 to 5 per 10 high-power field) are seen. In one case, the carcinoma was associated with a thymic cyst (3).

Clear cell carcinoma is considered to be a tumor of high-grade histology despite the slow growth in some cases. A review of the literature indicated that 9 of 13 patients (69 percent) either died of disease or had persistent disease at the time of follow-up (18). The differential diagnosis includes metastatic clear cell carcinoma

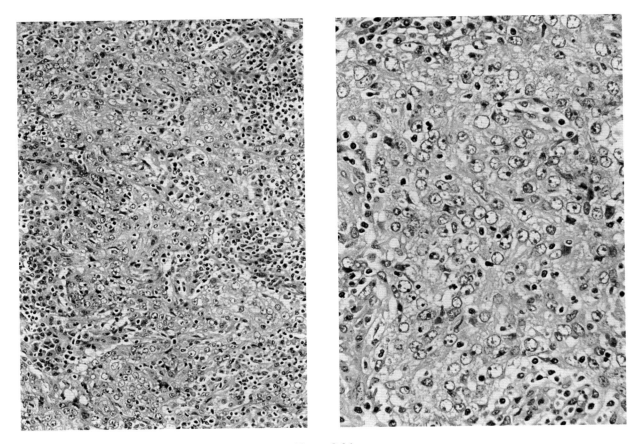

Figure 3-26

LYMPHOEPITHELIOMA-LIKE CARCINOMA

Left: The tumor consists of irregularly shaped, solid nests of polygonal cells with large vesicular nuclei and prominent nucleoli. The stroma is densely infiltrated by lymphocytes and plasma cells.

Right: Higher magnification of the same tumor shows cellular details. (Figs. 3-26 and 3-39 are from the same patient.)

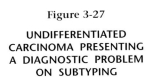

Figure 3-27

UNDIFFERENTIATED CARCINOMA PRESENTING A DIAGNOSTIC PROBLEM ON SUBTYPING

The individual tumor cells are somewhat similar to those shown in figure 3-26, although short spindle-shaped and infiltrating lymphocytes are few. This tumor may be subtyped as undifferentiated carcinoma or poorly differentiated spindle squamous carcinoma.

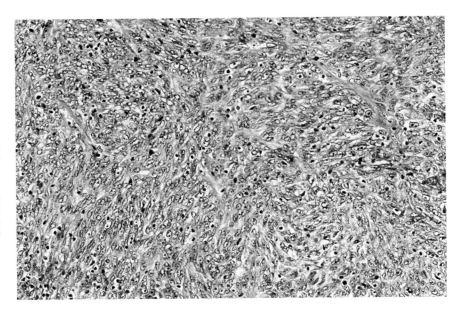

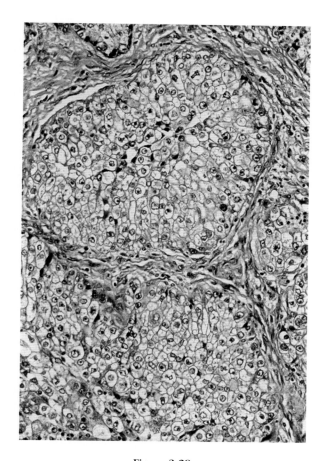

Figure 3-28

CLEAR CELL CARCINOMA

Solid tumor nests are composed of polygonal cells with abundant clear cytoplasm. (Courtesy of Dr. Hans Konrad Müller-Hermelink, Würzburg, Germany.)

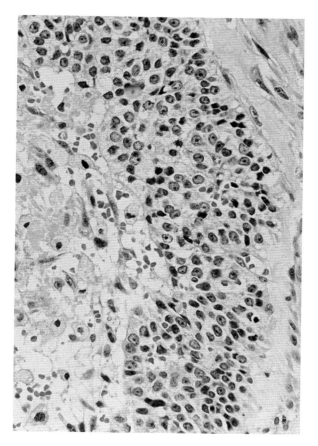

Figure 3-29

LARGE CELL CARCINOMA

The bulk of this tumor was necrotic, and only a thin layer of viable tumor cells remained at the extreme periphery. There are solid nests of polygonal cells with hyperchromatic nuclei and some prominent nucleoli. The left portion of the field is occupied by foamy histiocytes, which border an extensive area of coagulation necrosis.

from other organs, mediastinal seminoma, large B-cell lymphoma, parathyroid carcinoma, and predominantly epithelial (type B3) thymoma with a clear cell component (see fig. 2-55).

Large Cell Carcinoma (Undifferentiated Carcinoma in the WHO Classification)

Large cell carcinoma is a poorly differentiated carcinoma. Individual tumor cells are large and arranged in solid nests or display diffuse growth without sarcomatoid features, but show no differentiation microscopically toward any specific cell type, such as squamous cells, mucus-producing cells, or small neuroendocrine cells (figs. 3-29–3-31). In the lung, such carcinomas are designated large cell carcinoma. Lymphoepi-

thelioma-like carcinoma is considered to be a variety of large cell carcinoma. In the thymus, most large cell carcinomas are probably poorly differentiated squamous cell carcinomas ultrastructurally, but a few may be neuroendocrine in nature. Cases are few in number and the prognosis is usually poor. However, indolent behavior was noted in five undifferentiated large cell carcinomas of the thymus (cytokeratin positive, CD5 negative) associated with hyaline vascular type Castleman disease-like reaction (62). The indolent behavior was probably due to the host immune response. The differential diagnosis includes large cell carcinoma of the lung involving the mediastinum.

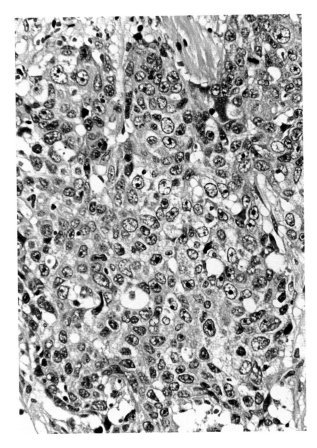

Figure 3-30

LARGE CELL CARCINOMA

There are large solid nests of large polygonal cells with round to oval vesicular nuclei and single distinct nucleoli, a small amount of pale stained cytoplasm, and ill-defined cell borders. There is no differentiation toward any particular cell type.

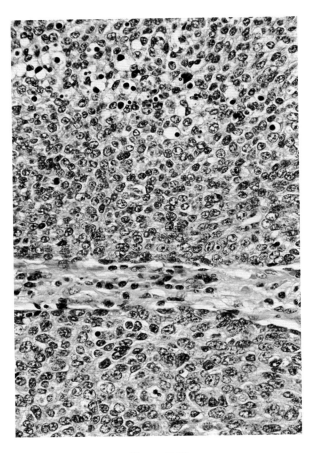

Figure 3-31

LARGE CELL CARCINOMA

In this tumor, although no definite keratinization or intercellular bridges are evident, the cellular details and arrangement suggest minimal squamous differentiation. There are many pyknotic cells in the center of a cell nest. The histology is similar to the poorly differentiated squamous cell carcinoma shown in figure 3-14, the primary tumor of which was shown in figure 3-9.

Sarcomatoid Carcinoma

The rare *sarcomatoid carcinoma* is composed in part of a carcinomatous element and in part of a sarcomatoid or sarcomatous element (80,95). This subtype includes *spindle cell carcinoma* and *carcinosarcoma*. The definition is different from that of sarcomatoid carcinoma in lung (91).

Grossly, the tumor is solid, often invasive, with foci of coagulation necrosis. It may be lobulated in part. Microscopically, the sarcomatoid or sarcomatous element displays spindle cells with oval, coarsely granular nuclei and inconspicuous nucleoli, arranged in bundles, a storiform pattern, or haphazardly. Mitotic figures are frequently seen. Separated from or within the

areas of the sarcomatoid or sarcomatous element are solid nests of large polygonal cells with oval, somewhat vesicular hyperchromatic nuclei, prominent nucleoli, and a moderate amount of cytoplasm, which may display differentiation toward squamous cells (fig. 3-32).

Suster and Moran (85) reported 16 cases of spindle cell thymic carcinoma, 12 of which had features of conventional spindle cell thymoma. In 2 cases, areas showing features of lymphoepithelioma-like carcinoma and anaplastic carcinoma were seen. Clinical follow-up of 8 patients showed aggressive biologic behavior with recurrence, metastasis, and death (5

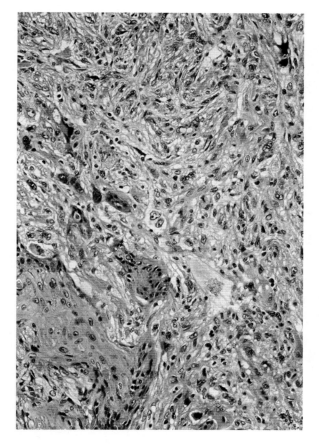

Figure 3-32

SARCOMATOID CARCINOMA

The tumor consists of solid nests of polygonal cells showing squamous differentiation, and surrounded by spindle cells with nuclear atypia and some bizarre tumor cells. There are no areas of specific mesenchymal differentiation. (Courtesy of Dr. Tetsuro Kodama, Utsunomiya, Japan.)

patients) within 5 years after diagnosis. The case shown in figure 2-74 as spindle cell thymoma with lung and liver metastases may be considered spindle cell carcinoma by some, but the nuclear atypia and mitotic activity are not sufficient to call this tumor spindle cell carcinoma.

Heterologous elements, such as rhabdomyomatous or osteosarcomatous areas, may be observed in the sarcomatoid element (carcinosarcoma). One thymic sarcomatoid carcinoma (carcinosarcoma) with myoid differentiation in the sarcomatous component was associated with a spindle cell thymoma (83). Rhabdomyoblastic cells may show cross striations and contain immunoreactive myoglobin (fig. 3-33)

(15,65,80). Cytokeratin is found not only in the carcinomatous elements but also in the spindle cells in some cases. In one case, some large and round rhabdomyoblastic cells showed immunoreactivity for cytokeratin (CK) 7 and CK8, using CAM5.2 and epithelial membrane antigen (15). The morphogenesis of this tumor is explained by the neoplastic metaplasia of the epithelial component to mesenchymal cells.

Sarcomatoid carcinoma is a high-grade malignant tumor. Tumor growth is rapid and metastatic spread is wide, resulting in a short patient survival period.

Carcinoma with t(15;19) Translocation

This subtype is included in the category of thymic carcinoma classified by the WHO (91). Carcinoma with translocation t(15;19)(q13;p13.1) is a rare aggressive and lethal carcinoma arising in supradiaphragmatic midline organs including the mediastinum of children and young adults (17,41,91). It resembles, microscopically, lymphoepithelioma-like, poorly differentiated squamous cell, mucoepidermoid, and undifferentiated large cell carcinomas.

CYTOLOGIC FINDINGS

Because of the many subtypes of thymic carcinoma, the cytologic findings are variable. Definite subtyping of the tumor is impossible unless characteristic features, such as keratinization, are identified. Core needle biopsy is preferred to fine needle aspiration cytology for diagnosis. It is impossible to determine from the cytology alone whether the tumor is primary in the thymus or metastatic to the mediastinum.

In cases of thymic carcinoma of low-grade histology, such as well-differentiated squamous cell carcinoma, basal cell carcinoma, and mucoepidermoid carcinoma, cellular atypia is mild to moderate and evidence of necrosis is minimal or absent (fig. 3-34) (14). In two cases of thymic basaloid carcinoma, the fine needle aspiration diagnosis was difficult and the differential diagnosis ranged widely; the cytologic diagnosis was poorly differentiated carcinoma in one and poorly differentiated adenocarcinoma in the other (68).

Distinguishing between invasive thymoma with nuclear atypia and thymic carcinoma may be difficult (71). In thymoma, immature (or cortical)

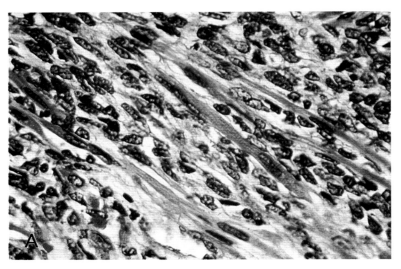

Figure 3-33

**SARCOMATOID CARCINOMA
WITH RHABDOMYOBLASTIC
DIFFERENTIATION**

A: The tumor consists of elongated cells with fibrillar eosinophilic cytoplasm and hyperchromatic nuclei. Cross striations are not evident in this field.

B: The upper half of the figure shows a single, large oval cell strongly immunoreactive for myoglobin surrounded by small tumor cells, which are negative for the marker. The lower half of the figure shows a single elongated tumor cell immunoreactive for myoglobin within the nonreactive spindle cell growth.

C: In another case, large round tumor cells have homogeneous to fibrillar eosinophilic cytoplasm. (Courtesy of Dr. Juan Rosai, Milan, Italy.)

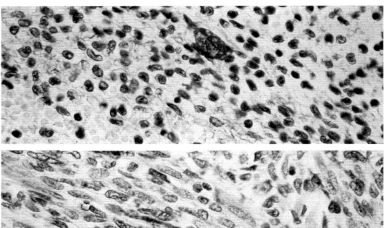

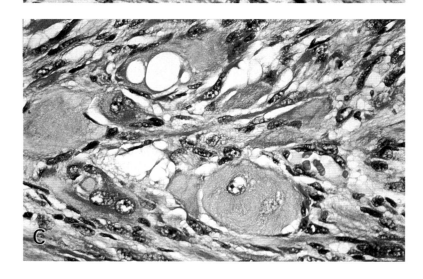

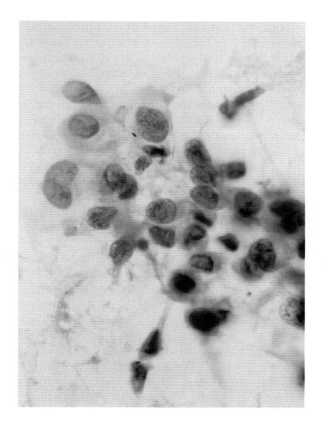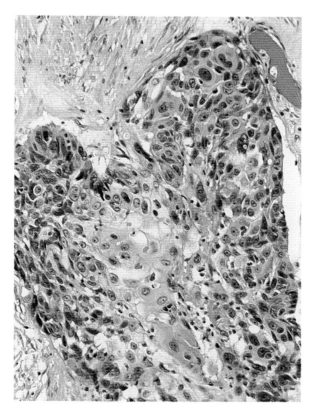

Figure 3-34

NEEDLE ASPIRATION CYTOLOGY OF SQUAMOUS CELL CARCINOMA OF THE THYMUS

Left: The cytology smear reveals a cell aggregate consisting of moderately large polygonal cells with varying sized hyperchromatic nuclei and a small to moderate amount of light green-stained cytoplasm. This most likely is consistent with squamous cell carcinoma.

Right: The resected anterior mediastinal tumor adherent to, but not invading, the lung has an irregularly shaped solid nest of atypical cells with a tendency to keratinization and somewhat sclerotic stroma. This is consistent with thymic squamous cell carcinoma. (Fig. 5A&B of Ebihara Y, Dilnur P. Cytology of the mediastinal tumors. Byori to Rinsho 2002:20:611.)

T cells may be detected by immunostaining of smears for CD1a; CD99 or terminal deoxynucleotidyltransferase (TdT) may be of help, although in type B3 thymoma lymphocytes are few. On the other hand, with carcinoma of high-grade histology, cellular atypia is marked, often with nuclear pleomorphism and hyperchromasia, nucleolar prominence, increased nuclear to cytoplasmic ratio, and a necrotic background (16).

IMMUNOHISTOCHEMICAL FINDINGS

Immunohistochemical analysis of thymic carcinoma should be done for both epithelial cells and lymphocytes. Most antibodies described in this section are reactive with formalin-fixed, paraffin-embedded tissue unless otherwise stated.

Since thymic carcinoma is an epithelial tumor, it is natural to expect that every tumor will react with antibodies against cytokeratins of various molecular weights and epithelial membrane antigen. This is, in fact, the case. Leu-7 (CD57) is positive in the majority of thymomas but negative in thymic squamous cell carcinoma in our experience (32). Since well- to moderately differentiated adenocarcinoma of the lung as well as small cell carcinoma immunostain for leu-7, this marker may be positive in some forms of thymic carcinoma.

Hishima et al. (25) reported that CD5, a type of receptor molecule that signals cell growth in T cells, was expressed immunohistochemically in epithelial cells of all of 7 thymic carcinomas (fig. 3-35), 2 of 5 atypical thymomas, but none

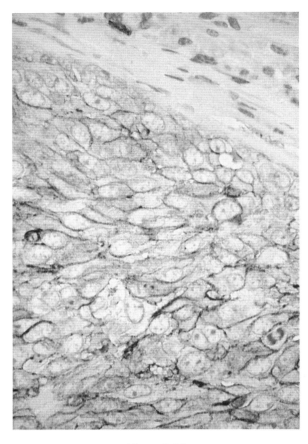

Figure 3-35

SQUAMOUS CELL CARCINOMA: CD5 IMMUNOSTAIN

All of the tumor cells show cytoplasmic membrane staining for CD5. A few lymphoid cells in the stroma are also positive.

of 11 typical thymomas or 43 carcinomas of other organs. Similar results were obtained by other investigators (13,89). Dorfman et al. (13), using a CD5 antibody (clone CD5/54/B4), reported that 9 of 9 thymic squamous cell carcinomas, 2 of 2 undifferentiated carcinomas, 2 of 4 lymphoepithelioma-like carcinomas, and 1 each of basaloid carcinoma, clear cell carcinoma, and unclassified thymic carcinoma, but none of 4 thymic small cell carcinomas was immunoreactive for CD5. None of 38 thymomas including 6 type B3 thymomas (well-differentiated thymic carcinoma of Müller-Hermelink et al.) was immunoreactive for CD5, although 2 of 3 thymic neoplasms with features borderline between thymic carcinoma and invasive thymoma were immunoreactive for CD5.

Hishima et al. (27) tested the immunoreactivity of CD70, a member of the tumor necrosis factor family that mediates the interaction between B and T lymphocytes on periodate-lysin paraformaldehyde (PLP)-fixed frozen tissue. They found that 7 of 8 thymic squamous cell carcinomas and 1 of 5 atypical thymomas showed positive immunoreactivity for CD70. None of 13 thymomas, 1 thymic carcinoid, and 24 intrathoracic malignant epithelial tumors of nonthymic origin including 17 lung cancers revealed a positive reaction.

Regarding the usefulness of thymic epithelial cell markers, Foxn1 and CD205 (DEC205), for the diagnosis of thymoma and thymic carcinoma (60), confirmatory study is needed (see chapter 2, Thymoma, Immunohistochemistry and Functional Correlation). Of 22 thymic carcinomas studied by Kuo (37), 4 of 10 squamous cell carcinomas and 7 of 8 adenosquamous carcinomas contained clusters of small tumor cells within the tumor nests. Small tumor cells constituted less than 1 percent of the entire tumor, and proved to be neuroendocrine cells by their immunoreactivity to neuron-specific enolase, chromogranin A, and/or synaptophysin. Some carcinoma cells other than the neuroendocrine small cells also displayed neuroendocrine markers in 68 percent of cases studied. Such frequent neuroendocrine differentiation in nonsmall cell thymic carcinoma has been reported by others (26,40).

Frequent KIT (CD117) overexpression in thymic carcinomas has been described by several authors (20,63). Recently, Nakagawa et al. (58) examined 50 thymomas and 20 thymic carcinomas for immunohistochemical markers. Immunoreactivity for KIT was noted in 1 each of type A and type B3 thymomas and 16 of 20 (80 percent) thymic carcinomas. CD5 was positive in 14 of 20 (70 percent) thymic carcinomas. At the same time, 20 squamous cell carcinomas of the lung invading the mediastinum were examined for expression of KIT and CD5: positive immunoreactivity was found in only 4 of 20 (20 percent) and 3 of 20 (15 percent), respectively; all 13 tumors that were positive for both KIT and CD5 were thymic carcinomas, and 13 tumors that were negative for both KIT and CD5 were lung carcinomas, indicating the usefulness of such markers in the differential diagnosis.

Analyses of surface phenotypes of infiltrating lymphocytes in thymic carcinoma, for which acetone, methyl benzoate, and xyline (AMeX) sections (cold acetone-fixed, paraffin-embedded sections) may be used (76), revealed no immature (or cortical) T cells but CD1a-negative, CD3-positive, and CD4- or CD8-positive mature T cells. The ratio of helper/inducer T cells to suppressor/cytotoxic T cells is the same as that seen in cancer of other organs (4,12,77). In other words, thymoma is a functional tumor with regard to migration from the bone marrow and maturation in the thymus of T cells, whereas thymic carcinoma has lost this function.

The CD1a-positive cells seen in thymic epithelial tumors are not only immature T cells but also Langerhans cells or interdigitating reticulum cells. The latter are present both within the tumor nests and the stroma, in clusters in areas showing medullary differentiation of thymoma, and scattered in other areas of thymoma and in thymic carcinoma (35). They can be demonstrated in formalin-fixed tissue by immunostaining for S-100 protein (see figs. 2-93, 2-94). S-100 protein–positive small lymphocytoid cells are also found in thymic tumors. The immunohistochemical profile of thymic carcinoma is summarized in Table 3-1.

MOLECULAR AND OTHER SPECIAL TECHNIQUES

Most of the data on genetic abnormalities of thymic carcinomas are single case reports. Squamous cell carcinoma is the most common type of thymic carcinoma. It shares genetic abnormalities with type B3 thymoma. Squamous cell carcinoma shows gains on chromosomes 1q, 17q, and 18 and losses on chromosomes 3p, 6, 16q, and 17p (see Table 2-8) (28,29,86,91,101).

Different results are reported by different investigators regarding p53 protein expression and gene mutation. Immunohistochemical expression of p53 protein was found in none of 8 noninvasive thymomas, only 1 of 9 invasive thymomas, and 14 of 19 thymic carcinomas (74 percent). Point mutations of the *p53* gene were recognized in only 2 of 18 thymic carcinomas (22). Another study on 12 noninvasive thymomas, 9 invasive/metastatic thymomas, and 13 thymic carcinomas indicated that all the tumors were immunoreactive for p53 protein,

and that the number of p53-positive tumor cells increased with the progression of the tumor from less than 10 percent (low expressor) to 10 to 50 percent (moderate expressor) to over 50 percent (high expressor) (90). This DNA sequencing study confirmed the presence of *p53* gene point mutations in all 10 cases examined, including 2 low expressor thymomas, suggesting that *p53* gene mutation is an early event in thymic tumorigenesis. In another study, however, mutation in the *p53* gene was not detected in 36 thymomas and 4 thymic carcinomas examined, suggesting no significant role for this gene in thymic tumorigenesis (23). Increased p53 protein expression was observed in all five carcinomas arising in the thymoma in one study (38).

Bcl-2 is positive in over 90 percent of thymic carcinomas, 40 percent of invasive thymomas, and no noninvasive thymomas (5). Bcl-2 is considered a good marker of the aggressiveness of thymic epithelial tumors.

The presence of *c-kit* gene mutation in thymic carcinoma has been studied by a few groups, because KIT (CD117) is often expressed in thymic carcinoma. Patients with a specific *c-kit* gene mutation are candidates for molecular target therapy by the specific tyrosine kinase inhibitor imatinib, which is the same strategy used for gastrointestinal stromal tumors (GIST). This gene mutation has not been detected so far in codons frequently mutated in GIST (63). One patient with KIT-positive thymic carcinoma with a mutated *c-kit* gene dramatically responded to imatinib therapy (82). Another potential therapeutic target is cyclooxygenase-2 (COX-2), which is strongly expressed immunohistochemically in all subtypes of thymomas and thymic carcinomas (72).

There is little genetic data for thymic carcinomas other than squamous cell carcinomas. Neuroendocrine carcinomas of the lung have been extensively studied but no comparable data are reported for thymic neuroendocrine carcinomas.

Rare carcinomas with the t(15;19) translocation have been reported in the mediastinum or other midline organs of young people (17). The histogenesis of this tumor type is unknown but it is a highly aggressive and lethal cancer. These tumors arise in the mediastinum but not from the thymus per se. As the name implies, translocation of t(15;19)(q13:p13.1) is a prerequisite

Table 3-1

POSITIVITY OF IMMUNOHISTOCHEMICAL MARKERS IN THYMIC CARCINOMA
(IN COMPARISON WITH THYMOMA AND CARCINOMA OF OTHER ORGANS)

Immuno-phenotypes	Thymic Carcinoma	Thymoma	Carcinomas of Other Organs	Reference
Epithelial cells				
CD5	70–100%[a]	0%, typical 50%, 4/8 atypical	15%[b]	13, 25, 58
CD70	90%	0%, typical 20%, 1/5 atypical	0%	27
CD117	>80%	4%	20%[b]	20, 58, 63
bcl-2	90%	0% noninvasive 40% invasive		5
CD57	rare[c]	frequent	some lung carcinomas	79
Lymphocytes				
CD1a, CD99, TdT[d]	0%	close to 100%	0%	4, 12, 79

[a]Excluding small cell carcinoma, four of which tested negative.
[b]Squamous cell carcinoma of the lung invading the mediastinum.
[c]Squamous cell carcinoma only, no other cell types tested.
[d]TdT = terminal deoxynucleotidyltransferase.

for diagnosis. The translocation generates *BRD4-NUT* fusion oncogenes.

PROGNOSTIC AND MALIGNANCY-ASSOCIATED FACTORS

Prognostic factors associated with thymic carcinoma include race, sex, age, immunologic status, performance status, therapeutic effects, TNM classification and stage, and factors associated with tumor malignancy. The last two are the most important for pathologists, and are assessed by relevant histologic, cytologic, molecular, and genetic factors.

TNM and Stage

The TNM classification and stage are not malignancy-associated factors but indicators of tumor progression. The TNM clinical classification has been proposed by the Union International Contre Cancer (UICC) (see Table 2-12) (96), and is based on the Masaoka system and its revised versions (46,79,93,99). It has been presented and discussed in chapter 2. Our comments made on the TNM classification of thymoma can also be applied to thymic carcinoma.

Based on a questionnaire survey on thymic epithelial tumors in Japan (33,34), thymic carcinoma cases were analyzed separately. Of histologically determined cases, there were 115 squamous cell carcinomas, 27 undifferentiated carcinomas, 18 small cell carcinomas of pure and combined types, 5 adenocarcinomas, 4 adenosquamous carcinomas, 2 mucoepidermoid carcinomas, 2 lymphoepithelioma-like carcinomas, and 1 clear cell carcinoma. Ten cases were in stage I; 11, stage II; 74, stage III; 26, stage IVa; and 61, stage IVb. Figure 3-36 shows the survival curves of 150 patients with thymic carcinoma followed according to tumor stage. The 5-year survival rates were 88.2, 51.7, and 37.6 percent for patients with stages I and II, stage III, and stage IV, respectively. These fairly good results were probably due to a large number of cases of squamous cell carcinoma, which is considered to be a low-grade malignancy.

Histologic Types

At the morphologic level, the most important prognostic factor is the histologic type of thymic carcinoma. Suster and Rosai (87) classified thymic carcinoma into low-grade and high-grade groups, as mentioned already (see Table 2-2). Accumulation of cases, particularly of mucoepidermoid carcinoma, a tumor of low-grade histology, has shown that the prognosis correlates with the degree of differentiation and cellular atypia (54).

Squamous cell carcinoma of the thymus behaves less aggressively than that of the lung. A patient with thymic squamous cell carcinoma

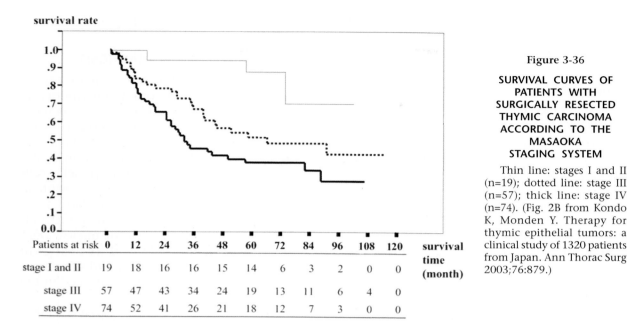

survival rate

Patients at risk	0	12	24	36	48	60	72	84	96	108	120
stage I and II	19	18	16	16	15	14	6	3	2	0	0
stage III	57	47	43	34	24	19	13	11	6	4	0
stage IV	74	52	41	26	21	18	12	7	3	0	0

survival time (month)

Figure 3-36

SURVIVAL CURVES OF PATIENTS WITH SURGICALLY RESECTED THYMIC CARCINOMA ACCORDING TO THE MASAOKA STAGING SYSTEM

Thin line: stages I and II (n=19); dotted line: stage III (n=57); thick line: stage IV (n=74). (Fig. 2B from Kondo K, Monden Y. Therapy for thymic epithelial tumors: a clinical study of 1320 patients from Japan. Ann Thorac Surg 2003;76:879.)

showing metastasis to the supraclavicular lymph nodes was cured by surgical resection and radiotherapy, and some tumors invading the lung were also cured by surgical resection and postoperative radiotherapy (78). Four of seven patients with squamous cell carcinoma reported by Truong et al. (92) were alive and well at 6 to 60 months postoperatively, while only three died of the disease at 7, 15, and 15 months. All six patients with pure squamous cell carcinoma reported by Kuo et al. (39) were alive for 13 to 43 months, one with disease. Every patient with well-differentiated squamous cell carcinoma among the consultation cases of Suster and Rosai (87) was alive. In contrast, the prognosis of patients with other histologic types, excluding the rare low-grade mucoepidermoid carcinoma and basaloid carcinoma, is extremely poor (73). These tumors are classified as high-grade by Suster and Rosai (87).

Degree of Histologic Differentiation and Cell Atypia

Squamous cell carcinoma occurring in any organ is subdivided into well, moderately, and poorly differentiated categories. This classification has not been adopted for thymic carcinoma, however, probably because of its rarity. Our experience suggests that large cell or poorly differentiated squamous cell carcinoma

without features of lymphoepithelioma-like carcinoma or without a small cell component shows marked proliferative activity and highly malignant behavior (see fig. 3-31). Such tumors should also be considered high grade. The dividing line between low- and high-grade squamous cell carcinoma needs to be clarified. In this regard, not only the degree of anaplasia and cell atypia but also the proliferative activity should be considered.

Lymphoepithelioma-like carcinoma is thought to be a poorly differentiated variety of squamous cell carcinoma by some investigators. Its highly malignant nature, as in the case of small cell carcinoma, has been proven by many investigators. Undifferentiated carcinoma of the nasopharynx (lymphoepithelioma-like carcinoma), however, can be cured by radiotherapy, even when metastases are present in lymph nodes of the superior cervical chain. If thymic lymphoepithelioma-like carcinoma is treated at a sufficiently early stage, then cure may also be possible. Clear cell carcinoma and sarcomatoid carcinoma are considered forms of poorly differentiated squamous cell carcinoma and are high-grade tumors with a poor prognosis.

The degree of cytologic atypia and the proliferative activity, which can be expressed as the mitotic index (percent mitoses), are also important parameters associated with malignancy.

In most cases, they are related to the degree of histologic differentiation: high-grade tumors often show marked individual cell atypia and increased mitotic activity.

Immunohistochemical Prognostic Factors

As described in the section on thymoma, diffuse expression in the cell membrane of β2-microglobulin, a light chain of human leukocyte antigen (HLA) class 1 and HLA-DR alpha-chain, appears to be associated with the grade of malignancy of thymoma and thymic squamous cell carcinoma. No studies have been done on other subtypes of thymic carcinomas.

The proliferative activity of tumor cells as assessed by proliferation-associated nuclear antigen (Ki-67) and by proliferating cell nuclear antigen (PCNA) is a good indicator of malignancy in many organs, and as expected, for thymic epithelial tumors as well. Although the number of thymic carcinoma cases studied are few, thymic carcinoma has a higher Ki-67 labeling index (16.55 ± 12.12 percent) than thymoma (type A, 1.16 ± 0.60; type AB, 4.51 ± 2.90; type B1, 4.72 ± 2.57; type B2, 6.41 ± 2.98; and type B3, 7.00 ± 3.15) (fig. 3-37) (24). A significant association ($P=0.007$) was found between the Ki-67 labeling index and survival of patients with thymic epithelial tumors (45 cases including 10 type B3 thymomas and 3 thymic carcinomas) (8). Further study is needed to clarify the relationship between the labeling index and the degree of malignancy in different histologic subtypes of thymic carcinoma.

Nuclear DNA Content and Histograms

As described in chapter 2, thymoma and thymic squamous cell carcinoma can be differentiated using a combination of mean nuclear DNA content and the presence of aneuploid stem cell lines (see fig. 2-102) (1). Thus far, such studies have not been done among subtypes of thymic carcinoma; however, together with studies of histogram patterns of DNA contents, such analyses are expected to be useful for separating low-grade and high-grade tumors. The difference in mean nuclear area of noninvasive thymoma, invasive thymoma, and thymic squamous cell carcinoma is significant, although there are certain overlaps among the groups (see fig. 2-101) (1). Survival curves according to

the histologic subtypes of thymic carcinoma are not available at present.

DIFFERENTIAL DIAGNOSIS

Distinguishing thymic carcinomas morphologically from the more common thymomas of the encapsulated and invasive types includes assessing not only the gross features, histologic structures, degree of cytologic atypia, and proliferative activity, but also including immunohistochemical analysis of both epithelial cells and lymphocytes to clarify cell type, proliferative activity, and function, particularly T-cell maturation. Sophisticated assessment methods include the determination of the nuclear DNA content of epithelial cells and its histogram pattern for evaluation of aneuploid stem lines. Abnormalities in genes may be revealed in the near future.

In thymic carcinoma as compared with thymoma, encapsulation is rare and appears limited to certain histologic types such as basaloid carcinoma, although capsule-like structures may be seen where the tumor reaches the capsule of the thymus, pleura, or pericardium. The borders of the carcinoma are usually irregularly nodular or scalloped as a result of invasive growth. Lobulation does not occur or is inconspicuous, and areas of coagulation necrosis vary in amount depending on the type of carcinoma. Cystic changes may be present in both thymoma and thymic carcinoma; calcification may be seen in the capsule of thymoma, but is almost always absent in carcinoma. The presence of typical perivascular spaces is characteristic of thymoma; however, structures resembling or suggestive of perivascular spaces may be seen in some thymic carcinomas, such as squamous cell and basaloid carcinoma.

Some type B3 thymomas reveal plump hyperchromatic nuclei, distinct round nucleoli, and frequent mitotic figures (10 or more per 10 high-power fields), similar to features seen in thymic carcinoma (45,69). The histologic features characteristic of thymoma and the presence of perivascular spaces may help to establish a diagnosis of thymoma. With regard to mitotic figures, no abnormal mitoses are seen in thymoma unless irradiated. Lymphocytes in thymoma also show mitotic activity, in which cell size may be of help in making the distinction

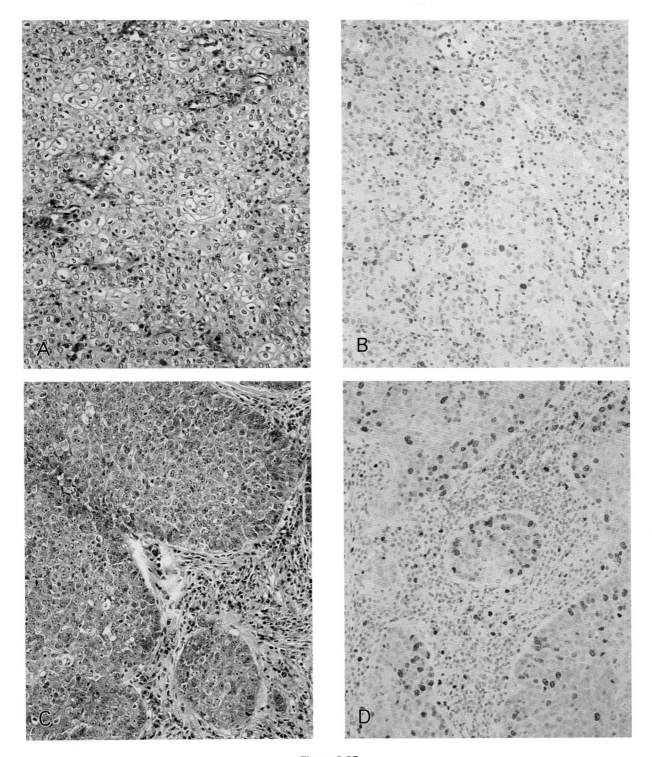

Figure 3-37

Ki-67 IMMUNOSTAINING IN TYPE B3 THYMOMA AND THYMIC CARCINOMA

Thymoma type B3 (A) contains scattered Ki-67-positive cells (approximately 10%) (B). Poorly differentiated squamous cell carcinoma (C) displays frequent Ki-67-positive cells (about 40%) (D).

from the mitotic figures of epithelial cells. The cell type can be confirmed by immunostaining for epithelial cell markers such as cytokeratin and surface phenotypes of lymphocytes by CD3 and CD45RO.

Although CD57 (leu-7) is often positive in thymoma and negative in squamous cell carcinoma, this epithelial cell marker is not useful for differentiating the two tumor types since it may be positive in other types of carcinoma, such as small cell neuroendocrine carcinoma. CD5 and CD70 are often positive in squamous cell carcinoma, and a few atypical (type B3) thymomas, but negative in other thymoma types (25,27).

The most important immunohistochemical findings for the differential diagnosis are TdT-, CD1a-, or CD99-positive immature (or cortical) T cells in thymoma and their virtual absence in thymic carcinoma (4,12). This finding indicates maintenance of the function of the thymic epithelium in thymoma and loss of this function in carcinoma. The absence of myasthenia gravis as a complication in patients with thymic carcinoma is probably related to this loss of function. T-cell subsets in thymic carcinoma are similar to those in cancers of other organs, consisting of either CD8- or CD4-positive mature T cells.

In rare cases, the differential diagnosis is difficult. This is expected, since in any organ, tumors on the histologic borderline between adenoma and carcinoma occur. Diagnosing thymic epithelial tumors as either thymoma or thymic carcinoma is difficult if there is a mixture of lymphocytes and epithelial cells with possible perivascular spaces, fine vasculature within aggregates of tumor cells (fig. 3-12), or if epithelial cells, outnumbering lymphocytes, display some nuclear atypia and proliferative activity (see fig. 2-40). In cases where thymic carcinoma develops from thymoma, features transitional between the two morphologies may be observed, making the histology difficult to interpret. In such cases, immunohistochemistry for lymphocyte surface markers helps in the diagnosis. If this is not possible, the presence of plasma cells and eosinophils favors a diagnosis of carcinoma.

Distinguishing thymic carcinoma from atypical carcinoid with moderate nuclear atypia, proliferative activity, and lack of typical features of carcinoid tumor such as rosettes may be difficult, since atypical carcinoid may simulate poorly differentiated carcinoma (see fig. 4-7). In such cases, Grimelius silver staining and immunostaining for neuroendocrine markers are essential for the diagnosis.

Differentiation from germ cell tumors is another consideration. Particular care should be exercised when establishing a diagnosis on the bases of a needle biopsy specimen. Dysgerminoma with minimal lymphocytic infiltration and embryonal carcinoma may mimic poorly differentiated or undifferentiated carcinoma, and choriocarcinoma may resemble poorly differentiated squamous cell carcinoma (see fig. 5-6). In such cases, immunohistochemical staining for placental alkaline phosphatase and beta-human chorionic gonadotropin must be done. The marked male predominance of malignant germ cell tumors should be borne in mind.

Diffuse large cell lymphoma with sclerosis may resemble undifferentiated carcinoma histologically. Diffuse large cell lymphoma can be differentiated by immunostaining for B-cell markers (see figs. 6-4, 6-7) (9,66).

In routine practice, thymic carcinoma must be differentiated from carcinoma of other organs metastatic to or involving the anterior mediastinum, particularly carcinoma of the neighboring organs such as the lung and malignant mesothelioma of the pleura. Grossly, differentiated squamous cell carcinoma of the thymus is quite different from that of the lung. Thymic squamous cell carcinoma has a much lower tendency to become necrotic, but often becomes sclerotic in the central portion of the tumor. Histologically, a radial arrangement or palisading of the tumor cells at the periphery of cell nests is not common in thymic carcinoma, and abrupt keratinization simulating Hassall corpuscles may be seen. Moderately prominent round nucleoli are found more frequently in thymic than in pulmonary squamous cell carcinoma.

In some cases, the distinction between thymic and lung carcinomas depends largely or entirely upon the location of the primary tumor and lymph node metastases. This is true for poorly differentiated squamous cell carcinoma, mucoepidermoid carcinoma, adenocarcinoma, small cell neuroendocrine carcinoma, clear cell carcinoma, and sarcomatoid carcinoma.

Staining for thyroid transcription factor-1 (TTF-1) and surfactant apoprotein has potential use in distinguishing between pulmonary and thymic cancer (53,59,64,67). TTF-1 is present in about 75 percent of pulmonary adenocarcinomas and in a smaller percentage of large cell carcinomas (25 percent) and squamous cell carcinomas (10 percent), and is absent in cancer of other sites including the thymus, excluding the thyroid gland. CD5 and CD70 immunohistochemistry is promising for differentiating primary and metastatic carcinomas involving the thymus, since, as already stated, carcinomas arising from other organs do not express CD5 and CD70 (25,27). Analysis of larger numbers of tumors will be required to confirm these findings. A high frequency of KIT (CD117) expression in thymic carcinomas (58) was described in the section on immunohistochemistry. CT evaluation and a history of smoking may also help in establishing a diagnosis of primary lung carcinoma. Abnormalities in oncogenes and suppressor genes may be useful in the future.

TUMOR SPREAD AND METASTASIS

The routes and patterns of local tumor spread and distant metastases are identical to those in thymoma, although the frequency is much higher in thymic carcinoma. Therefore, the same TNM classification and staging system can be applied to thymic cancer. Since lymph node metastasis is rare in thymoma, lymphatic involvement within the thymus is also rare; however, it is occasionally recognized in cases of thymic carcinoma (fig. 3-38). Since we have seen a case of thymic squamous cell carcinoma with supraclavicular lymph node metastasis without obvious anterior mediastinal node involvement, a detailed analysis of the lymphatic tumor spread in thymic carcinoma may serve for the definition of N1 in TNM system. The most frequent sites of metastases are lymph nodes (mediastinal, cervical, and axillary), followed by bone, lung, liver, and brain.

TREATMENT

The treatment of choice for patients with thymic carcinoma depends upon the stage of the disease and the tumor histology. The relevance of TNM classification and staging is at present under discussion (see chapter 2). For treatment purposes, Suster and Rosai (87) divided thymic carcinomas into two groups: those with low-

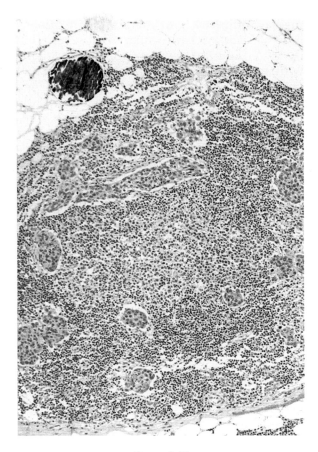

Figure 3-38

LYMPHATIC EXTENSION OF THYMIC SQUAMOUS CELL CARCINOMA WITHIN THYMIC TISSUE

Small, irregularly shaped solid tumor nests are present within the thymic tissue, which was near the primary tumor. A calcified Hassall corpuscle is evident.

grade and those with high-grade histology. For tumors with low-grade histology, resection followed by radiotherapy is reported to be sufficient in most resectable cases. We feel that if the tumor is localized within the thymus and completely resected, postoperative radiotherapy may not be necessary. However, complete removal of the thymus with tumor is mandatory, since lymphatic spread may be present within the thymus. On the other hand, most patients with advanced low-grade and high-grade tumors have an unfavorable outcome even with a combination of surgery, radiation, and chemotherapy. High-grade tumors must be detected while still confined to within the anterior mediastinum, without metastasis. Treatment results in our cases are similar to those reported by Suster and Rosai, except for some patients with squamous cell carcinoma who have had an unfavorable outcome.

Kondo and Monden (34) reported therapeutic results of 1,320 thymic epithelial tumors compiled from 115 institutions in Japan. The 5-year survival rates of patients whose thymic carcinoma was totally resected, subtotally resected, and inoperable were 67, 30, and 24 percent, respectively; the rates of those with thymoma were 93, 64, and 36 percent, respectively. Fifty-one percent of patients developed recurrence after total resection of the tumor. Kondo and Monden concluded that total resection is the most important positive prognostic factor in the treatment of thymic epithelial tumors.

PROGNOSIS

The prognosis of patients with thymic carcinoma depends on the histologic type, degree of differentiation, stage of the disease, and so forth, and has been described briefly in the foregoing section on prognostic and malignancy-associated factors. Because of the rarity of cases, no further statement can be made at present, including comparisons of various histologic types.

ASSOCIATION OF EPSTEIN-BARR VIRUS WITH DEVELOPMENT OF THYMIC EPITHELIAL TUMORS

Because of the presence in the thymus of undifferentiated carcinoma with features of lymphoepithelioma-like carcinoma, which is indistinguishable histologically from nasopharyngeal undifferentiated carcinoma, an association with the Epstein-Barr virus (EBV) has been suspected. Lymphoepithelioma-like carcinoma is now understood to be a poorly differentiated form of squamous cell carcinoma since it contains desmosomes, tonofibrils, and cytokeratins.

The association of EBV with thymic lymphoepithelioma-like carcinoma was first reported by Leyvraz et al. in 1985 (44). They clarified the serologic profile: the presence of EBV-associated nuclear antigen in the carcinoma cells and a high level of the viral genome in the DNA, suggesting a role of EBV in the genesis of thymic carcinoma. In

1988, another case was reported by Dimery et al. (11), who stated that EBV was causally related to the development of thymic lymphoepithelioma-like carcinoma, since an EBV-hybridizing fragment was present in the tumor DNA genome but absent in the DNA of peripheral blood lymphocytes.

The association of EBV was investigated in 26 thymic epithelial tumors, including 8 noninvasive and 13 invasive thymomas and 5 thymic carcinomas (49). A homogeneous terminal structure in the viral DNA was determined in a single case of lymphoepithelioma-like thymic carcinoma, indicating clonal growth (fig. 3-39, top), whereas this was absent in thymoma or cancers of other histologic types. In addition, in situ hybridization for EBV-encoded small RNA (EBER) was positive in a majority of the lymphoepithelioma-like carcinoma cells (fig. 3-39, bottom). Lymphoepithelioma-like thymic carcinoma may represent a unique pathologic entity distinct from EBV-negative thymic epithelial tumors.

Weiss et al. (94) found that of 14 cases of extranasopharyngeal lymphoepithelioma (3 palatine tonsil, 1 oral floor, 1 pyriform sinus, 4 skin, 4 lung, and 1 uterine cervix), only 1 lung cancer showed a positive in situ hybridization signal for the EBV genome. They concluded that despite the histologic similarity, most lymphoepithelioma-like carcinomas probably have a pathogenesis different from that of nasopharyngeal lymphoepithelioma. No lymphoepithelioma-like thymic carcinomas were included in their series, however.

A review of the literature indicates that approximately 47 percent of thymic lymphoepithelioma-like carcinomas are associated with EBV, as demonstrated by EBER in situ hybridization or DNA analysis (6,81,91,97). EBV is almost always positive in this type of thymic carcinoma occurring in children and young adults. The EBV-positive rate is lower in adults over the age of 30 years, and the presence or absence of EBV does not seem to have prognostic significance (91).

Although the authors did not find an association of EBV in 21 thymomas, there is a report indicating that all of 3 thymomas and 3 of 5 thymic lymphoid hyperplasias in a Hong Kong study were positive for the EBV genome by Southern blot analysis using the BamH1-W fragment as the EBV-DNA probe (51). Such a

Figure 3-39

LYMPHOEPITHELIOMA-LIKE CARCINOMA WITH HOMOGENEOUS TERMINAL STRUCTURE OF EPSTEIN-BARR VIRUS (EBV) DNA AND POSITIVE IN SITU HYBRIDIZATION FOR EPSTEIN-BARR VIRUS ENCODED RNA (EBER)

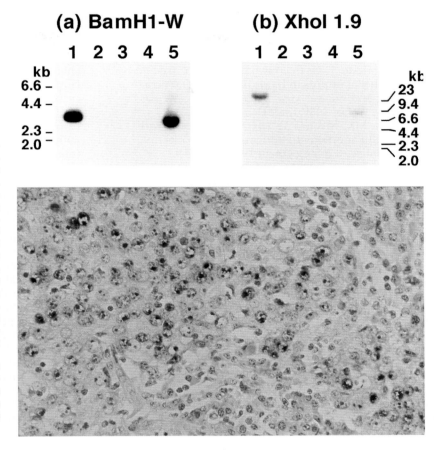

Top: DNA extracted from cultured cell lines and fresh autopsy material from a lymphoepithelioma-like carcinoma was subjected to Southern blot hybridization after BamH1-W digestion. As probes, 32P-labeled BamH1-W (detecting an internal repetitive sequence) and XhoI 1.9 (detecting a terminal repetitive sequence) fragments were used in (a) and (b), respectively. 1: Raji cell; 2: Ramos cell; 3, 4, and 5: tissues of spleen, liver, and liver metastasis from the autopsy case, respectively. (Fig. 3 from Matsuno Y, Mukai K, Uhara H, et al. Detection of Epstein-Barr virus DNA in a Japanese case of lymphoepithelioma-like thymic carcinoma. Jpn J Cancer Res 1992;83:129.)

Bottom: In situ hybridization on paraffin sections using an oligonucleotide probe for EBER reveals positive signals in a majority of tumor cells. No signals were seen in control sections treated with RNase.

high incidence of EBV association in thymic lesions may be due to the endemic nature of EBV in the studied area or a genetic predisposition of the population to EBV infection. However, the EBV-DNA detected could well have been present in the infiltrating lymphocytes and not in the epithelial cells, and therefore, the clonality of the positive cells must be confirmed in this study. Indeed, a recent report indicated that none of 78 thymomas in a Taiwanese study

showed a detectable EBV genome, whereas 6 of 21 thymic carcinomas displayed nuclear signals within the tumor cells by in situ polymerase chain reaction and/or RNA in situ hybridization. In another tumor, signals were displayed not within the tumor cells but within lymphocytes (6). Another report also disclosed that none of 14 noninvasive thymomas or 7 invasive thymomas had detectable EBER1 in Chinese patients in Taiwan (97).

REFERENCES

1. Asamura H, Nakajima T, Mukai K, Noguchi M, Shimosato Y. Degree of malignancy of thymic epithelial tumors in terms of nuclear DNA content and nuclear area. An analysis of 39 cases. Am J Pathol 1988:133:615-22

2. Babu MK, Nirmala V. Thymic carcinoma with glandular differentiation arising in a congenital thymic cyst. J Surg Oncol 1994;57:277-9.

3. Chalabreysse L, Etienne-Mastroianni B, Adeleine P, Cordier J-F, Greenland T, Thivolet-Bejui F. Thymic carcinoma: a clinicopathological and Immunohistological study of 19 cases. Histopathology 2004;44:367-74.

4. Chan JK, Tsang WY, Seneviratne S, Pau MY. The MIC2 antibody 013. Practical application for the study of thymic epithelial tumors. Am J Surg Pathol 1995;19:1115-23.

5. Chen FF, Yan JJ, Jin YT, Su IJ. Detection of bcl-2 and p53 in thymoma: expression of bcl-2 as a reliable marker of tumor aggressiveness. Hum Pathol 1996;27:1089-92.

6. Chen PC, Pan CC, Yang AH, Wang LS, Chiang H. Detection of Epstein-Barr virus genome within thymic epithelial tumours in Taiwanese patients by nested PCR, PCR in situ hybridization, and RNA in situ hybridization. J Pathol 2002;197:684-8.

7. Choi WW, Lui YH, Lau WH, Crowley P, Khan A, Chan JK. Adenocarcinoma of the thymus: report of two cases, including a previously undescribed mucinous subtype. Am J Surg Pathol 2003;27:124-30.

8. Commin CE, Messerini L, Novelli L, Boddi V, Dini S. Ki-67 antigen expression predicts survival and correlates with histologic subtype in the WHO classification of thymic epithelial tumors. Int J Surg Pathol 2004;12:395-400.

9. Davis RE, Dorfman RF, Warnke RA. Primary large-cell lymphoma of the thymus: a diffuse B-cell neoplasm presenting as primary mediastinal lymphoma. Hum Pathol 1990;21:1262-8.

10. Di Tommaso L, Kuhn E, Kurrer M, et al. Thymic tumor with adenoid cystic carcinoma like features. A clinicopathologic study of 4 cases. Am J Surg Pathol 2007;31:1161-7.

11. Dimery IW, Lee JS, Blick M, Pearson G, Spitzer G. Hong WK. Association of the Epstein-Barr virus with lymphoepithelioma of the thymus. Cancer 1988;61:2475-80

12. Dorfman DM, Pinkus GS. CD99 (p30/32^{MIC2}) immunoreactivity in the diagnosis of thymic neoplasms and mediastinal lymphoproliferative disorders. A study of paraffin sections using monoclonal antibody 013. Appl Immunohistochem 1996;4:34-42.

13. Dorfman DM, Shahsafaei A, Chan JK. Thymic carcinomas, but not thymomas and carcinomas of other sites, show CD5 immunoreactivity. Am J Surg Pathol 1997;21:936-40.

14. Ebihara Y, Dilnur P. [Cytology of the mediastinal tumors.] Byori to Rinsho 2002;20:608-13. [In Japanese.]

15. Eimoto T, Kitaoka M, Ogawa H, et al. Thymic sarcomatoid carcinoma with skeletal muscle differentiation: report of two cases, one with cytogenetic analysis. Histopathology 2002;40:46-57.

16. Finley JL, Silverman JF, Strausbauch PH, et al. Malignant thymic neoplasms: diagnosis by fine-needle aspiration biopsy with histologic, immuno-histochemical, and ultrastructural confirmation. Diagn Cytopathol 1986;2:118-25.

17. French CA, Miyoshi I, Aster JC, et al. BRD4 bromodomain gene rearrangement in aggressive carcinoma with translocation t(15;19). Am J Pathol 2001;159:1987-92.

18. Hasserjian RP, Klimstra DS, Rosai J. Carcinoma of the thymus with clear-cell features. Report of eight cases and review of the literature. Am J Surg Pathol 1995;19:835-41.

19. Hattori H. High-grade thymic carcinoma other than basaloid or mucoepidermoid type could be associated with multilocular thymic cyst: report of two cases. Histopathology 2003;43:501-2.

20. Henley JD, Cummings OW, Loehrer PJ Sr. Tyrosine kinase receptor expression in thymomas. J Cancer Res Clin Oncol 2004;130:222-4.

21. Henry K. Mucin secretion and striated muscle in the human thymus, Lancet 1966;1:183-5.

22. Hino N, Kondo K, Miyoshi T, Uyama T, Monden Y. High frequency of p53 protein expression in thymic carcinoma but not in thymoma. Br J Cancer 1997;76:1361-6.

23. Hirabayashi H, Fujii Y, Sakaguchi M, et al. p16INK4, pRB, p53 and cyclin D1 expression and hypermethylation of CDKN2 gene in thymoma and thymic carcinoma. Int J Cancer 1997;73:639-44.

24. Hiroshima K, Iyoda A, Toyozaki T et al. Proliferative activity and apoptosis in thymic epithelial neoplasms. Mod Pathol 2002;15:1326-32.

25. Hishima T, Fukayama M, Fujisawa M, et al. CD5 expression in thymic carcinoma. Am J Pathol 1994;145:268-75

26. Hishima T, Fukayama M, Hayashi Y, et al. Neuroendocrine differentiation in thymic epithelial tumors with special reference to thymic carcinoma and atypical thymoma. Hum Pathol 1998;29:330-8.

27. Hishima T, Fukayama M, Hayashi Y, et al. CD70 expression in thymic carcinoma. Am J Surg Pathol 2000;24:742-6

28. Inoue M, Starostik P, Zettl A, et al. Correlating genetic aberrations with World Health Organization-defined histology and stage across the spectrum of thymomas. Cancer Res. 2003;63:3708-15.

29. Inoue M, Marx A, Zettl A, Ströbel P, Müller-Hermelink HK, Starostik P. Chromosome 6 suffers frequent and multiple aberrations in thymoma. Am J Pathol 2002;161:1507-13.

30. Kirchner T, Müller-Hermelink HK. New approaches to the diagnosis of thymic epithelial tumors. Prog Surg Pathol 1989;10:167-89

31. Kirchner T, Schalke B, Buchwald J, Ritter M, Marx A, Müller-Hermelink HK. Well-differentiated thymic carcinoma. An organotypical low-grade carcinoma with relationship to cortical thymoma. Am J Surg Pathol 1992;16:1153-69.

32. Kodama T, Watanabe S, Sato Y, Shimosato Y, Miyazawa N. An immunohistochemical study of thymic epithelial tumors. I. Epithelial component. Am J Surg Pathol 1986;10:26-33.

33. Kondo K, Monden Y. [A questionnaire about thymic epithelial tumors in Japan.] Nippon Gekagakkai Zasshi 2001;15:633-42. [In Japanese.]

34. Kondo K, Monden Y. Therapy for thymic epithelial tumors: a clinical study of 1,320 patients from Japan. Ann Thorac Surg 2003;76:878-85.

35. Kondo K, Mukai K, Sato Y, Matsuno Y, Shimosato Y, Monden Y. An immunohistochemical study of thymic epithelial tumors. III. The distribution of interdigitating reticulum cells and S-100 beta-positive small lymphocytes. Am J Surg Pathol 1990;14:1139-47.

36. Kornstein MJ, Curran WJ Jr, Turrisi AT 3rd, Brooks JJ. Cortical versus medullary thymomas: a useful morphologic distinction? Hum Pathol 1988;19:1335-9.

37. Kuo TT. Frequent presence of neuroendocrine small cells in thymic carcinoma: a light microscopic and immunohistochemical study. Histopathology 2000;37:19-26.

38. Kuo TT, Chan JK. Thymic carcinoma arising in thymoma is associated with alterations in immunohistochemical profile. Am J Surg Pathol 1998;22:1474-81.

39. Kuo TT, Chang JP, Lin FJ, Wu WC, Chang CH. Thymic carcinomas: histopathological varieties and immunohistochemical study. Am J Surg Pathol 1990;14:24-34.

40. Lauriola L, Erlandson RA, Rosai J. Neuroendocrine differentiation is a common feature of thymic carcinoma. Am J Surg Pathol 1998;22:1059-66.

41. Lee AC, Kwong YI, Fu KH, Chan GC, Ma L, Lau YL. Disseminated mediastinal carcinoma with chromosomal translocation (15;19). A distinctive clinicopathologic syndrome. Cancer 1993;72:2273-6.

42. Leong AS, Brown JH. Malignant transformation in a thymic cyst. Am J Surg Pathol 1984;8:471-5.

43. Levine GD, Rosai J. Thymic hyperplasia and neoplasia: a review of current concepts. Hum Pathol 1978;9:495-515.

44. Leyvraz S, Henle W, Chahinian AP, et al. Association of Epstein-Barr virus with thymic carcinoma. N Engl J Med. 1985;312:1296-9

45. Marino M, Müller-Hermelink HK. Thymoma and thymic carcinoma. Relation of thymoma epithelial cells to the cortical and medullary differentiation of thymus. Virchows Arch A Pathol Anat Histopathol 1985;407:119-49.

46. Masaoka A, Monden Y, Nakahara K, Tanioka T. Follow-up study of thymomas with special reference to their clinical stages. Cancer 1981;48:2485-92.

47. Matsuno Y, Morozumi N, Hirohashi S, Shimosato Y, Rosai J. Papillary carcinoma of the thymus: report of four cases of a new microscopic type of thymic carcinoma. Am J Surg Pathol 1998;22:873-80.

48. Matsuno Y, Mukai K, Noguchi M, Sato Y, Shimosato Y. Histochemical and immunohistochemical evidence of glandular differentiation in thymic carcinoma. Acta Pathol Jpn 1989;39:433-8.

49. Matsuno Y, Mukai K, Uhara H, et al. Detection of Epstein-Barr virus DNA in a Japanese case of lymphoepithelioma-like thymic carcinoma. Jpn J Cancer Res 1992;83:127-30.

50. Matsuo T, Hayashida R, Kobayashi K, Tanaka Y, Ohtsuka S. Thymic basaloid carcinoma with hepatic metastasis. Ann Thorac Surg 2002;74:579-82.

51. McGuire LJ, Huang DP, Teoh R, Arnold M, Wong K, Lee CK. Epstein-Barr virus genome in thymoma and thymic lymphoid hyperplasia. Am J Pathol 1988;31:385-90.

52. Mizukami Y, Kurumaya H, Yamada T, et al. Thymic carcinoma involving the thyroid gland: report of two cases. Hum Pathol 1995;26:576-9.

53. Mizutani Y, Nakajima T, Morinaga S, et al. Immunohistochemical localization of pulmonary surfactant apoproteins in various lung tumors. Special reference to nonmucus producing lung adenocarcinomas. Cancer 1988;61:532-7

54. Moran CA, Suster S. Mucoepidermoid carcinomas of the thymus. A clinicopathologic study of six cases. Am J Surg Pathol 1995;19:826-34.

55. Moran CA, Suster S, El-Naggar A, Luna MA. Carcinomas arising in multilocular thymic cysts of the neck: a clinicopathological study of three cases. Histopathology 2004;44:64-8.

56. Morinaga S, Sato Y, Shimosato Y, Shinkai T, Tsuchiya R. Multiple thymic squamous cell carcinomas associated with mixed type thymoma. Am J Surg Pathol 1987;11:982-8.

57. Müller-Hermelink HK, Marino M, Palestro G, Schumacher U, Kirchner T. Immunohistological evidence of cortical and medullary differentiation in thymoma. Virchows Arch A Pathol Anat Histopathol 1985;408:143-61.

58. Nakagawa K, Matsuno Y, Kunitoh H, Maeshima A, Asamura H, Tsuchiya R. Immunohistochemical KIT (CD117) expression in thymic epithelial tumors. Chest 2005;128:140-4.

59. Nicholson AG, McCormick CJ, Shimosato Y, Butcher DN, Sheppard MN. The value of PE-10, a monoclonal antibody against pulmonary surfactant, in distinguishing primary and metastatic lung tumours. Histopathology 1995;27:57-60.

60. Nonaka D, Henley JD, Chirboga L, Lee Y. Diagnostic utility of thymic epithelial markers CD205 (DEC205) and Foxn1 in thymic epithelial neoplasms. Am J Surg Pathol 2007;31:1038-44.

61. Nonaka D, Klimstra D, Rosai J. Thymic mucoepidermoid carcinomas: a clinicopathologic study of 10 cases and review of the literature. Am J Surg Pathol 2004;28:1526-31.

62. Nonaka D, Rodriguez J, Rollo JL, Rosai J. Undifferentiated large cell carcinoma of the thymus associated with Castleman disease–like reaction: a distinctive type of thymic neoplasm characterized by an indolent behavior. Am J Surg Pathol 2005;29:490-5.

63. Pan CC, Chen PC, Chiang H. KIT (CD117) is frequently overexpressed in thymic carcinomas but is absent in thymomas. J Pathol 2004;202:375-81.

64. Pecciarini L, Cangi MG, Doglioni C. Identifying the primary sites of metastatic carcinoma: the increasing role of immunohistochemistry. Current Diag Pathol 2001;7. 168-75.

65. Okudela K, Nakamura N, Sano J, Ito T, Kitamura H. Thymic carcinosarcoma consisting of squamous cell carcinomatous and embryonal rhabdomyosarcomatous components. Report of a case and review of the literature. Pathol Res Pract. 2001;197:205-10.

66. Perrone T, Frizzera G, Rosai J. Mediastinal diffuse large-cell lymphoma with sclerosis. A clinicopathologic study of 60 cases. Am J Surg Pathol 1986;10:176-91.

67. Pomplun S, Wotherspoon AC, Shah G, Goldstraw P, Lada G, Nicholson AG. Immunohistochemical markers in the differentiation of thymic and pulmonary neoplasms. Histopathology 2002;40:152-8.

68. Posligua L, Ylagan L. Fine-needle aspiration cytology of thymic basaloid carcinoma: case studies and review of the literature. Diag Cytopathol 2006;34:358-66.

69. Quintanilla-Martinez L, Wilkins EW Jr. Choi N, Efird J, Hug E, Harris NL. Thymoma. Histologic subclassification is an independent prognostic factor. Cancer 1994;74:606-17.

70. Ra SH, Fishbein MC, Baruch-Oren T, et al. Mucinous adenocarcinoma of the thymus. Report of 2 cases and review of the literature. Am J Surg Pathol 2007;31:1330-6.

71. Riazmontazer N. Bedayat C, Izadi B. Epithelial cytologic atypia in a fine needle aspirate of an invasive thymoma. A case report. Acta Cytol 1992;36:387-90.

72. Rieker RJ, Joos S, Mechtersheimer G, et al. COX-2 upregulation in thymomas and thymic carcinomas. Int J Cancer 2006;119:2063-70.

73. Ritter JH, Wick MR. Primary carcinomas of the thymus gland. Semin Diagn Pathol 1999;16:18-31.

74. Rosai J, Levine GD. Tumors of the thymus. Atlas of Tumor Pathology, 2nd Series, Fascicle 13, Washington, D.C.: Armed Forces Institute of Pathology; 1976:35-37, 50-101, 177-80.

75. Rosai J, Sobin LH. Histologic typing of tumours of the thymus. World Health Organization international histological classification of tumours, 2nd ed. New York: Springer; 1999.

76. Sato Y, Mukai K, Watanabe S, Goto M, Shimosato Y. The AMeX method. A simplified technique of tissue processing and paraffin embedding with improved preservation of antigens for immunostaining. Am J Pathol 1986;125:431-5.

77. Sato Y, Watanabe S, Mukai K, et al. An immunohistochemical study of thymic epithelial tumors: II. Lymphoid component. Am J Surg Pathol 1986;10:862-70.

78. Shimosato Y, Kameya T, Nagai K, Suemasu K. Squamous cell carcinoma of the thymus. An analysis of eight cases. Am J Surg Pathol 1977;1:109-21.

79. Shimosato Y, Mukai K. Tumors of the mediastinum. Atlas of Tumor Pathology, Third Series, Fascicle 21, Washington, D. C.: Armed Forces Institute of Pathology; 1997.

80. Snover DC, Levine GD, Rosai J. Thymic carcinoma. Five distinctive histological variants. Am J Surg Pathol 1982;6:451-70.

81. Stephan JL, Galambrun C, Boucheron S, Varlet F, Delabesse E, Macintyre E. Epstein-Barr virus-positive undifferentiated thymic carcinoma in a 12-year-old white girl. J Pediatr Hematol Oncol 2000;22:162-6.

82. Strobel P, Hartmann M, Jakob A, et al. Thymic carcinoma with overexpression of mutated KIT and the response to imatinib. N Engl J Med 2004;350:2625-6.

83. Suarez Vilela D, Salas Valien JS, Gopnzalez Moran MA, Izquierdo Garcia F, Riera Velasco JR. Thymic carcinosarcoma associated with a spindle cell thymoma: an immunohistochemical study. Histopathology 1992;21:263-8.

84. Suster S, Moran CA. Primary thymic epithelial neoplasms showing combined features of thymoma and thymic carcinoma. A clinicopathologic study of 22 cases. Am J Surg Pathol 1996;20:1469-80.

85. Suster S, Moran CA. Spindle cell thymic carcinoma: clinicopathologic and immunohistochemical study of a distinctive variant of primary thymic epithelial neoplasm. Am J Surg Pathol 1999;23:691-700.

86. Suster S, Moran CA. The mediastinum. In Weidner N, Cote RJ, Suster S, Weiss LM, eds. Modern surgical pathology. Philadelphia: Saunders; 2003:439-504.

87. Suster S, Rosai J. Thymic carcinoma. A clinicopathologic study of 60 cases. Cancer 1991;67:1025-32.

88. Takahashi F, Tsuta K, Matsuno Y, et al. Adenocarcinoma of the thymus: mucinous subtype. Hum Pathol 2005;36:219-223.

89. Tateyama H, Eimoto T, Tada T, Hattori H, Murase T, Takino H. Immunoreactivity of a new CD5 antibody with normal epithelium and malignant tumors including thymic carcinoma. Am J Clin Pathol 1999;111:235-40.

90. Tateyama H, Eimoto T, Tada T, et al. p53 protein expression and p53 gene mutation in thymic epithelial tumors. An immunohistochemical and DNA sequencing study. Am J Clin Pathol 1995;104:375-81.

91. Travis WD, Brambilla E, Müller-Hermelink HK, Harris CC, eds. World Health Organization Classification of Tumours. Pathology and genetics of tumours of the lung, pleura, thymus and heart. Lyon: IARC Press; 2004.

92. Truong LD, Mody DR, Cagle PT, Jackson-York GL, Schwartz MR, Weeler TM. Thymic carcinoma. A clinicopathologic study of 13 cases. Am J Surg Pathol 1990;14:151-66

93. Tsuchiya R, Koga K, Matsuno Y, Mukai K, Shimosato Y. Thymic carcinoma: proposal for pathological TNM and staging. Pathol Int 1994;44:505-12.

94. Weiss LM, Movahed LA, Butler AE, et al. Analysis of lymphoepithelioma and lymphoepithelioma-like carcinoma for Epstein-Barr viral genomes by in situ hybridization. Am J Surg Pathol 1989;13:625-31.

95. Wick MR, Scheithauer BW, Weiland LH, Bernatz PE. Primary thymic carcinomas. Am J Surg Pathol 1982;6:613-30

96. Wittekind Ch, Greene FL, Henson DE, Hutter RV, Sobin LH, eds. TNM supplement. A commentary on uniform use, 3rd ed. New York: Wiley-Liss; 2003:118-9.

97. Wu TC, Kuo TT. Study of Epstein-Barr virus early RNA 1 (EBER1) expression by in situ hybridization in thymic epithelial tumors of Chinese patients in Taiwan. Hum Pathol 1993;24:2235-8.

98. Yamakawa Y, Masaoka A, Hashimoto T, et al. A tentative tumor-node-metastasis classification of thymoma. Cancer 1991;68:1984-7.

99. Yaris N, Nas Y, Cobanoglu U, Yavuz MN. Thymic carcinoma in children. Pediatr Blood Cancer 2006;47:224-7.

100. Yonemori K, Tsuta K, Tateishi U, et al. Diagnostic accuracy of CT-guided percutaneous cutting needle biopsy for thymic epithelial tumors. Clin Radiology 2006;61:771-5.

101. Zettl A, Strobel P, Wagner K, et al. Recurrent genetic aberrations in thymoma and thymic carcinoma. Am J Pathol 2000;157:257-66.

4 THYMIC NEUROENDOCRINE CARCINOMAS

Neuroendocrine neoplasms of the mediastinum include lesions derived from neuroendocrine elements within the thymus, from paraganglionic rests, or from misplaced embryonal structures within the mediastinum. Thymic neuroendocrine carcinomas are the most common neuroendocrine neoplasms of this anatomic region (59).

Thymic neuroendocrine carcinomas (NECs) are malignant thymic epithelial tumors that are predominantly or exclusively composed of neuroendocrine cells (52,65). They include *well-differentiated NECs (carcinoid tumor)* and *poorly differentiated NECs*. Poorly differentiated tumors include large cell NEC and small cell carcinoma of neuroendocrine type, but do not include ordinary thymic carcinomas. The latter may contain scattered or aggregated neuroendocrine cells (22,31,36). Also not included are neurogenic tumors with neuroendocrine features, for example, cytokeratin-negative paragangliomas. Paragangliomas are described separately. Neuroendocrine differentiation can be revealed by immunohistochemical staining for chromogranin A, synaptophysin, and neural cell adhesion molecule (NCAM [CD56]), or by the detection of neuroendocrine granules ultrastructurally.

Controversy surrounds the classification of NECs, that is, where to position carcinoid tumor, small cell carcinoma, and large cell NEC. In the lung, small cell carcinoma and carcinoid tumors are placed separately under the category of malignant epithelial tumors, whereas large cell NEC is categorized as a variant of large cell carcinoma (65). Criteria for subtyping NECs vary according to investigators. This Fascicle follows the criteria and classification proposed in the second edition of the World Health Organization (WHO) Histological Typing of Thymic Tumors (52), placing these three tumors in the category of neuroendocrine carcinomas, although the most recent edition of the WHO classification includes NECs under the category of thymic carcinoma (65).

Carcinoid tumors are designated as well-differentiated NEC because the patient outcome is poor. Even encapsulated or minimally invasive tumors may at times show local recurrence, distant metastasis, and even death due to tumor years after resection (12,14,42,43). No standardized nomenclature has been established, however, and some investigators still use the term carcinoid tumor.

Moran and Suster (43) divided NECs by grade of malignancy (degree of differentiation) into low-grade (well-differentiated), intermediate-grade (moderately differentiated) and high-grade (poorly differentiated) tumors. These tumors display an increasing degree of cellular atypia and mitotic activity (less than 3, 3 to 10, and more than 10 per 10 mitoses high-power fields). These features correspond roughly to typical/atypical carcinoid, atypical carcinoid with cellular and architectural atypia and increased mitotic activity, and large cell NEC and small cell carcinoma, respectively. Moran and Suster also found features transitional between carcinoid tumor and small cell carcinoma, which are only rarely encountered in carcinoid tumors of other organs. The presence of transitional features is controversial and remains to be verified.

In the spectrum of neuroendocrine carcinomas, classic carcinoid tumor occupies one end, and highly malignant small cell carcinoma occupies the opposite end. Between these two entities, there are carcinoid tumor with cellular and architectural atypia and large cell NEC.

WELL-DIFFERENTIATED NEUROENDOCRINE CARCINOMA (CARCINOID TUMOR)

Well-differentiated neuroendocrine carcinoma (WDNEC) (*carcinoid tumor*) is a well-differentiated tumor composed of a uniform population of cells growing in organoid nests, rosettes, glands, ribbons, and festoons, and in which neuroendocrine differentiation can be demonstrated immunohistochemically or ultrastructurally (52). It is of low-grade to intermediate-grade malignancy.

Until 1972, the tumor was referred to by such terms as epithelial thymoma, mediastinal branchial adenoma, parathyroid adenoma, and unclassified mediastinal tumor. Kay and Wilson (26) described an adrenocorticotropic hormone (ACTH)-secreting thymoma in a patient with Cushing syndrome in 1970, the histology and ultrastructure of which were typical of carcinoid tumor, but they refrained from labeling it "carcinoid." This was understandable, since most investigators at that time held the prevailing view that one should hesitate to make a diagnosis of carcinoid tumor unless it was of intestinal origin. In fact, even tumors of bronchial origin were classified as bronchial adenomas. In 1966, at the National Cancer Center Hospital in Tokyo, an anterior mediastinal tumor with features typical of carcinoid tumor with rosettes was not diagnosed as carcinoid tumor but diagnosed as probable parathyroid adenoma.

Rosai and Higa (49) described eight anterior or anterosuperior mediastinal tumors in 1972 and reviewed eight other cases reported previously under various names. They considered such tumors to be endocrine neoplasms of thymic origin that were "related to carcinoid tumors" of other organs, such as those of the gastrointestinal tract, lung, gallbladder, bile duct, and pancreas. In a separate communication, Rosai et al. (50) described three cases of "mediastinal endocrine neoplasm in patients with multiple endocrine adenomatosis," which were histologically identical to the eight cases described separately and were regarded as neoplasms belonging to the carcinoid tumor family. Although they did not designate these cases as carcinoid tumors of the thymus, these two reports were considered to represent the first documented categorization of carcinoid tumor of the thymus as a distinct entity. Thereafter, several reports appeared describing carcinoid tumors (21,37,62,71,74), and accumulation of more cases during the last decade has made it possible to characterize the morphology, function, and behavior of these tumors and to distinguish them from carcinoid tumors of other organs (12,14,16,27,39,41,43).

Atypical carcinoid tumors of the lung were defined originally by Arrigoni et al. in 1972 (2). Such tumors had: 1) increased mitotic activity, with one mitotic figure per 1 to 2 high-power fields (5 to 10 per 10 high-power fields); 2) foci of coagulation necrosis; 3) nuclear pleomorphism, hyperchromatism, and increased nuclear to cytoplasmic ratio; and 4) hypercellularity and disorganized architecture. Travis et al. (67), after univariate and multivariate analyses of various parameters concerning carcinoid tumors of the lung, revised Arrigoni's criteria, changing the number of mitotic figures in atypical carcinoid tumors to 2 to 10 mitoses per 10 high-power fields (2 mm^2) or the presence of foci of necrosis. Travis et al. suggested that pleomorphism, cellularity, and vascular invasion are more subjective findings and not significant on multivariate analysis. These criteria for atypical carcinoid tumors have been adopted by the WHO histologic typing of thymic tumors (52,65)

Most carcinoid tumors of the thymus contain small punctate necrotic foci in large solid nests and have some mitotic activity, and are similar histologically to atypical carcinoid tumor of the bronchus (18,43,69). Typical carcinoid tumors with low mitotic activity and without necrosis are practically nonexistent in the thymus. The presence of necrosis may be due to the size of the tumor, which is usually much larger than carcinoid tumor of the bronchus. In order to avoid confusion with the nomenclature used for tumors in other organs, it is better not to use the term "atypical carcinoid tumor" in the thymus, although the term "atypia" can be used to describe some carcinoid tumors with cellular and/or architectural atypia and more frequent mitotic figures than those defined for bronchial carcinoid (53,67).

Histogenesis

Carcinoid tumors of the intestine and bronchi were thought to arise from the neuroendocrine cells present in organs believed to be of neural crest (neuroectoderm) origin. This hypothesis was advocated in the 1960s and 1970s by Pearse et al. (47) and the tumors were called APUDomas (APUD indicating amine precursor uptake and decarboxylation). Later, however, it was demonstrated that neuroendocrine cells in the aerodigestive tract do not migrate from the neural crest, but come from the primitive epithelial cells originally present in those organs (48,55).

This hypothesis can also be applied to carcinoid tumor (WDNEC) of the thymus. Argyrophil and argentaffin cells are present in the thymus of chickens, pigeons, and reptiles (19), and argyrophil cells (49) and immunoreactive calcitonin-containing cells may be found in human thymuses and are the presumed cells of origin of thymic neuroendocrine tumors. It is difficult, however, to prove the presence of Kulchitsky cells of the diffuse endocrine system in the human thymus. If in situ development and differentiation of neuroendocrine cells also occur in the human thymus, then the presence in the thymus of carcinoid tumor and small cell carcinoma with neuroendocrine features and combined forms of neuroendocrine and non-neuroendocrine tumors (described later), as well as the frequent presence of neuroendocrine cells in ordinary thymic carcinomas (22,31,36), can be easily understood.

Clinical Findings

Carcinoid tumors of the thymus comprise 2 to 4 percent of all anterior mediastinal neoplasms; occur in almost all age groups between 16 and 100 years of age, with a predilection for adults between 40 and 60 years; and are more common in males (ratio, 3 to 1) (12,14,18,43). Carcinoid tumors vary from 2 to 20 cm in greatest dimension. About one third of the patients are asymptomatic, and the tumors are found incidentally on chest roentgenograms for other reasons. The remaining patients have nonspecific symptoms resulting from the anterior mediastinal mass, including chest pain, cough, and dyspnea. Weight loss is noted in some patients.

In one study of 80 patients with carcinoid tumors, 22 percent had symptoms and signs related to endocrine abnormalities, including 6 percent (5 patients) with Cushing syndrome (43). The most frequent endocrine abnormalities were multiple endocrine neoplasia type 1 (MEN 1), affecting primarily the pituitary gland, pancreas, and parathyroid glands and occasionally resulting in Zollinger-Ellison syndrome. MEN type 2 occurred rarely and affected thyroid C cells, the adrenal medulla, and the parathyroid glands (5,6,37,43,50,57,71). These studies confirm that carcinoid tumor of the thymus is often a part of the MEN syndrome, and it is reported that MEN 1-related carcinoid tumors constitute approximately 25 percent of all thymic carcinoid tumors (63). In a prospective study of 85 patients with MEN 1, 7 developed

thymic carcinoid tumor during the mean follow-up period of 8 years (17).

In addition to reports of thymic carcinoid tumor associated with Cushing syndrome (13,32,57), there is a reported case of thymic carcinoid tumor associated with acromegaly due to the ectopic secretion of growth hormone-releasing hormone (GHRH) in which immunoreactive GHRH, vasoactive intestinal polypeptide, and somatostatin were seen in the tumor cells (6). Also reported is a case of thymic carcinoid tumor associated with acromegaly and Cushing syndrome due to the ectopic production of GHRH and ACTH, with immunoreactive GHRH, ACTH, and neuropeptide Y in tumor cells (25).

The carcinoid syndrome is rarely associated with carcinoid tumors of the lung, unless there are metastases to distant organs, such as the liver. We are not aware of any case of pure mediastinal carcinoid tumor associated with the carcinoid syndrome, even among those with hematogenous metastasis. There was a single report of a patient with poorly differentiated carcinoma of the thymus closely admixed with neuroendocrine and spindle cell sarcomatous components, who developed typical carcinoid syndrome with skin flushing and increased urinary 5-hydroxyindolacetic acid when the tumor recurred after surgical resection. The tumor cells were positive for cytokeratin, chromogranin A, synaptophysin, protein gene product 9.5 (PGP9.5), and Grimelius silver stain, and contained abundant electron-dense granules of 100 to 300 nm (46).

At the National Cancer Center Hospitals in Tokyo and Kashiwa, Japan, there were 12 cases of carcinoid tumor during the period between 1965 and 1999 (9 men and 3 women aged 34 to 74 years). No patients had endocrine manifestations. During the same period, more than 300 cases of thymoma and thymic carcinoma were resected in the same institutions. A questionnaire survey in Japan found 41 thymic carcinoid tumors (3.1 percent) among 1,320 thymic epithelial and neuroendocrine tumors (thymoma, 82.8 percent; thymic carcinoma, 14.1 percent) (29). Of the 41 patients, 30 were males and 11 were females, ranging in age from 13 to 70 years. There are no data regarding endocrine abnormalities.

Nonfunctional thymic carcinoid tumors, such as those not associated with Cushing syndrome, are often large and easily detected by routine

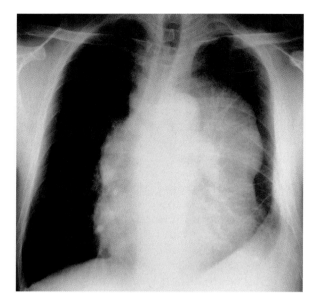

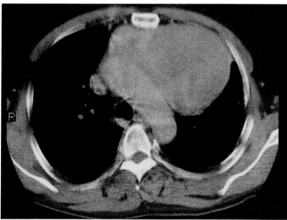

Figure 4-1

CARCINOID TUMOR

Top: Posterior-anterior chest roentgenogram reveals a large tumorous density overlapping the left pulmonary hilus, with the convexity toward the left lung. The contents of the mediastinum are displaced toward the right lung. There is pleural thickening on the left.

Bottom: Computerized tomography (CT) at the level of the aortic arch discloses a clearly defined tumorous density, which displaces the superior vena cava and ascending aorta to the right and compresses the lungs bilaterally. (Fig. 3-140 from Fascicle 21, Third Series.) (Figs. 4-1, 4-2, 4-9, 4-15, and 4-20 are from the same patient.)

chest X ray. They present as a large, radiopaque, noncystic anterior mediastinal mass projecting into the pleural space unilaterally or bilaterally (fig. 4-1). On the other hand, thymic carcinoid

tumors associated with Cushing syndrome may be so small that they are undetectable by routine posterior-anterior and lateral chest roentgenograms. In such cases, computerized tomography (CT) is useful. Among the 5 cases associated with Cushing syndrome reported by Wick et al. (71), only 1 tumor was identified on routine chest X ray, 2 were found at autopsy, and 2 by CT. Of the total 15 cases, 5 showed osteoblastic bone metastasis, which was disclosed by skeletal survey roentgenograms and radionuclide bone scans.

Gross Findings

Functional carcinoid tumors may be as small as 1.3 cm (71), but nonfunctional tumors are often large when detected, encapsulated or circumscribed, with a pale tan to gray-white, solid cut surface, with or without scattered pinhead-sized areas of necrosis (figs. 4-2, 4-3). Irregular areas of coagulation necrosis or hemorrhage may also be present. The tumor frequently adheres to, and at times invades, surrounding organs or tissue, such as the pleura, pericardium, lung, and adventitia of the major vessels. Fibrous bands producing lobulation of the tumor, as are often seen in thymoma, are not present. Two independent tumors within a single thymus have been described in a few instances; however, the possibility of an intrathymic lymphatic metastasis should always be kept in mind, since lymph node metastasis is not rare.

Microscopic Findings

Carcinoid tumors, particularly classic examples, are made up of solid organoid nests, rosettes, and festoons of small to medium-sized, uniform polygonal cells, and less frequently, spindle cells. They have centrally located, round to oval, finely granular nuclei with stippled chromatin, thin nuclear membranes, and inconspicuous or small nucleoli, and a small to moderate amount of lightly eosinophilic, finely granular cytoplasm (fig. 4-4). The stroma is scanty and delicately vascular. Mitotic figures are often few in number but as many as 21 per 10 high-power fields have been seen (fig. 4-5) (69). Central, punctate coagulation necrosis is found within large cell nests in almost all cases (fig. 4-4D). Foci of coagulation necrosis and mitotic activity of 2 to 10 per 10 high-power fields are features of "atypical carcinoid,"

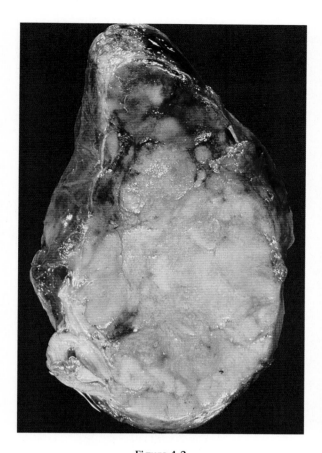

Figure 4-2

CARCINOID TUMOR

Horizontal section of a carcinoid tumor reveals encapsulation with thin fibrous tissue and a granular to faintly lobulated, yellowish tan, medullary cut surface with no recognizable areas of necrosis.

and tumors with 11 or more mitotic figures are considered to be poorly differentiated large cell NEC by Travis et al. (66,67). Whether or not the criteria for classifying neuroendocrine tumors of the lung can be adopted for the thymus is questionable and requires future investigation. For the time being, it may be better not to use the term "atypical" in the thymus, unless the carcinoid tumor is combined with areas showing features of poorly differentiated or undifferentiated carcinoma, as stated earlier.

Wick et al. (71,72) described four additional histologic patterns in thymic carcinoid tumors: 1) a very sclerotic stroma, compressing the tumor cell clusters, and occasionally producing an "Indian file" cell arrangement; 2) a cribriform pattern; 3) sheet-like masses of tumor cells with a scanty

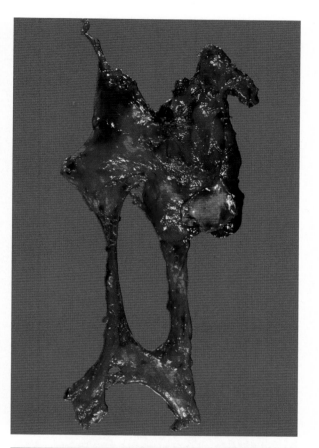

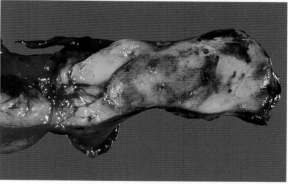

Figure 4-3

CARCINOID TUMOR

Top: Posterior aspect of a surgically resected thymus with tumors in the right lobe. The membranous tissue with a smooth surface attached to the right lobe is a portion of the pericardium.

Bottom: Horizontal section of the thymus reveals a thinly encapsulated tumor with a pale tan congested surface showing yellow streaks of necrosis. Three smaller tumors were present in the same lobe, and multiple lymph nodes with metastases in the mediastinum and neck were removed at the same time. (Figs. 4-3 and 4-4 are from the same patient.)

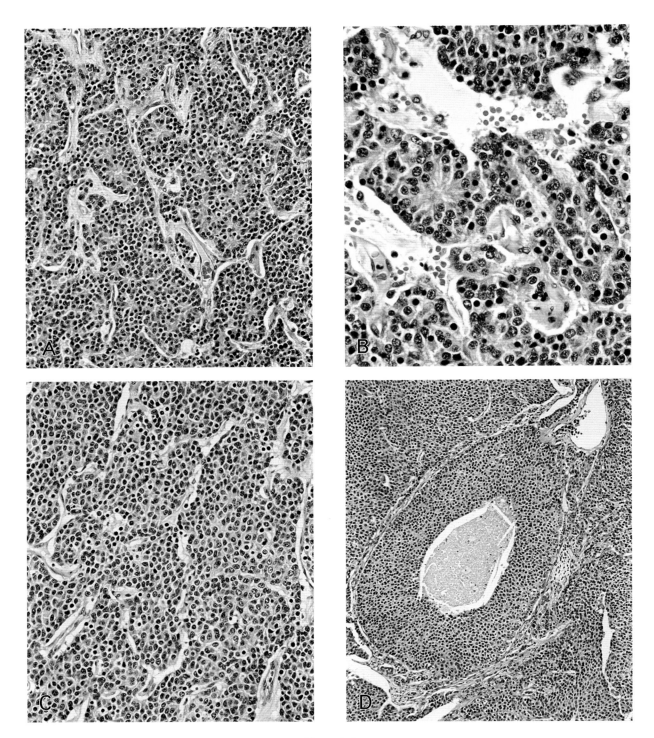

Figure 4-4

HISTOLOGY OF CARCINOID TUMOR

A,B: Irregularly shaped nests of tumor cells with round to oval bland nuclei, inconspicuous nucleoli, and finely granular cytoplasm are closely associated with delicate blood vessels. Rosettes are evident.

C: Metastasis in a lymph node is composed of slightly larger cells with a few mitotic figures, without rosette formation.

D: A focus of punctate coagulation necrosis is seen in the center of a tumor nest.

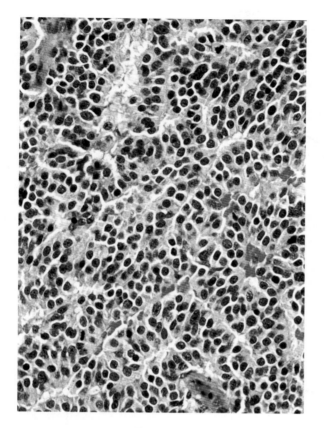

Figure 4-5

CARCINOID TUMOR WITH MITOTIC FIGURES

Two mitotic figures, one at the right upper corner and one at the left lower corner of the figure, are evident in this high-power view of an area with histologic features typical of carcinoid tumor.

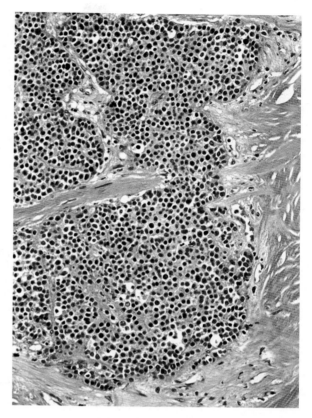

Figure 4-6

CARCINOID TUMOR WITH SCLEROTIC STROMA

Marked sclerosis and hyalinization of the stroma are evident. Tumor cells in the right upper corner appear to be undergoing atrophy due probably to impaired blood supply.

vascular stroma showing only a vaguely organoid cellular arrangement; and 4) the classic carcinoid tumor pattern, but with focal collections of intracellular brown-gray granular pigment, which is periodic acid–Schiff (PAS) positive and appears to be lipofuscin (figs. 4-6–4-8). Sclerotic stroma and lipofuscin-like intracellular pigment may indicate a longstanding tumor. A cribriform pattern indicates aggregates of rosette-like, small acinar or glandular structures (fig. 4-9) or the presence of small foci of liquefaction necrosis within the cell nests. Glandular structures, which could well be rosettes with exaggerated lumens, are seen not only in carcinoid tumor but also in combined small cell carcinoma (see fig. 4-30). A vaguely organoid pattern may simply indicate a lesser degree of differentiation and greater proliferative activity of the tumor cells, the presence of

which indicates the intermediate-grade, moderately differentiated NEC of Moran and Suster (43). A cervical lymph node metastasis in one case showed a histology similar to medullary carcinoma of the thyroid (fig. 4-7C). In that case, the primary tumor in the mediastinum removed 12 years earlier was composed in part of classic carcinoid tumor (fig. 4-7A) and in part of poorly differentiated tumor with a less organoid arrangement (fig. 4-7B). This case may be an example of classic carcinoid tumor (WD-NEC), which showed malignant progression to intermediate-grade (moderately differentiated) NEC and then to high-grade (poorly differentiated) large cell NEC (43). Sustentacular cells (3) are considered to be an organoid arrangement marker, but are identified only infrequently in thymic carcinoid tumor (fig. 4-10).

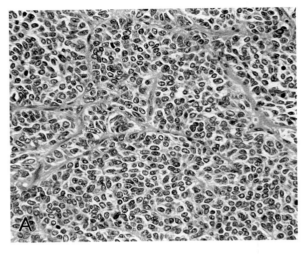

Figure 4-7

CARCINOID TUMOR WITH STRUCTURAL AND CELLULAR ATYPIA

A: In the primary tumor, nests of polygonal to oval tumor cells are closely associated with blood vessels.

B: In other areas, larger tumor cells with an increased nuclear to cytoplasmic ratio and an increased number of mitotic figures grow diffusely, as in undifferentiated carcinoma or malignant lymphoma.

C: A recurrent tumor in a lymph node, which was found 12 years later, shows a further increase in cellular atypia. (Courtesy of Dr. Tadakazu Shimoda, Tokyo.) (Figs. 4-7 and 4-17 are from the same patient.)

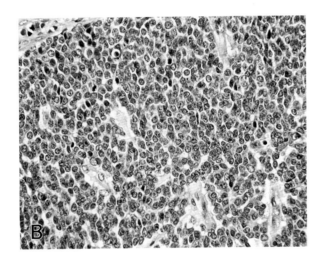

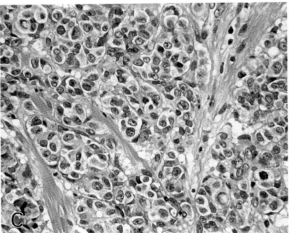

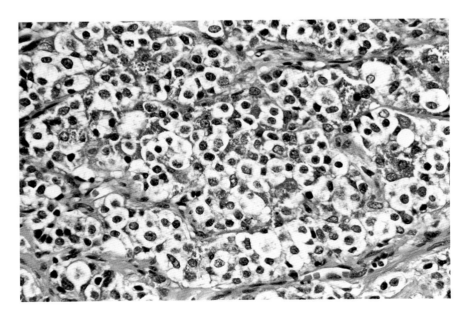

Figure 4-8

CARCINOID TUMOR WITH LIPOFUSCIN-LIKE PIGMENT

The tumor cells possess ballooned, clear cytoplasm, which contains coarsely granular gray-brown pigment.

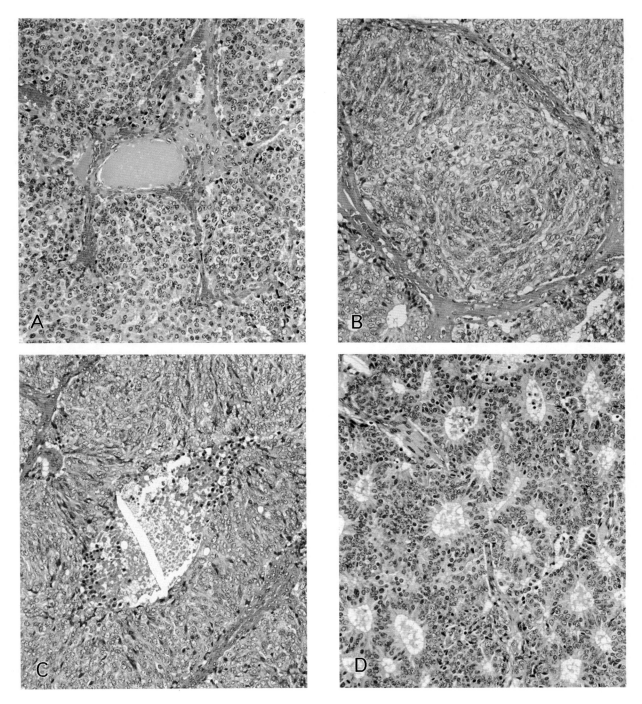

Figure 4-9

CARCINOID TUMOR WITH SPINDLE CELLS AND GLANDULAR STRUCTURES

A: Large solid nests are composed of round to polygonal cells with vesicular nuclei, small nucleoli, and a small amount of cytoplasm. This tumor could be diagnosed as carcinoid tumor with cellular atypia.

B: In other areas, cell nests consist of short spindle cells arranged in whorls, which are adjacent to areas with glandular structures.

C: Punctate central necrosis is seen in a large tumor nest made of short spindle cells.

D: Many well-defined glandular structures are present in other areas. This tumor was positive for chromogranin A, somatostatin, and α-hCG. The Grimelius stain was also positive, but Alcian blue-periodic acid–Schiff (ABPAS) was negative.

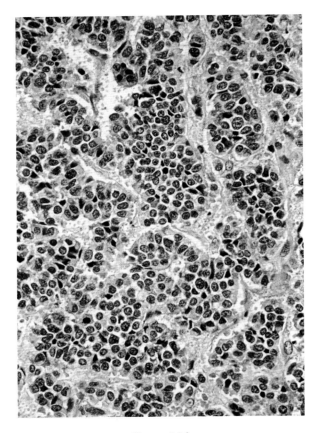

Figure 4-10

CARCINOID TUMOR WITH SUSTENTACULAR CELLS

Solid tumor cell nests are bordered in some areas by spindle, triangular, or stellate cells. These cells were S-100 protein positive immunohistochemically. (Figs. 4-10 and 4-24 are from the same patient.)

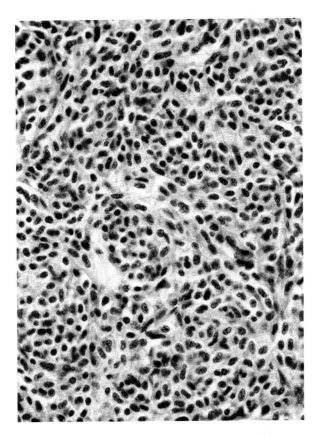

Figure 4-11

SPINDLE CELL CARCINOID TUMOR

The tumor shows diffuse growth. Ill-defined bundles of short spindle cells have oval finely granular nuclei, inconspicuous nucleoli, and finely granular cytoplasm. (Courtesy of Dr. Tetsuro Kodama, Utsunomiya, Japan.)

Histologic Variants

There are several histologic variants of carcinoid tumor: spindle cell type, pigmented type, carcinoid with amyloid, oncocytic type, mucinous stroma type, angiomatoid type, and combinations of these variants. These variants are rare, except for the spindle cell and oncocytic types.

Spindle Cell Carcinoid. Spindle-shaped tumor cells are considered to be a component of classic thymic carcinoid tumor (figs. 4-9B,C, 4-11) (74). If the tumor is predominantly or entirely made up of spindle cells that are often arranged in bundles, as in a spindle cell carcinoid tumor of the periphery of the lung, the thymic tumor is designated as a spindle cell carcinoid tumor (fig. 4-11) (32,39). This may cause diagnostic difficulties.

Pigmented Carcinoid. There are two types of pigmented carcinoid: one harboring melanin-containing dendritic melanocytes within tumor cell nests and melanophages in tumor nests and fibrovascular stroma (23,32,34), and another showing melanin-containing carcinoid tumor cells and melanophages (28). Pigmented cells stain with the Fontana-Masson stain and are negative with iron stains (28). Pigmented cells are positive for S-100 protein but negative for melanoma antigen HMB45 (32). The tumor cells are either of the classic type or spindle shaped, and cases associated with Cushing syndrome have been described (32,34). Since dendritic melanocytes are also found in thymoma (see fig. 2-64), the presence of such cells within neuro-endocrine tumors is to be expected. Pigmented

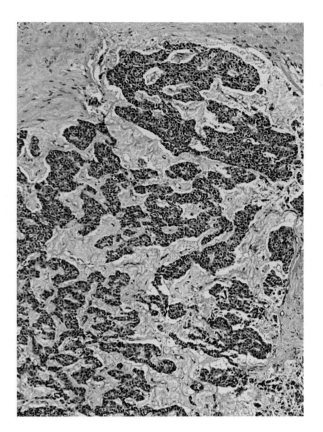 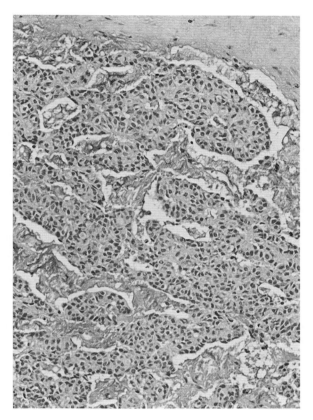

Figure 4-12

CARCINOID TUMOR WITH MUCINOUS STROMA

Left: Abundant extracellular connective tissue type mucin is present in the stroma, giving a false impression of "mucinous (or goblet cell) carcinoid tumor" as seen in the appendix and ovary.

Right: Alcian blue stain. (Figs. 4-12 and 4-18 are from the same patient.)

carcinoid tumors with intracellular melanin or lipofuscin are also described (53,74).

Carcinoid with Amyloid Stroma (Extrathyroidal Medullary Carcinoma). This is a rare tumor and is similar to medullary carcinoma with amyloid stroma of the thyroid gland. Component cells are immunoreactive for calcitonin (52,72).

Oncocytic Carcinoid. This tumor is similar to oncocytic carcinoid tumor of the bronchus, and is made up of vaguely organoid nests, cords, and ribbons of large to medium-sized polygonal cells. These cells have abundant eosinophilic granular cytoplasm, round to oval nuclei, and occasional prominent nucleoli. Cytoplasmic granularity is due to the presence of numerous mitochondria. Among 22 carcinoid tumors with prominent oncocytic features reported, 2 were associated with MEN 1 and 1 with Cushing syndrome (41).

Carcinoid with Mucinous Stroma. This is also a rare variant in which abundant extracellular connective tissue mucin is present in the stroma (fig. 4-12), giving an appearance of mucinous carcinoma, but there is no cytoplasmic mucus (58). Stromal mucin is not a product of the tumor cells and this subtype is a different tumor from mucinous or goblet cell carcinoid of the appendix and ovary. Goblet cell carcinoid arising in a mature teratoma of the mediastinum has been reported (35).

Angiomatoid Carcinoid. This variant is characterized by the presence of blood-filled cystic spaces which are lined not by endothelial cells but by tumor cells (40).

Carcinoid with Sarcomatous Changes. This rare variant is a mixture of a carcinoid element and a sarcomatous element, and is clinically a highly aggressive tumor (30,46). It is not a collision of

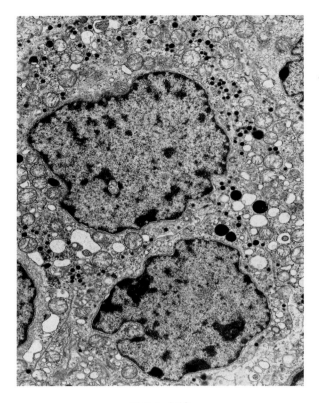

Figure 4-13

ULTRASTRUCTURE OF CARCINOID TUMOR WITH ECTOPIC PRODUCTION OF ADRENOCORTICOTROPIC HORMONE (ACTH)

Many neurosecretory granules of about 160 nm in diameter are evident in the cytoplasm of the tumor cells. The mitochondria and smooth endoplasmic reticulum are moderately developed. The patient developed Cushing syndrome, and laboratory data indicated ectopic production of ACTH. (Fig. 3-154 from Fascicle 21, Third Series.)

Cushing syndrome. Membrane-bound dense–core granules of 150 to 500 nm in diameter, which are of the neurosecretory type, are always present and often abundant (fig. 4-13). Cellular attachments of the desmosomal type may be present, but are often poorly developed. Cytoplasmic fibrils, probably intermediate filaments, may be arranged in whorls, usually in the Golgi areas. A basal lamina can be identified, although it is scanty (74).

Cytologic Findings

Fine needle aspiration cytology in conjunction with imaging and immunocytochemistry is diagnostic for thymic carcinoid tumor. Aspirates consist of single or loosely cohesive, medium-sized cells with round to oval finely granular (salt and pepper) nuclei and scanty but finely granular cytoplasm. Interspersed are some larger cells with moderate to abundant granular cytoplasm (70) or densely clumped chromatin and prominent nucleoli (44). Characteristic optically clear, paranuclear inclusion-like spaces with a semicircular or discoid appearance can be demonstrated with the Romanowsky stain; these correspond to aggregates of intermediate filament and are immunoreactive for cytokeratin (16). Oil red-O stained lipid-rich tumor cells have been reported (56).

Figure 4-14 shows the histology, Grimelius stain, and imprint smear of thymic carcinoid tumor metastatic to the lung. Tumor cells in imprint smears possess uniform, round to oval, granular or vesicular nuclei; small nucleoli; a small amount of pale-stained cytoplasm; and indistinct cell borders.

Immunohistochemical Findings (Including Functional Correlation with Paraneoplastic Syndrome)

The argentaffin reaction with the Fontana-Masson stain is negative in thymic carcinoid tumor, as in bronchial carcinoid tumor. The argyrophil reaction with the Grimelius stain is variably positive (figs. 4-14, 4-15).

As in carcinoid tumors at other locations, the cells of thymic carcinoid tumor immunostain for neuron-specific enolase (NSE), chromogranin A, synaptophysin, and NCAM/CD56 with variable intensity (figs. 4-16–4-19). Serotonin has been demonstrated focally in a few cases (74), but gastrin-releasing peptide (GRP) has not.

two unrelated tumors, rather the sarcomatous element is considered to be due to dedifferentiation or divergent development from a common precursor. It may show fibrosarcomatous, myoid, osseous, or chondroid differentiation.

Ultrastructural Findings

In most thymic carcinoid tumors, centrally located nuclei contain evenly dispersed chromatin and inconspicuous nucleoli. The cytoplasm contains variable numbers of mitochondria and Golgi apparatuses. The rough endoplasmic reticulum is often abundant, and there is a moderate amount of smooth endoplasmic reticulum in some cases, particularly those complicated by

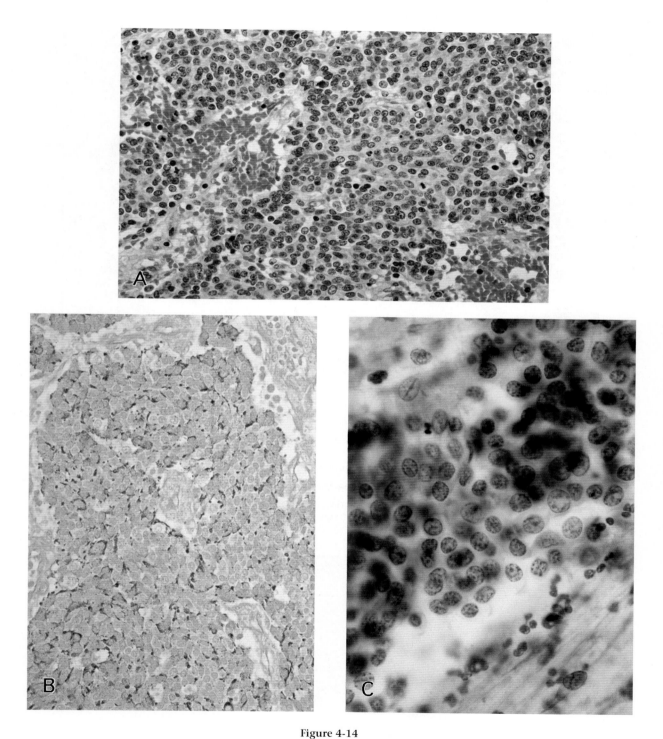

Figure 4-14

THYMIC CARCINOID TUMOR METASTATIC TO LUNG

A: Histology of carcinoid tumor metastatic to the lung.

B: Grimelius stain reveals eccentrically located reaction products in many tumor cells.

C: Imprint smear of the metastatic tumor shows a piled-up aggregate of medium-sized cells with uniform, oval to round, granular to vesicular nuclei; small nucleoli; a small amount of pale-stained cytoplasm; and ill-defined cell borders. (Courtesy of Drs. Tamiko Takemura and Tsunekazu Hishima, Tokyo, Japan.)

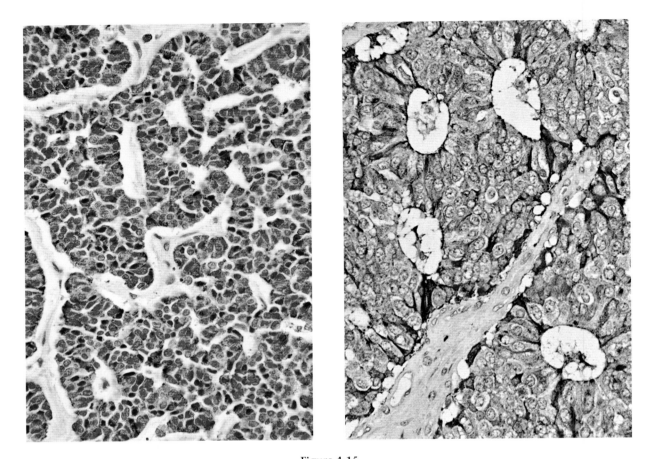

Figure 4-15

CARCINOID TUMOR WITH ARGYROPHILIA

Left: The tumor cells in trabeculae or festoons show marked argyrophilia with the Grimelius stain.
Right: Tumor cells arranged in glandular structures are frequently positive for the Grimelius stain.

Figure 4-16

CARCINOID TUMOR IMMUNOREACTIVE FOR NEURON-SPECIFIC ENOLASE (NSE)

The tumor cells show variable cytoplasmic staining for NSE.

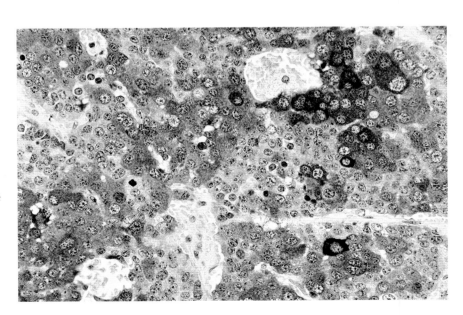

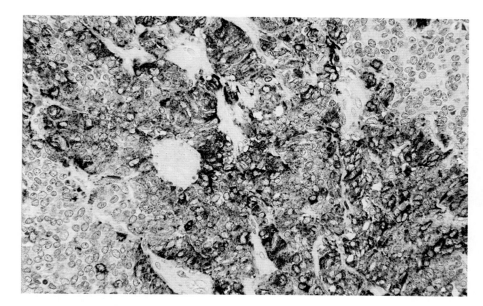

Figure 4-17

CARCINOID TUMOR IMMUNOREACTIVE FOR CHROMOGRANIN A

Many tumor cells are immunoreactive for chromogranin A.

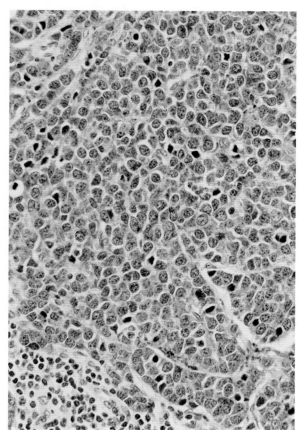
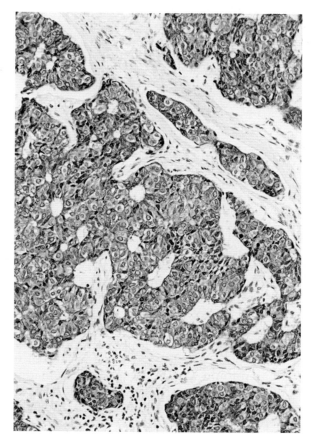

Figure 4-18

CARCINOID TUMORS IMMUNOREACTIVE FOR SYNAPTOPHYSIN

Left: The cytoplasm of the tumor cells stains moderately for synaptophysin.
Right: Tumor cells arranged in a glandular pattern are strongly immunoreactive for synaptophysin.

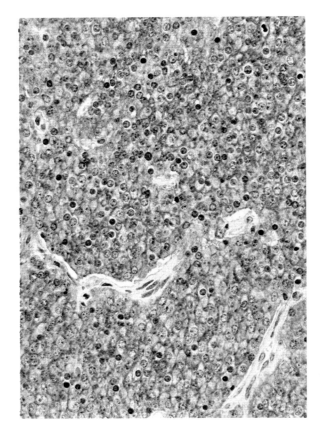

Figure 4-19

CARCINOID TUMOR IMMUNOREACTIVE FOR NEURAL CELL ADHESION MOLECULE (NCAM)

The cell membrane of almost all the tumor cells are strongly immunoreactive for NCAM (immunostaining after cold acetone fixation and paraffin embedding).

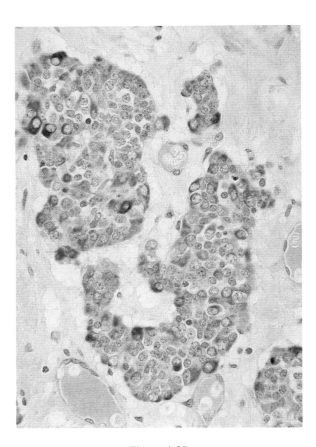

Figure 4-20

CARCINOID TUMOR IMMUNOREACTIVE FOR SOMATOSTATIN

The tumor cells, particularly those at the periphery of the nests, are strongly immunoreactive for somatostatin.

Somatostatin is frequently detected (fig. 4-20) (74). A study of five tumors revealed the presence of NSE in two, chromogranin A in two, ACTH in two, calcitonin in one, neurotensin in three, and cholecystokinin in all five (21). In all five cases, more than two hormones were detected immunohistochemically. Calcitonin gene-related peptide, gastrin, somatostatin, substance P, and serotonin were not demonstrated in any of these cases. In another study of eight atypical carcinoid tumors, all were positive for cytokeratin, NSE, synaptophysin, and chromogranin A; five were positive for calcitonin (69).

Although intracytoplasmic immunoreactive ACTH is detected in some carcinoid tumors clinically associated with Cushing syndrome (fig. 4-21C), it is difficult to prove the presence of ACTH

immunohistochemically in other cases. In such cases, radioimmunoassay of an extract of tumor tissue confirms the presence of the peptide. In a case of thymic carcinoid tumor with Cushing syndrome, the ACTH-positive granules were present only in a few tumor cells (24). This finding was explained by either the prompt secretion of the product or the presence of only a few cells capable of ACTH production.

The following is an example of a case in which ACTH was produced by the tumor. Eighteen months after surgical resection of a thymic carcinoid tumor producing ACTH (fig. 4-21), pulmonary metastasis developed. Laboratory data disclosed hypernatremia, hypokalemia, and elevated blood ACTH and cortisol levels (419.8 pg/mL and 60 µg/dL, respectively). The patient had a rapid downhill course and died

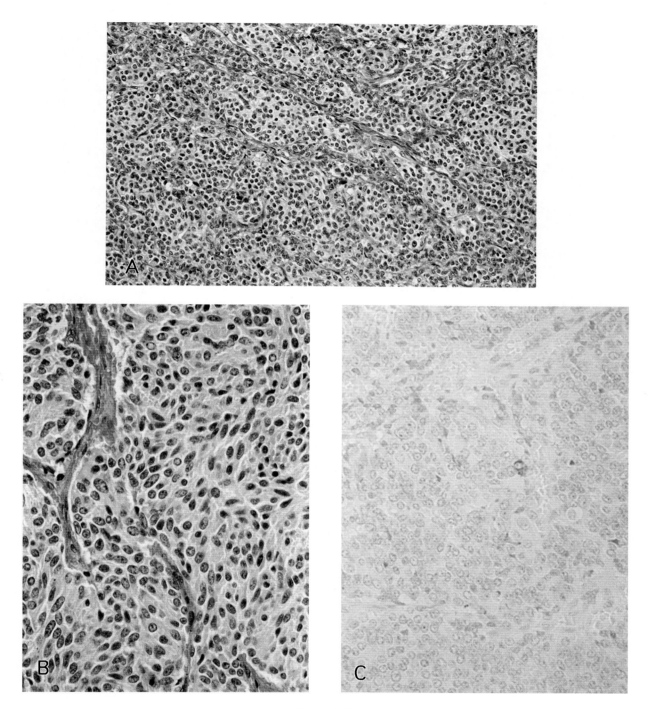

Figure 4-21

CARCINOID TUMOR WITH ECTOPIC ACTH PRODUCTION

A,B: Low-power (A) and high-power (B) views of a mediastinal tumor composed of nests of polygonal to short spindle cells with round to oval nuclei and finely granular cytoplasm supported by delicate blood vessels. Initially, the tumor was silent endocrinologically, but showed signs of ACTH production when it recurred. However, ACTH could not be demonstrated immunohistochemically in either the primary or the metastatic tumor. (Courtesy of Dr. Koji Chihara, Shizuoka, Japan.)

C: Another carcinoid tumor associated with Cushing syndrome. The patient was a 50-year-old male with a 3-cm, largely encapsulated, invasive anterior mediastinal tumor. A few cells are immunoreactive for ACTH.

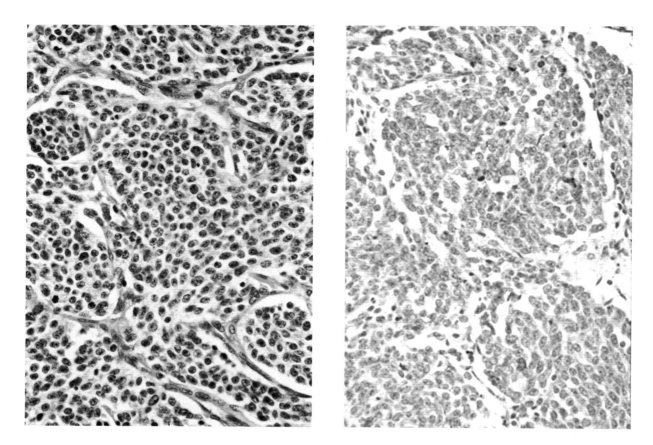

Figure 4-22

CARCINOID TUMOR PRODUCING BETA-HUMAN CHORIONIC GONADOTROPIN (β-HCG)

Left: The oval tumor cells with slight nuclear atypia and distinct nucleoli are intimately associated with delicate blood vessels.
Right: The cytoplasm is variably immunostained for β-hCG. There are no features of choriocarcinoma. (Courtesy of Dr. Toru Kameya, Shizuoka, Japan.)

of widespread metastases to lung, heart, liver, kidney, pituitary gland, muscle, and bone. The tumor tissue at autopsy contained 26,000 pg/g of ACTH. ACTH, however, could not be demonstrated immunohistochemically either in the surgically resected primary tumor or in the metastatic lesions obtained at autopsy. The tumor showed strong immunohistochemical positivity for NSE, moderate positivity for chromogranin A, and Grimelius argyrophilia, and only focal positivity for cytokeratin, synaptophysin, and S-100 protein (sustentacular cells only).

A rare case of thymic carcinoid tumor containing a significantly high level of calcitonin, whole human chorionic gonadotropin (hCG), and parathyroid hormone (PTH) was reported (60). The tumor was unresectable and systemic metastases developed 10 months after explorato-

ry thoracotomy. The surgically obtained tumor had the histology of carcinoid tumor (fig. 4-22). Grimelius argyrophilia was noted, as well as positive immunostaining for NSE, chromogranin A, PGP9.5 and β-hCG (fig. 4-22, right); calcitonin, PTH, parathyroid hormone-related protein (PTHrP), calcitonin gene-related peptide, ACTH, GRP, serotonin, and pancreatic polypeptide were negative, and there were no features of choriocarcinoma. The surgically obtained tumor tissue contained 9,600 mIU/g wet weight hCG (whole), 140 ng/g wet weight calcitonin, and 66 μg/g wet weight NSE. Midregion PTH was 83 ng/g wet weight; C-terminal PTH, 1.7 ng/g wet weight; and N-terminal PTH was undetectable. The autopsy revealed diffuse parathyroid hyperplasia and multiple islet cell tumors of the pancreas. MEN type 1 associated with thymic

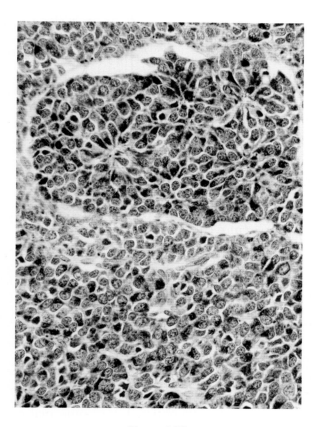

Figure 4-23

**CARCINOID TUMOR IMMUNOREACTIVE
FOR CYTOKERATIN**

The tumor cells in both solid nests and rosettes show intense immunoreactivity for low molecular weight cytokeratin (by CAM5.2) in the paranuclear region. (Courtesy of Dr. Noboru Mohri, Tokyo, Japan.)

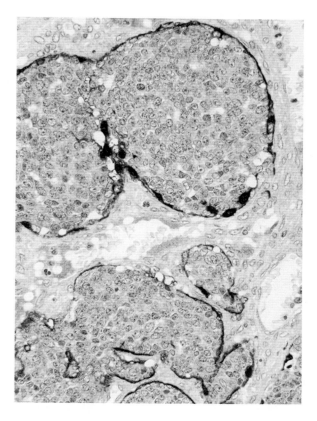

Figure 4-24

**CARCINOID TUMOR WITH S-100
PROTEIN–POSITIVE SUSTENTACULAR CELLS**

The solid tumor cell nests are bordered by elongated cells, which stain intensely for S-100 protein. The nests with sustentacular cells were limited to small areas of the primary tumor, and were not evident in tumor that recurred 10 years later.

carcinoid tumor was considered, although the pituitary gland was not examined.

Apart from bioactive substances, NCAM is always detected in thymic carcinoid tumor (fig. 4-19). With regard to cytoskeletal components, tumor cells contain low molecular weight cytokeratin, which often shows dot-like immunostaining with CAM5.2 or AE1/3 in the paranuclear region (fig. 4-23), probably corresponding to whorls of cytoplasmic fibrils. S-100 protein–positive sustentacular cells may be present focally in primary classic carcinoid tumors (figs. 4-10, 4-24), but are absent in the metastatic tumors examined thus far. Therefore, it is believed that sustentacular cells may be lost during the growth of the tumor, along with loss of an organoid arrangement.

With regard to proliferative activity, cells positive for proliferating cell nuclear antigen (PCNA) are frequently found even in a tumor with only occasional mitotic figures. In such tumors, the frequency of stained nuclei is higher in areas composed of more atypical cells. Staining may be absent in some rosettes (fig. 4-25), indicating that rosette-forming tumor cells may have reduced proliferative activity. Labeling indices of proliferation-associated nuclear antigen (Ki-67) in 11 thymic carcinoid tumors varied from 0.0 to 6.1 percent, and no correlation between the indices and prognosis or lymph node metastasis was found (18). Indices in two patients who died of tumor were 1.8 and 0.0 percent.

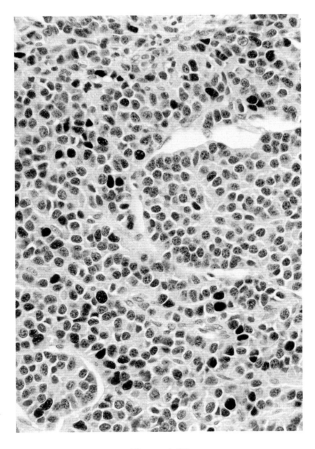

Figure 4-25

CARCINOID TUMOR IMMUNOREACTIVE WITH PROLIFERATING CELL NUCLEAR ANTIGEN (PCNA)

Slightly less than half of the tumor cells show nuclear staining for PCNA, but only a few positive cells are noted in areas with rosettes. (Courtesy of Dr. Noboru Mohri, Tokyo, Japan.)

Molecular and Other Special Diagnostic Techniques

No proven genetic information common to thymic carcinoid tumor (WDNEC) in general and of diagnostic and prognostic significance is available. In one study, 10 male patients from eight families with thymic carcinoid associated with MEN 1 and without Cushing syndrome were studied (63). Mutation analysis for genotype/phenotype correlation in the families with clustering of the tumor revealed mutations in different exons/introns of the *MEN1* gene. Loss of heterozygosity (LOH) was studied in seven cases to look for genetic abnormalities: no LOH occurred in the *MEN1* region, but LOH occurred in the 1p region of two tumors. From these results, as well as the male preponderance in this series, the authors suggested the involvement of modifying genes in addition to the *MEN1* gene and involvement of a putative tumor suppressor gene in 1p.

DNA ploidy pattern was analyzed in 8 of 12 thymic carcinoid tumors by laser scanning cytometry (18). Only 1 tumor was considered to be aneuploid; the other 7 tumors were diploid. The patient with the aneuploid tumor had multiple metastases to lymph nodes (pN3) at the time of surgery, but remains alive without an apparent recurrent tumor almost 4 years after surgery. Among the 7 patients with diploid tumors, 3 were pN0, 1 was pN1, 2 were pN2, and 1 was pN3.

Differential Diagnosis

If tumor cells are arranged in the characteristic organoid pattern, the diagnosis of thymic carcinoid tumor is easy. If the organoid pattern is vague, areas typical of carcinoid tumor should be sought by examination of multiple sections. Immunohistochemistry should be performed to exclude poorly differentiated carcinoma, malignant lymphoma, and some germ cell tumors, as well as to disclose the presence of neuroendocrine markers. Occasional diagnostic difficulty is encountered when individual cells are large and more atypical than the usual carcinoid tumor cells (figs. 4-7, 4-26). Such tumors are called "atypical" carcinoid tumors or moderately differentiated NECs by some pathologists, but it is better to designate them as nonsmall cell neuroendocrine carcinoma or large cell NEC, unless features of typical carcinoid tumor are evident elsewhere. Neuroendocrine markers are more strongly and more diffusely expressed in carcinoid tumor (WDNEC) than in poorly differentiated NEC of large cell or small cell type.

Where to draw the line between carcinoid tumor and poorly differentiated small cell or large cell NEC is controversial. Travis et al. (66) defined large cell NEC of the lung, which is discussed in detail in the following section. Their definition can be largely applied to thymic tumors except for the number of mitoses, since up to 21 mitoses per 10 high-power fields may be seen in thymic tumors with features characteristic of carcinoid tumor.

Thyroid transcription factor-1 (TTF-1) was reported to be positive in 19 of 20 pulmonary carcinoid tumors but negative in 3 thymic carcinoid tumors and 50 intestinal carcinoid tumors (45), and it may be used for differentiation from pulmonary carcinoid tumor. Thymic carcinoid tumor should be differentiated from metastatic carcinoid tumor from other organs, such as the lung and gastrointestinal tract, particularly when TTF-1 is negative. In such cases, information regarding preoperative imaging and surgical findings is of great help for the differential diagnosis. Paraganglioma can be differentiated from thymic carcinoid tumor by the histologic patterns in most cases, but in some cases, immunohistochemistry for low molecular weight cytokeratin, which is negative in paraganglioma, is needed.

Type B3 thymoma may mimic thymic carcinoid tumor if the former has a rosette-like structure or is composed of short spindle cells with finely granular cytoplasm. Rosette-like structures in thymoma are devoid of central lumens and are frequently associated with lymphocytes; rosettes in carcinoid tumors often possess lumens and are not infiltrated with lymphocytes. In a difficult case, immunohistochemical analysis of tumor cells and lymphocytes is helpful for diagnosis. Rarely, structures resembling perivascular spaces are seen in carcinoid tumor; these are often artifacts.

When the immunohistochemical findings are still inconclusive, the presence of neurosecretory granules disclosed by electron microscopy is diagnostic. Some thymic carcinoid tumors produce unknown bioactive substances whose presence cannot yet be verified.

Treatment and Prognosis

The standard treatment for thymic carcinoid tumor has not been established, but the first choice is surgical removal of the neoplasm with regional lymph node dissection, since anterior mediastinal and cervical lymph nodes are the frequent sites of metastasis. There is no standard in lymph node dissection, since lymphatic flow in the anterior mediastinum and its surroundings has not yet been fully understood, and it may depend on the location of the tumor. If the tumor is pT1 at stage I (see Tables 2-10 to 2-13), adjuvant therapy may

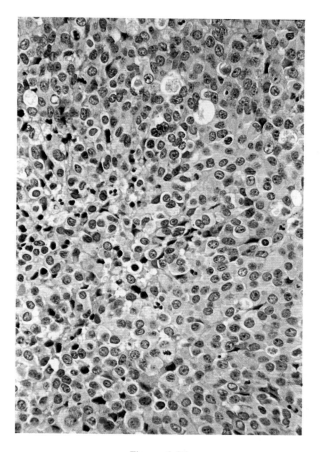

Figure 4-26

CARCINOID TUMOR WITH AREAS OF STRUCTURAL AND CELLULAR ATYPIA

Diffuse growth of moderately large cells with round to oval finely granular nuclei, small nucleoli, and a moderate amount of ground-glass cytoplasm. A few mitotic figures and frequent pyknotic cells are present. Grimelius argyrophilia was evident. The tumor was inoperable and the patient died 2 years later with widespread metastases. (Courtesy of Dr. Tetsuro Kodama, Utsunomiya, Japan.)

not be needed, but if the tumor is pT2 at stage I or higher, postoperative radiotherapy, with or without chemotherapy, is indicated. Needless to say, if curative surgery cannot be performed or if lymph node metastasis is detected, adjuvant therapy must be considered.

The prognosis of patients with Cushing syndrome is invariably poor. Even without such a syndrome, the prognosis of patients with thymic carcinoid tumor is worse than previously believed, in comparison with patients with carcinoid tumor of other organs (71). Of 15 patients, 11 had metastases and 8 of these were either dead or likely to die from the tumor. Of 4 patients without metastases, 2 died of Cushing syndrome and 2 survived without recurrence for 1 year after surgery.

A study of 14 treated patients with atypical carcinoid tumors revealed a poor prognosis for patients with large tumors (6 to 20 cm) (12). The overall survival rates were 46 percent and 31 percent at 3 and 5 years, respectively; however, all the patients died of disease within 109 months as a result of local progression, local relapse, distant metastases, or a combination of these. The median survival periods were 71, 30, and 5 months for patients who had total resection, partial resection, and simple biopsy, respectively. In a large series of 80 cases of carcinoid tumor, clinical follow-up was obtained in 50 patients (43). Overall survival was approximately 60 percent at 5 years and approximately 25 percent at 10 years. Patients with low-grade tumors (typical carcinoid) had 5- and 10-year disease-free survival rates of 50 percent and 9 percent, respectively; those with intermediate-grade tumors (atypical carcinoid) had 20 percent and 0 percent, respectively; and those with high-grade tumors (small cell carcinoma and large cell NEC) had a 5-year survival rate of 0 percent. The results were distinctly worse than those for patients with pulmonary carcinoid and NEC (4,67). It was concluded that the behavior of thymic neuroendocrine carcinoma seems to correlate with the histologic grade and degree of differentiation of the tumor (43).

Regarding the 40 cases of carcinoid tumor collected by a questionnaire survey in Japan (29), invasion of the lung was seen in 40 percent; pericardium, 30 percent; brachiocephalic artery, 25 percent; and superior vena cava, 10 percent. Lymph node metastasis was seen in 25 percent of cases, and the recurrence and 5-year survival rates after grossly complete removal of the tumor were 64 percent and 85 percent, respectively. Of 11 carcinoid tumors surgically resected at the National Cancer Center Hospitals in Tokyo and Kashiwa, tumors had invaded surrounding structures in 4 cases, lymph node metastases were detected in 6, recurrence occurred in only 2, and the 5-year survival rate was 82 percent. Even with recurrence, the clinical course was generally protracted, and one patient was still alive 4 years after the local recurrence. Two patients, both of whom had stage IV tumors at the time of diagnosis, died of systemic metastasis. The reason for better survival in Japan than in other countries is unknown.

Frequent sites of metastasis include mediastinal lymph nodes, cervical lymph nodes, lung, bone, and liver (15,43). Bone metastases are often osteoblastic.

POORLY DIFFERENTIATED NEUROENDOCRINE CARCINOMAS

Large cell NEC and small cell carcinoma of neuroendocrine type are included in this category.

Large Cell Neuroendocrine Carcinoma

Histologically, *large cell NEC* of the thymus is similar to the lung cancer of the same name. The histologic criteria of pulmonary large cell NEC (66) have been adopted for the mediastinal counterpart: 1) organoid nesting, trabecular, palisading, and rosette-like patterns; 2) increased mitoses (11 or more per 10 high-power fields, average 60); 3) features of nonsmall cell carcinoma; 4) frequent necrosis; and 5) neuroendocrine differentiation by immunohistochemistry or electron microscopy. Compared to carcinoid tumors, individual tumor cells are larger and organoid histologic structures are less distinct. However, distinction between the two tumors may be difficult, as discussed in the previous section.

Reported cases of large cell NEC are few and some appear to have been diagnosed as atypical carcinoid tumor or NEC. The prognosis of patients is generally poor (7,9,27,43). Individual tumor cells are large and polygonal, with a low nuclear to cytoplasmic ratio, often large vesicular nuclei, and prominent nucleoli. Pleomorphic or giant tumor cells may be seen. In a reported case, mitotic figures ranged from 19 to 26 per 10 high-power fields and areas similar to those seen in carcinoid tumors were noted (9). Tumor cells were strongly positive for NSE, chromogranin A, and low molecular weight (by CAM5.2) and broad spectrum (by AE1/3) cytokeratins. The patient died 2 years and 2 months after incomplete removal of the tumor. Cases with areas similar to carcinoid tumor may be diagnosed by some pathologists as carcinoid tumor with atypia (anaplasia).

An illustrative case of thymic large cell NEC is described. An anterior mediastinal tumor was disclosed by CT in a 61-year-old woman (fig. 4-27A). Malignant thymic tumor was the diagnosis obtained by needle core biopsy, most likely atypical carcinoid tumor. The tumor was adherent to the visceral pleura of the right upper lobe of the lung, and combined resection was performed with resection of metastases to the mediastinal and supraclavicular lymph nodes. The tumor was circumscribed, but nonencapsulated, with an ivory colored, irregularly lobulated surface including small pale yellow opaque areas of necrosis (fig. 4-27B). The tumor invaded the lung parenchyma. Histologically, it consisted of solid nests of medium-sized polygonal cells with vesicular hyperchromatic nuclei, some distinct nucleoli, and a small to moderate amount of cytoplasm. Mitotic figures were frequent (30 per 10 high-power fields). Although the palisading of tumor cells at the periphery of the tumor nests was not conspicuous, occasional rosettes were noted (fig. 4-27C). Metastases were found in 33 of 41 lymph nodes examined. Cells immunoreactive for bcl-2, leu-7, chromogranin A, synaptophysin, S-100 protein, carcinoembryonic antigen (CEA), hCG, PGP9.5, cytokeratins (by CAM5.2 and 34βE12), and c-kit (fig. 4-27D) were scattered. NCAM, NSE, somatostatin, serotonin, calcitonin, pancreatic polypeptide, and ACTH were negative. Ki-67-positive cells were found in about 10 percent of tumors. The patient is on antitumor chemotherapy for recurrent cancer 14 months postoperatively.

Small Cell Carcinoma of Neuroendocrine Type

Thymic *small cell carcinoma* is characterized by diffuse growth and solid nests of small polygonal to spindle cells with finely granular nuclei, inconspicuous nucleoli, scanty cytoplasm, and ill-defined cell borders. Rosettes and extensive areas of coagulation necrosis may be present (fig. 4-28). In some cases, tumors with features of small cell carcinoma have well-differentiated areas with a carcinoid histology (27,43,73,75).

The features of neuroendocrine tumors presented in the literature include dense core granules of 100 to 200 nm or 200 to 500 nm in diameter depending upon the type of tumor reported (fig. 4-29), and the presence of immunoreactive NSE, chromogranin A, synaptophysin, NCAM, and brain gut amine and peptide hormones (fig. 4-28C) (64,66). In the lung, the typical histology of small cell carcinoma, without ultrastructural or immunohistochemical evidence of neuroendocrine features, is sufficient to categorize a tumor as small cell carcinoma (of neuroendocrine type), since the presence of neuroendocrine features is difficult to prove in 20 to 30 percent of cases. This is in contrast to the criteria for large cell NEC, in which the presence of neuroendocrine features is required for diagnosis. Although evidence of neuroendocrine differentiation is usually found in thymic small cell carcinoma on ultrastructural or immunohistochemical examination (52,65), neurosecretory granules are few in number and often difficult to find (fig. 4-29), and the intensity and extent of positive immunoreactivity for neuroendocrine markers are much less than in carcinoid tumors. Investigations of the neuroendocrine properties of this tumor are still insufficient, and no standardized definition of neuroendocrine small cell carcinoma has yet been given.

Since dense core granules may not be neurosecretory granules but small lysosomes or exocrine granules, immunoelectron microscopy is necessary to prove the granules to be of neurosecretory type. Not only their morphology but also their location, often beneath the cell membrane or within cytoplasmic processes, are important for identification in routine practice. A few amine and peptide hormones have been identified, including ACTH in the tumor of a case of thymic small cell carcinoma associated with Cushing syndrome (20,51). Therefore, care must be exercised in the use of the term neuroendocrine carcinoma.

Small cell carcinoma, neuroendocrine type, of the thymus has been reported occasionally in the world literature but there has been no unequivocal case similar to small (oat) cell carcinoma of the lung reported in the National Cancer Center Hospital of Tokyo over the last 40 years, except three consultation cases, one pure small cell carcinoma of the thymus and two combined small cell carcinomas. The case of pure small cell carcinoma was in a 71-year-old female, who underwent complete resection of a 7.5 x 5.0 x 2.0 cm anterior mediastinal tumor (Masaoka stage II) followed by 50 Gy of irradiation. Ten months later the patient developed multiple

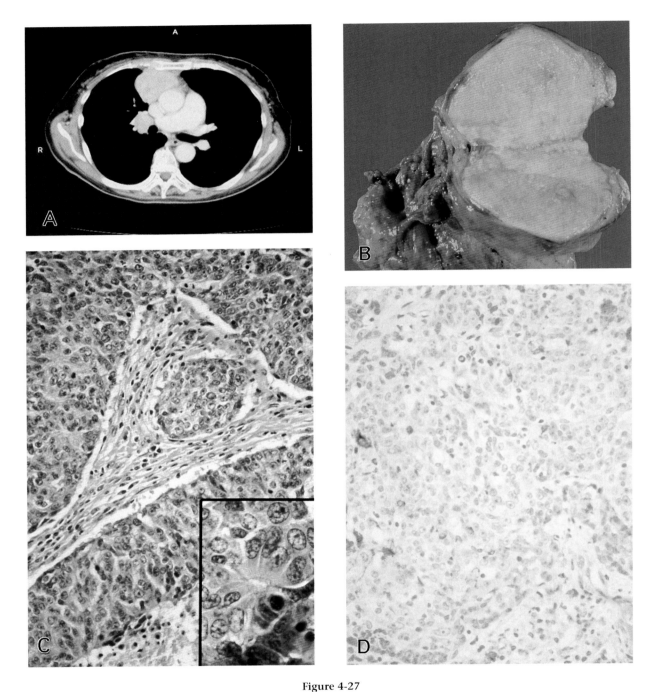

Figure 4-27

LARGE CELL NEUROENDOCRINE CARCINOMA

A: CT reveals a 53 x 44 mm, well-defined, anterior mediastinal tumor in which a small low density area suggestive of cystic degeneration is present. Also present is a mediastinal metastatic node on the right side, which extends to the right supraclavicular region. Invasion into the lung parenchyma is not apparent.

B. The anterior mediastinal tumor shows a well-circumscribed, granular or irregularly lobulated cut surface, with pale yellow areas of necrosis. The tumor is present largely within the thymus.

C. Histologically, the tumor consists of solid nests of small to medium-sized polygonal cells with hyperchromatic vesicular nuclei, some distinct nucleoli, and small to moderate amounts of cytoplasm. The inset reveals a rosette.

D. Immunohistochemically, scattered cells are chromogranin A positive. (Courtesy of Dr. Toru Kameya, Shizuoka, Japan.)

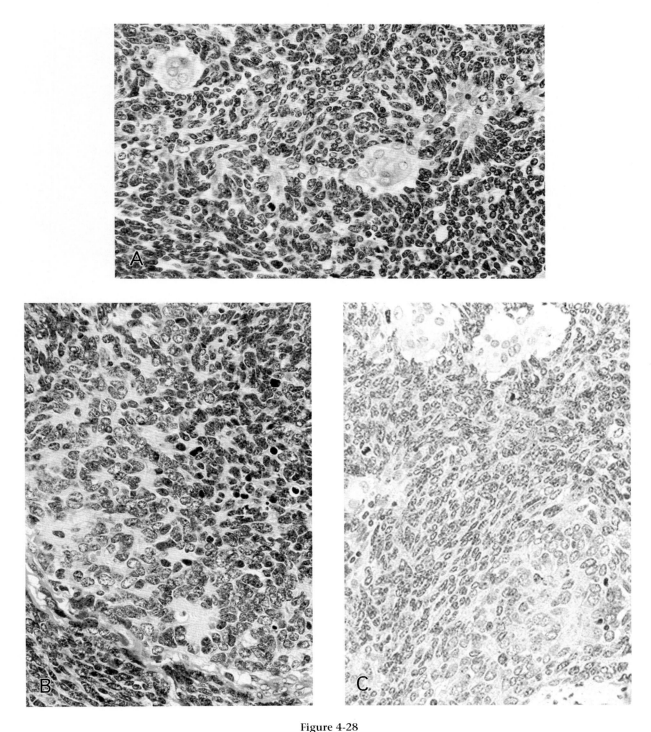

Figure 4-28

SMALL CELL CARCINOMA

A: The tumor cells diffusely infiltrate and engulf non-neoplastic thymic epithelial cells. They have scanty cytoplasm with ill-defined cell borders and nuclei with finely granular chromatin and inconspicuous nucleoli.

B: Higher magnification reveals a few rosettes.

C: Some large tumor cells are weakly positive for synaptophysin. Chromogranin A was negative. (Courtesy of Dr. Keiko Ishii, Matsumoto, Japan.)

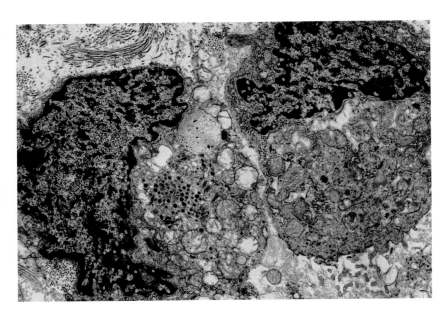

Figure 4-29

ULTRASTRUCTURE OF SMALL CELL CARCINOMA

Only a few tumor cells, as shown here, contain neurosecretory granules. (Fig. 11 from Truong LD, Mody DR, Cagle PT, Jackson-York GL, Schwartz MR, Wheeler TM. Thymic carcinoma. A clinicopathologic study of 13 cases. Am J Surg Pathol 1990;14:163.)

implantation metastases in the right pleural cavity with effusion, which contained tumor cells with features of small cell carcinoma. The NSE level in the pleural fluid was 40 ng/mL (normal: less than 10 ng/mL). There was no tumor in the lung. Histologically, the tumor was a typical small cell carcinoma with a few rosettes, frequent mitotic figures, and small scattered foci of necrosis. Immunohistochemically, NSE was positive focally, synaptophysin was positive in a few cells, but cytokeratin, chromogranin A, GRP, and somatostatin were negative (fig. 4-28).

Combined Small Cell Carcinoma. A combination of small cell carcinoma and squamous cell carcinoma appears to be more frequent in the thymus than in the lung. One of four cases reported by Truong et al. (68), and all of three cases (two with squamous cell carcinoma and one with adenosquamous carcinoma) reported by Kuo et al. (33) were combined small cell carcinomas. Dense core granules are rare and cases with positive immunohistochemical neuroendocrine markers are limited in number, suggesting that epithelial characteristics predominate over neuroendocrine characteristics in many thymic combined small cell carcinomas. Since NSE is not neuron specific in other organs, and is the only neuroendocrine marker shown in some reported cases of thymic combined small cell carcinoma, its reactivity in other subtypes of thymic carcinoma should be tested. Thymic small cell carcinoma, which is called neuroendocrine by many investigators,

shows a lower frequency of neuroendocrine markers than small cell carcinoma of the lung. Some cases may not be neuroendocrine carcinomas but poorly differentiated squamous cell carcinomas with small tumor cells. More detailed investigation is necessary before categorizing such cases as neuroendocrine.

A case that was difficult to diagnose is shown in figure 4-30. An anterior mediastinal tumor demonstrating limited invasion into the upper lobe of the lung was resected. The tumor was composed of solid nests of small short spindle cells, frequent rosette-like structures, and small areas with glandular structures. Mitotic figures were easily found. Special stains disclosed an absence of epithelial mucin and the presence of immunoreactive NSE and a secretory component. NCAM and chromogranin A could not be demonstrated. This may have been a rare case of combined small cell carcinoma and adenocarcinoma of the thymus, considering similar features were seen in a case of carcinoid tumor (see figs. 4-9, 4-15, right). The fact that NSE was the only neuroendocrine marker in this case, however, cannot exclude the possibility of poorly differentiated adenocarcinoma predominantly composed of small tumor cells.

Another case shown in figure 4-31 is also problematic diagnostically, and histologically may or may not be a combined small cell carcinoma. This anterior mediastinal tumor invaded the left upper lobe of the lung, pericardium,

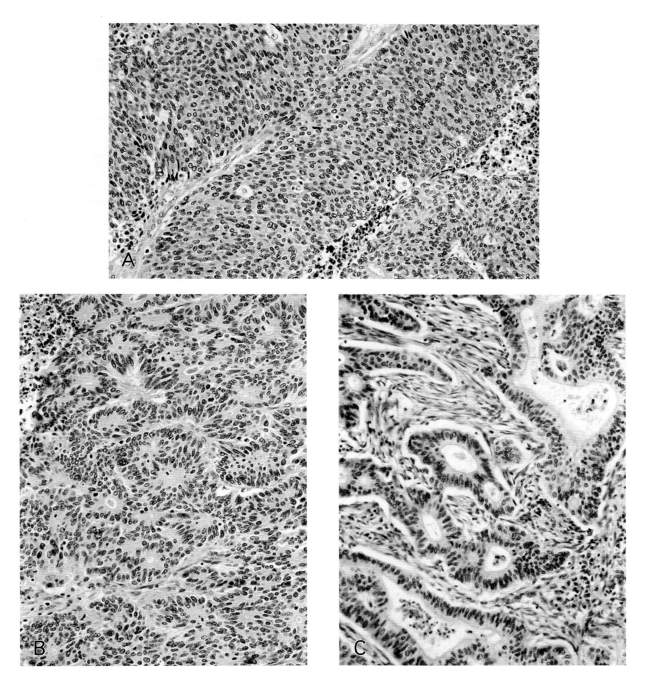

Figure 4-30

POSSIBLE COMBINED SMALL CELL AND ADENOCARCINOMA OF PROBABLE THYMIC ORIGIN

A: Solid nests of the tumor consist of small short spindle cells with oval, finely granular nuclei and scanty cytoplasm. A single rosette is seen. The histology is similar to small cell carcinoma of the lung.

B: In some areas, frequent rosettes are present.

C: In a small area, glandular structures are lined by columnar cells. The ABPAS stain revealed no epithelial mucin and only a glycocalyx is present at the luminal border of the cells.

Immunohistochemically, NSE was positive, but no other neuroendocrine markers were detected, including NCAM, chromogranin A, and synaptophysin. This could be poorly differentiated adenocarcinoma of small tumor cell type. (Courtesy of Dr. Shinji Masuda, Takaoka, Japan.)

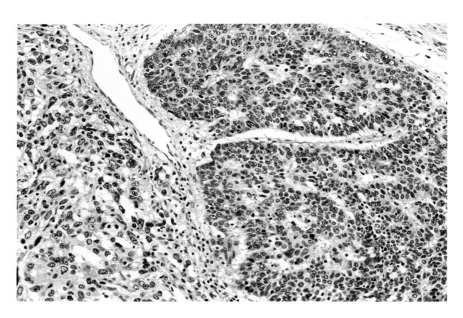

Figure 4-31

PROBABLE COMBINED SMALL CELL AND LARGE CELL CARCINOMA

Small cell carcinoma with rosettes is on the right and large cell carcinoma on the left. The area with small cell carcinoma shows characteristic finely granular nuclei, and that with the large cell component, vesicular nuclei with distinct nucleoli. A possibility of adenocarcinoma of small tumor cell type cannot be excluded. (Courtesy of Dr. Yoshiro Tachiyama, Hiroshima, Japan.)

and left brachiocephalic vein. It consisted in part of rosette-like or small glandular structures composed of small tumor cells and in part of irregularly arranged medium-sized tumor cells with vesicular nuclei and small nucleoli. Immunohistochemically, the tumor cells were positive for NSE and weakly positive for chromogranin A. The Grimelius stain revealed no argyrophilia. This case could also be poorly differentiated adenocarcinoma with scattered neuroendocrine type tumor cells.

Histogenesis

The cell of origin of poorly differentiated NECs is not known but is probably the same as that of carcinoid tumors (WDNEC), that is, primitive epithelial cells present in the thymus.

Cytologic Findings

We have no experience with needle aspiration cytology of poorly differentiated NEC, both small cell carcinoma and large cell NEC. The cytologic findings are probably identical to those in the pulmonary counterpart.

Immunohistochemical Findings

Because of the small number of cases reported and encountered, it is difficult to make a general statement concerning the immunoreactivity of the tumor cells of poorly differentiated NECs. From the definition of large cell NEC, the tumor cells should react with low molecular weight cytokeratin and at least one neuroendocrine marker, such as chromogranin A, synaptophysin, NCAM (CD56), or brain-gut peptide, excluding NSE and CD57 (leu-7). The latter two markers are nonspecific and react with not only neuroendocrine cells but also some non-neuroendocrine cells. From our experience with lung tumors, it is assumed that fewer cells are reactive with chromogranin A, synaptophysin, and NCAM in large cell NEC than carcinoid tumor. Frequent overexpression of c-kit in pulmonary large cell NEC is reported (1), but it is not a useful marker for thymic tumors, since some non-neuroendocrine type thymic carcinomas are also immunoreactive for c-kit (see the section on thymic carcinoma immunohistochemistry).

In small cell carcinoma, tumor cells reactive with chromogranin A and synaptophysin may be difficult to find except, if present, in areas with features of carcinoid tumor. Immunoreactivity for NCAM is expected to be present in poorly differentiated NEC but must be confirmed at that time. Reactivity to low molecular weight cytokeratin is either minimal or absent except in areas with features of carcinoid tumor. CK20 is negative in most pulmonary small cell carcinomas and in a few of the tested thymic poorly differentiated NECs of small cell type, while TTF-1 is positive in many pulmonary small cell carcinomas and some extrapulmonary small cell carcinomas. This indicates that both CK20 and TTF-1 are of limited value for diagnosing thymic tumors (8,10), although further study is needed for TTF-1.

Molecular and Other
Special Diagnostic Techniques

Because of the rarity of thymic poorly differentiated NECs, there is no information available regarding genetics or other molecular changes related to the oncogenesis of and susceptibility to these tumors, and which would be of diagnostic and prognostic significance.

Differential Diagnosis

Poorly differentiated NEC of the thymus should be distinguished from pulmonary large cell NEC and small cell carcinoma metastatic to the mediastinum. For this purpose, clinical data such as imaging and surgical findings are most important. The usefulness of TTF-1 is unclear at present. Differentiation from other thymic carcinomas requires a detailed histologic examination and immunostaining for neuroendocrine markers, since thymic carcinoma may contain groups of synaptophysin-positive tumor cells and scattered chromogranin A-positive cells.

Prognosis and Malignancy-Associated Factors

As already stated, the prognosis of patients with both small cell carcinoma and large cell NEC is poor, and worse than that for carcinoid tumor. Recurrences are common; all reported patients have died of the tumor between 1 and 4 years after diagnosis (7,15,27,42,43). In contrast to the very poor prognosis of patients with small cell carcinoma of the lung, many of whom die within 1 to 2 years of diagnosis, there is a longer average survival time for patients with thymic small cell carcinoma of both pure and combined types. This indicates that some thymic small cell carcinomas are different from small cell carcinoma of the lung, and either are morphologically and biologically related to carcinoid tumor (43,75) or are related to poorly differentiated squamous cell carcinoma of small cell type.

In a large series of 87 cases of large cell NEC of the lung, the overall 5-year survival rate was 57 percent (61). Five-year survival rates of patients with stages I, II, III, and IV were 67, 75, 45, and 0 percent, respectively. There was no statistically significant difference between the overall survival rate of patients with large cell NEC and those with other poorly differentiated nonsmall cell lung cancers. The outcome for those with stage I large cell NEC was poorer than that for patients with the same stage of other poorly differentiated nonsmall cell lung cancers (61).

Treatment

Although TNM classification and staging are important factors for determining treatment, intense postoperative adjuvant therapy, either irradiation, chemotherapy, or combined radiochemotherapy, should be instituted for patients with tumors in every stage, even stage II, aiming at longer survival and ultimate cure. In cases in which the histologic or cytologic diagnosis has been established with aspiration cytology or needle biopsy, preoperative chemotherapy may be indicated. Treatment strategy will be standardized after accumulation of more cases.

COMBINED THYMIC EPITHELIAL TUMORS (INCLUDING NEUROENDOCRINE CARCINOMAS)

Combined thymic epithelial tumors include tumors showing a combination of distinct subtypes of thymoma and thymic carcinoma or NEC. Excluded from this category are tumors with combinations of two or more thymoma subtypes, such as type B2 and B3 thymoma; tumors showing a mixture of thymic carcinoma subtypes, such as thymic carcinoma with areas of squamous cell carcinoma and areas of lymphoepithelioma-like carcinoma; and combined small cell carcinoma.

Combined thymic epithelial tumors may be called *composite thymoma-thymic carcinoma, mixed neuroendocrine carcinoma and thymoma*, and other related terms. In order to make a diagnosis of combined thymic epithelial tumor, both components must be clearly recognizable on hematoxylin and eosin (H&E)-stained sections. The amount or percentage occupied by each component should be recorded in the diagnosis.

The classification and definition of combined thymic epithelial tumors in the most recent WHO classification (65) are confusing. In the table of tumor categories, combined thymic epithelial tumors are placed in the category of thymic carcinoma, and this may be due to a mistake in the printing. In the text, cases with a combination of thymoma subtypes such as

B2 and B3 thymomas, and combined small cell carcinoma are described as examples of combined thymic epithelial tumors. Thymoma is known to display different subtypes in a single tumor, and such cases should be designated as composite thymoma but not as combined thymic epithelial tumor.

Combined thymic epithelial tumors are rare. A combination of thymoma and thymic carcinoma is occasionally seen (see figs. 3-17, 3-18, 3-24). The most frequent combination is type B3 thymoma and squamous cell carcinoma (see fig. 3-18). Some thymic squamous cell and adenosquamous carcinomas have a small cell carcinoma component (31,33). These are not combined thymic epithelial tumors, but are combined small cell carcinomas. Combined B2/B3 thymoma is placed in the category of combined thymic epithelial tumors by some investigators (65), but this interpretation is not acceptable. A combination of two or more distinct thymoma subtypes is due to malignant progression of thymoma or of low-grade NEC into higher-grade tumors, or due to bidirectional differentiation of multipotential thymic epithelial precursor cells. Collision of two different tumors occurs rarely.

Grossly, two different components may or may not be recognized. Microscopically, a recognizable transition between the two components may or may not be observed.

The case shown in figure 4-32 is probably a combined carcinoid tumor (WDNEC) and thymoma in an elderly man (18,53). The tumor was encapsulated and 4 cm in greatest dimension (fig. 4-32A). Microscopically, lobulation by fibrous septa was apparent. The tumor consisted of typical carcinoid tumor cells forming rosettes; solid nests of larger tumor cells with finely granular eosinophilic cytoplasm resembling oncocytes; and polygonal to oval epithelial cells arranged in nests and sheets with frequent dilated perivascular spaces resembling epithelial cell-predominant (type B3) thymoma (fig. 4-32B–D). The Grimelius silver reaction was positive only in the rosette-forming and oncocytoid cells. NSE was positive in limited areas, and rare cells containing pancreatic polypeptide and calcitonin were found. NCAM, chromogranin A, synaptophysin, somatostatin, GRP, serotonin, and ACTH were negative. Electron microscopic examination of paraffin-embedded tissue dem-

onstrated that some cells were equipped with tonofibrils and desmosomes but not with membrane-bound electron–dense granules, whereas other cells contained electron-dense granules of the neurosecretory type without features of thymic epithelial cells. This case suggested a combination of carcinoid tumor (WDNEC) and thymoma. The presence of such a tumor in the thymus indicates that the neoplasm developed from primitive multipotential (or bipotential) cells, supporting the concept of the histogenesis of carcinoid tumor described previously (55).

Another somewhat similar case of combined thymoma and carcinoid tumor was recently reported. The patient was a 42-year-old Japanese woman; an anterior mediastinal tumor invading the pericardium and lung was surgically resected (54). The tumor was lobulated and consisted largely of small oval cells with or without small nucleoli and scattered terminal deoxynucleotidyltransferase (TdT), CD1a-, and CD99-positive lymphocytes. Areas with squamoid features suggestive of B3 thymoma were also noted. Perivascular spaces were frequently dilated. In other lobules, there were frequent Hassall corpuscle–like squamous pearls surrounded by small oval epithelial cells (fig. 3-33A). Since the serum NSE was elevated to 110 ng/dL preoperatively, immunostaining for chromogranin A, synaptophysin, NSE, and NCAM (CD56) was done, all of which were strongly positive in small nests at the periphery of the tumor lobules without Hassall corpuscle-like pearls (fig. 4-33C). Close examination of such lobules on H&E-stained sections showed that individual tumor cells with positive neuroendocrine markers at the periphery of the lobules were smaller than thymoma cells and resembled carcinoid tumor cells (fig. 4-33B). Electron microscopic study also confirmed the presence of small dense core granules in the cytoplasm of a few tumor cells. Although these two cases were included in the section of combined thymic epithelial tumor, they are more correctly diagnosed as type B3 thymoma with focal neuroendocrine differentiation.

A case of combined spindle cell thymoma and carcinoid tumor was reported by Cho et al. (11), which was associated with pure red cell aplasia. In this case, a large carcinoid tumor was surrounded by a spindle cell thymoma.

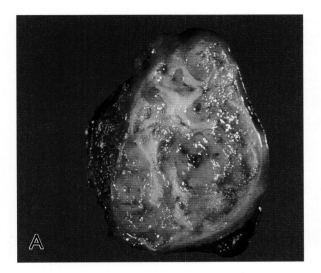

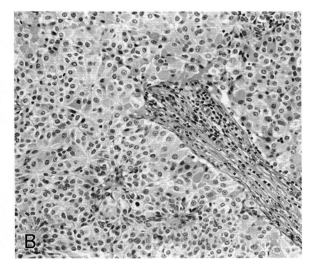

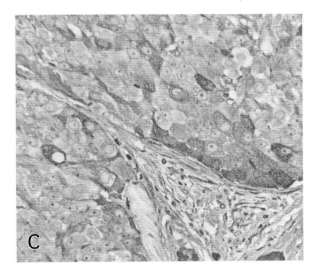

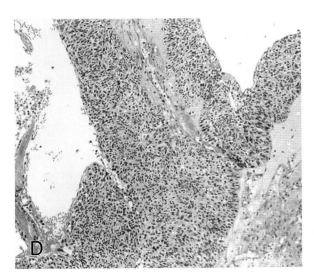

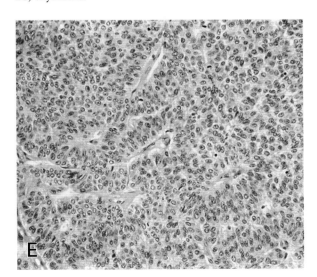

Figure 4-32

TYPE B3 THYMOMA WITH NEUROENDOCRINE DIFFERENTIATION (WITH FEATURES OF CARCINOID TUMOR)

A: Grossly, the tumor is completely encapsulated and partly lobulated.

B: The tumor is incompletely lobulated by fibrous septa. It is composed of oval to polygonal cells with oval nuclei and small but distinct nucleoli forming rosettes. Some tumor cells possess abundant eosinophilic cytoplasm and resemble oncocytes.

C: Grimelius stain of an area similar to that shown in B discloses a positive reaction in the cytoplasm, stronger in the cells bordering the cell nests.

D: In some areas, there are cystic spaces and perivascular spaces with a few lymphoid cells. Palisading tumor cells line the perivascular space.

E: In other areas, oval to short spindle tumor cells with distinct nucleoli show diffuse growth and palisading around blood vessels, resembling predominantly epithelial (type B3) thymoma.

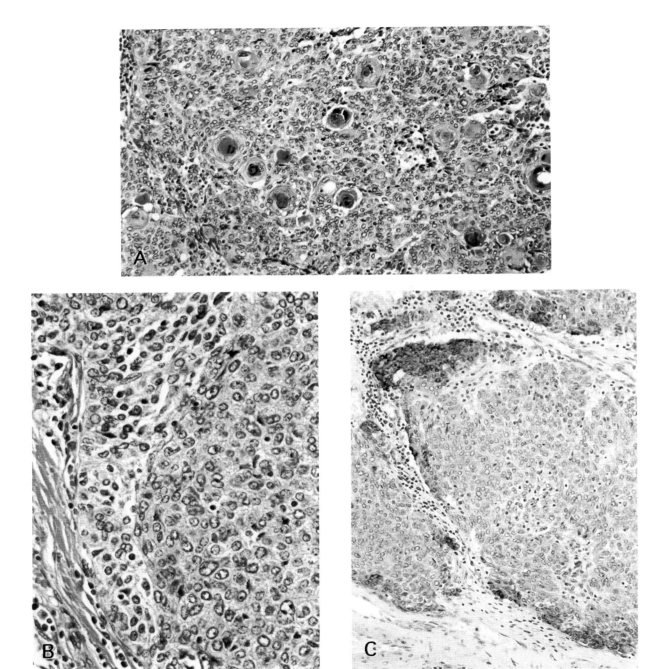

Figure 4-33

TYPE B3 THYMOMA WITH NEUROENDOCRINE DIFFERENTIATION (WITH FEATURES OF CARCINOID TUMOR)

A: The tumor is lobulated and composed largely of small oval/polygonal cells with scattered lymphocytes. In some lobules, there are many Hassall corpuscle–like structures. This variant has been described as thymoma with squamous cell (Hassall corpuscle) differentiation.

B: High-power view of the periphery of a lobule reveals a band of small cells resembling carcinoid tumor cells, which are clearly distinguishable from thymoma cells.

C: Small nests at the periphery of tumor lobules are strongly positive for chromogranin A. A similar staining pattern was obtained by immunostaining for synaptophysin, neuron-specific enolase (NSE), and neural cell adhesion molecule (NCAM). (Courtesy of Dr. Junichi Shiraishi, Tokyo, Japan.)

Coexistence of thymoma in the right lobe and carcinoid tumor in the left lobe of the thymus has been reported (38). A case of carcinoid tumor with divergent sarcomatoid differentiation was also reported (30). It was composed of nests of carcinoid tumor cells in a sarcomatous stroma characterized by fibrosarcoma-like spindle cells with areas of chondroid and osseous differentiation. Areas with features of carcinoid tumor were reported to be positive for NSE, vimentin, and cytokeratin. This neoplasm was weakly positive for synaptophysin and somatostatin, and negative for chromogranin A, ACTH, and calcitonin. Ultrastructurally, the spherical dense core granules of neurosecretory type were much smaller than those in the carcinoid tumor.

The prognosis of patients with combined thymic epithelial tumors is determined by the most aggressive component.

REFERENCES

1. Araki K, Ishii G, Yokose T, et al. Frequent overexpression of the c-kit in large cell neuroendocrine carcinoma of the lung. Lung Cancer 2003;40:173-80.
2. Arrigoni MG, Woolner LB, Bernatz PE. Atypical carcinoid tumors of the lung. J Thorac Cardiovasc Surg 1972;64:413-21.
3. Barbareschi M, Frigo B, Mosca L, et al. Bronchial carcinoids with S-100 positive sustentacular cells. A comparative study with gastrointestinal carcinoids, pheochromocytomas and paragangliomas. Pathol Res Pract 1990;186:212-22.
4. Beasley MB, Thunnissen FB, Brambilla E, et al. Pulmonary atypical carcinoid: predictors of survival in 106 cases. Hum Pathol 2000;31:1255-65.
5. Birnberg FA, Webb WR, Selch MT, Gamsu G, Goodman PC. Thymic carcinoid tumors with hyperparathyroidism. AJR Am J Roentgenol 1982;139:1001-4.
6. Boix E, Pico A, Pinedo R, Aranda I, Kovacs K. Ectopic growth hormone-releasing hormone secretion by thymic carcinoid tumour. Clin Endocrinol (Oxf) 2002;57:131-4.
7. Chalabreysse L, Etienne-Mastroianni B, Adeleine P, Cordier JF, Greenland T, Thivolet-Bejui F. Thymic carcinoma: a clinicopathological and immunohistological study of 19 cases. Histopathology 2004;44:367-74.
8. Chan JK, Suster S, Wenig BM, Tsang WY, Chan JB, Lau AL. Cytokeratin 20 immunoreactivity distinguishes Merkel cell (primary cutaneous neuroendocrine) carcinomas and salivary gland small cell carcinomas from small cell carcinomas of various sites. Am J Surg Pathol 1997;21:226-34.
9. Chetty R, Batitang S, Govennder D. Large cell neuroendocrine carcinoma of the thymus. Histopathology 1997;31:274-6.
10. Cheuk W, Kwan MY, Suster S, Chan JK. Immunostaining for thyroid transcription factor 1 and cytokeratin 20 aids the distinction of small cell carcinoma from Merkel cell carcinoma, but not pulmonary from extrapulmonary small cell carcinomas. Arch Pathol Lab Med 2001;125:228-31.
11. Cho KJ, Ha CW, Koh JS, Zo JI, Jang JJ. Thymic carcinoid tumor combined with thymoma—neuroendocrine differentiation in thymom? J Korean Med Sci 1993;8:458-63.
12. de Montpreville VT, Macchiarini P, Dulmet E. Thymic neuroendocrine carcinoma (carcinoid): a clinicopathologic study of fourteen cases. J Thorac Cardiovasc Surg 1996;111:134-41.
13. de Perrot M, Spiliopoulos A, Fischer S, Totsch M, Keshavjee S. Neuroendocrine carcinoma (carcinoid) of the thymus associated with Cushing's syndrome. Ann Thorac Surg 2002;73:675-81.
14. Fukai I, Masaoka A, Fujii Y, et al. Thymic neuroendocrine tumor (thymic carcinoid): a clinicopathologic study in 15 patients. Ann Thorac Surg 1999;67:208-11.
15. Gal AA, Kornstein MJ, Cohen C, Duarte IG, Miller JI, Mansour KA. Neuroendocrine tumors of the thymus: a clinicopathological and prognostic study. Ann Thorac Surg 2001;72:1179-82.
16. Gherardi G, Marveggio C, Placidi A. Neuroendocrine carcinoma of the thymus: aspiration biopsy, immunocytochemistry, and clinicopathologic correlates. Diag Cytopathol 1995;12:158-64.
17. Gibril F, Chen YJ, Schrump DS, et al. Prospective study of thymic carcinoids in patients with multiple endocrine neoplasia type 1. J Clin Endocrinol Metab. 2003;88:1066-81.
18. Goto K, Kodama T, Matsuno Y, et al. Clinicopathologic and DNA cytometric analysis of carcinoid tumors of the thymus. Mod Pathol 2001;14:985-94.
19. Hakânson R, Larsson LI, Sundler F. Peptide and amine producing endocrine-like cells in the chicken thymus. A chemical, histochemical and electron microscopic study. Histochemistry 1974;39:25-34.

20. Hekimgil M, Hamulu F, Cagirici U, et al. Small cell neuroendocrine carcinoma of the thymus complicated by Cushing's syndrome. Report of a 58-year-old woman with a 3-year history of hypertension. Pathol Res Pract 2001;197:129-33.

21. Herbst WM, Kummer W, Hoffmann W, Otto H, Heym C. Carcinoid tumors of the thymus. An immunohistochemical study. Cancer 1987;60:2465-70.

22. Hishima T, Fukayama M, Hayashi Y, et al. Neuroendocrine differentiation in thymic epithelial tumors with special reference to thymic carcinoma and atypical thymoma. Hum Pathol 1998;29:330-8

23. Ho FC, Ho JC. Pigmented carcinoid tumour of the thymus. Histopathology 1977;1:363-9.

24. Huntrakoon M, Lin F, Heitz PU, Tomita T. Thymic carcinoid tumor with Cushing's syndrome. Report of a case with electron microscopic and immunoperoxidase studies for neuron-specific enolase and corticotropin. Arch Pathol Lab Med 1984;108:551-4.

25. Jansson JO, Svensson J, Bengtsson BA, et al. Acromegaly and Cushing's syndrome due to ectopic production of GHRH and ACTH by a thymic carcinoid tumour: in vitro responses to GHRH and GHRP-6. Clin Endocrinol (Oxf) 1998;48:243-50.

26. Kay S, Wilson MA. Ultrastructural studies of an ACTH-secreting thymic tumor. Cancer 1970;26:445-52.

27. Klemm KM, Moran CA. Primary neuroendocrine carcinomas of the thymus. Semin Diag Pathol 1999;16:32-41.

28. Klemm KM, Moran CA, Suster S. Pigmented thymic carcinoids: a clinicopathological and immunohistochemical study of two cases. Mod Pathol 1999;12:946-8.

29. Kondo K, Monden Y. A questionnaire about thymic epithelial tumors in Japan. Nippon Gekagakkai Zasshi 2001;15:633-42. (in Japanese with English abstract)

30. Kuo TT. Carcinoid tumor of the thymus with divergent sarcomatoid differentiation: report of a case with histogenetic consideration. Hum Pathol 1994;25:319-23.

31. Kuo TT. Frequent presence of neuroendocrine small cells in thymic carcinoma: a light microscopic and immunohistochemical study. Histopathology 2000;37:19-26.

32. Kuo TT. Pigmented spindle cell carcinoid tumour of the thymus with ectopic adrenocorticotropic hormone secretion: report of a rare variant and differential diagnosis of mediastinal spindle cell neoplasms. Histopathology 2002;40:159-65.

33. Kuo TT, Chang JP, Lin FJ, Wu WC, Chang CH. Thymic carcinomas: histopathological varieties and immunohistochemical study. Am J Surg Pathol 1990;14:24-34.

34. Lagrange W, Dahm HH, Karstens J, Feichtinger J, Mittermayer C. Melanocytic neuroendocrine carcinoma of the thymus. Cancer 1987;59:484-8.

35. Lancaster KJ, Liang CY, Myers JC, McCabe KM. Goblet cell carcinoid arising in a mature teratoma of the mediastinum. Am J Surg Pathol 1997;21:109-13.

36. Lauriola L, Erlandson RA, Rosai J. Neuroendocrine differentiation is a common feature of thymic carcinoma. Am J Surg Pathol 1998;22: 1059-66.

37. Marchkevsky AM, Dikman SH. Mediastinal carcinoid with an incomplete Sipple's syndrome. Cancer 1979;43:2497-501.

38. Mizuno T, Masaoka A, Hashimoto T, et al. Coexisting thymic carcinoid tumor and thymoma. Ann Thorac Surg 1990;50:650-2.

39. Moran CA, Suster S. Spindle-cell neuroendocrine carcinomas of the thymus (spindle-cell thymic carcinoid): a clinicopathologic and immunohistochemical study of seven cases. Mod Pathol 1999;12:587-91.

40. Moran CA, Suster S. Angiomatoid neuroendocrine carcinoma of the thymus: report of a distinctive morphological variant of neuroendocrine tumor of the thymus resembling a vascular neoplasm. Hum Pathol 1999;30:635-9.

41. Moran CA, Suster S. Primary neuroendocrine carcinoma (thymic carcinoid) of the thymus with prominent oncocytic features: a clinicopathologic study of 22 cases. Mod Pathol 2000;13:489-94.

42. Moran CA, Suster S. Thymic neuroendocrine carcinomas with combined features ranging from well-differentiated (carcinoid) to small cell carcinoma. A clinicopathologic and immunohistochemical study of 11 cases. Am J Clin Pathol 2000;113:345-50.

43. Moran CA, Suster S. Neuroendocrine carcinomas (carcinoid tumor) of the thymus. A clinicopathologic analysis of 80 cases. Am J Clin Pathol 2000,114:100-10.

44. Nichols GL, Hopkins MB, Geisinger KR. Thymic carcinoid. Report of a case with diagnosis by fine needle aspiration biopsy. Acta Cytol 1997;41:1839-44.

45. Oliveira AM, Tazelaar HD, Myers JL, Erickson LA, Lloyd RV. Thyroid transcription factor-1 distinguishes metastatic pulmonary from well-differentiated neuroendocrine tumors of other sites. Am J Surg Pathol 2001;25:815-9.

46. Paties C, Zangrandi A, Vassallo G, Rindi G, Solcia E. Multidirectional carcinoma of the thymus with neuroendocrine and sarcomatoid components and carcinoid syndrome. Pathol Res Pract 1991 187:170-7.

47. Pearse AG, Polak JM, Heath CM. Polypeptide hormone production by "carcinoid" apudomas and their relevant ctyochemistry. Virchow Arch B Cell Pathol 1974;16:95-109.

48. Pictet RL, Rall LB, Phelps P, Rutter WJ. The neural crest and the origin of the insulin-producing and other gastrointestinal hormone-producing cells. Science 1976;191:191-2.

49. Rosai J, Higa E. Mediastinal endocrine neoplasm, of probable thymic origin, related to carcinoid tumor. Clinicopathologic study of 8 cases. Cancer 1972;29:1061-74.

50. Rosai J, Higa E, Davie J. Mediastinal endocrine neoplasm in patients with multiple endocrine adenomatosis. A previously unrecognized association. Cancer 1972;29:1075-83.

51. Rosai J, Levine GD. Tumors of the thymus. Atlas of Tumor Pathology, 2nd Series, Fascicle 13. Washington, D.C.: Armed Forces Institute of Pathology; 1976.

52. Rosai J, Sobin LH. Histologic typing of tumours of the thymus. World Health Organization international histological classification of tumours, 2nd ed. New York: Springer-Verlag; 1999.

53. Shimosato Y, Mukai K. Tumors of the mediastinum, Atlas of Tumor Pathology, 3rd Series, Fascicle 21, Washington, D.C.: Armed Forces Institute of Pathology; 1997.

54. Shiraishi J, Nomori H, Orikasa H, Mori T, Yamazaki K. Atypical thymoma (WHO B3) with neuroendocrine differentiation: report of a case. Virchows Arch 2006;449:234-7.

55. Sidhu GS. The endodermal origin of digestive and respiratory tract APUD cells. Histopathologic evidence and a review of the literature. Am J Pathol 1979;96:5-20.

56. Smith NL, Finley JL. Lipid-rich carcinoid tumor of the thymus gland: diagnosis by fine-needle aspiration biopsy. Diagn Cytopathol 2001;25:130-3.

57. Sugiura H, Morikawa T, Itoh K, et al. thymic neuroendocrine carcinoma: a clinicopathologic study in four patients. Ann Thorac Cardiovasc Surg 2000;6:304-8.

58. Suster S, Moran CA. Thymic carcinoid with prominent mucinous stroma. Report of a distinctive morphologic variant of thymic neuroendocrine neoplasm. Am J Surg Pathol 1995;19:1277-85.

59. Suster S, Moran CA. Neuroendocrine neoplasms of the mediastinum. Am J Clin Pathol 2001;115[Suppl]: S17-27.

60. Takayama T, Kameya T, Inagaki K, et al. MEN type 1 associated with mediastinal carcinoid producing parathyroid hormone, calcitonin and chorionic gonadotropin. Pathol Res Pract 1993;189:1090-6.

61. Takei H, Asamura H, Maeshima A, et al. Large cell neuroendocrine carcinoma of the lung: a clinicopathologic study of eighty-seven cases. J Thoracic Cardiovasc Surg 2002;124:285-92.

62. Tanaka T, Tanaka S, Kimura H, Ito J. Mediastinal tumor of thymic origin and related to carcinoid tumor. Acta Pathol Jpn 1973;24:413-26.

63. Teh BT, Zedenius J, Kytola S, et al. Thymic carcinoids in multiple endocrine neoplasia type 1. Ann Surg 1998;228:99-105.

64. Tome Y, Hirohashi S, Noguchi M, et al. Immunocytologic diagnosis of small-cell lung cancer in imprint smears. Acta Cytol 1991;35:485-90.

65. Travis WD, Brambille E, M ller-Hermelink HK, Harris CC, eds. World Health Organization Classification of Tumours. Pathology and genetics of tumours of the lung, pleura, thymus and heart. Lyon: IARC Press; 2004.

66. Travis WD, Linnoila RI, Tsokos MG, et al. Neuroendocrine tumors of the lung with proposed criteria for large-cell neuroendocrine carcinoma. An ultrastructural, immunohistochemical, and flow cytometric study of 35 cases. Am J Surg Pathol 1991;15:529-53.

67. Travis WD, Rush W, Flieder DB, et al. Survival analysis of 200 pulmonary neuroendocrine tumors with clarification of criteria for atypical carcinoid and its separation from typical carcinoid. Am J Surg Pathol 1998;22:934-44.

68. Truong LD, Mody DR, Cagle PT, Jackson-York GL, Schwartz MR, Weeler TM. Thymic carcinoma. A clinicopathologic study of 13 cases. Am J Surg Pathol 1990;14:151-66.

69. Valli M, Fabris GA, Dewar A, et al. Atypical carcinoid tumour of the thymus: a study of eight cases. Histopathology 1994;24:371-5.

70. Wang DY, Kuo SH, Chang DB, et al. Fine needle aspiration cytology of thymic carcinoid. Acta Cytol 1995;39:423-7.

71. Wick MR, Carney JA, Bernatz PE, Brown LR. Primary mediastinal carcinoid tumors. Am J Surg Pathol 1982;6:195-205.

72. Wick MR, Rosai J. Neuroendocrine neoplasms of the mediastinum. Semin Diagn Pathol 1991;8:35-51.

73. Wick MR, Scheithauer BW. Oat cell carcinoma of the thymus. Cancer 1982;49:1652-7.

74. Wick MR, Scheithauer BW. Thymic carcinoid. A histologic, immunohistochemical, and ultrastructural study of 12 cases. Cancer 1984;53:475-84.

75. Wick MR, Scheithauer BW, Weiland LH, Bernatz PE. Primary thymic carcinomas. Am J Surg Pathol 1982;6:613-30.

5 GERM CELL TUMORS

DEFINITION AND CLASSIFICATION

A *germ cell tumor* is believed to develop from a germ cell during the process of maturation of a primordial germ cell into a gamete. It can arise not only in the gonad but also in the midline of the body, such as in the intracranial pineal region, anterior mediastinum, retroperitoneum, and sacrococcygeal region, where germ cells migrate during embryogenesis and sometimes become misplaced (ectopic germ cells). Since the thymus is located in the midline of the thorax, it is easily understood that a germ cell tumor may develop within, or in the proximity of, the thymus. In fact, almost all mediastinal germ cell tumors are found either within or adjacent to the thymus. Rare occurrences in the posterior mediastinum or within the pericardial sac have been reported (5,52,62). Although this "misplacement" theory in which mediastinal germ cell tumors originate from ectopic primordial germ cells is supported by recent genetic and epigenetic data (10,12,57,58), and is generally believed to be so, it has not yet been proven in every tumor. Some mediastinal germ cell tumors could well originate from somatic cells, such as the primordial cells of the thymus (25,74), i.e., through anaplasia of the primitive thymic epithelial cells to form totipotential cells. In support of this theory, Kaplan et al. (28) reported that "extragonadal teratomas arise mitotically from diploid cells and no heterosexual (XX) tumors were seen in males, which would be expected in parthenogenetic tumors."

Every form of germ cell tumor occurs in the mediastinum: teratoma (mature, immature, and with a secondary malignant component), seminoma (germinoma), embryonal carcinoma, yolk sac tumor (endodermal sinus tumor), choriocarcinoma, and mixed germ cell tumor. Table 5-1 shows the classification of germ cell tumors based on the modified World Health Organization (WHO) system (66,70). We are not aware of any reported cases of spermatocytic seminoma in the mediastinum, however.

INCIDENCE AND CLINICAL FEATURES

Mediastinal germ cell tumors are rare neoplasms, accounting for about 15 percent of all mediastinal cysts and tumors (62,74). They occur at all ages, although there is a bimodal age distribution, with one peak in infancy and another in childhood/adolescence (41). In infants and children less than 8 years of age, teratoma and yolk sac tumor make up almost all of the germ cell tumors. There is no sex predilection for teratoma but a female predominance for yolk sac tumor (ratio, 4 to 1) (58). All of the malignant nonseminomatous germ cell tumors in older patients in one series occurred in males (58).

The anterior mediastinum is the most frequent site of extragonadal germ cell tumors. Fewer germ cell tumors of the mediastinum, however, were surgically resected during the past 41 years at the National Cancer Center Hospital, Tokyo,

Table 5-1

MODIFIED WORLD HEALTH ORGANIZATION CLASSIFICATION OF GERM CELL TUMORS[a]

Tumors of One Histologic Type
  Seminoma
  Spermatocytic seminoma
  Embryonal carcinoma
  Yolk sac tumor (adult type)
  Yolk sac tumor (childhood type)
  Teratoma
    Mature
    Immature
    With a secondary malignant component
  Choriocarcinoma

Mixed Germ Cell Tumors
  Embryonal carcinoma and mature or immature teratoma
  Yolk sac tumor and mature or immature teratoma
  Seminoma and teratoma
  Seminoma and embryonal carcinoma
  Choriocarcinoma and embryonal carcinoma
  Choriocarcinoma and teratoma
  Choriocarcinoma and seminoma

[a]Section from Table 47-3 from Ulbright TM. Testicular and paratesticular tumors. In: Sternberg's diagnostic surgical pathology, 4th ed. Mills SE, Carter D, Greenson JK, Oberman HA, Reuter V, Stoler MH, eds. Philadelphia: Lippincott Williams & Wilkins; 2004:2170.

Table 5-2

SURGICALLY RESECTED GERM CELL TUMORS[a]

	No. of Cases (Age)	
	Male	Female
One histologic type		
MT (or with IMT)[b]	26 (6-54)[c]	34(11-72)
(with Ca or Sa)	0	0
Sem	2 (19, 21)	0
Em	0	0
YST	1 (23)	0
Cho	2 (15, 22)	0
Mixed germ cell tumors		
MT + YST	1 (58)	0
MT + Em	1 (27)	0
MT +I MT +YST	2 (15, 25)	0
MT + IMT + Sem + Ad	1 (17)	0
MT+ IMT + Ad + CaSa + NB	1 (39)	0
IM T+ Sem	1 (17)	0
IMT + Sem + Ad	1 (24)	0
IMT + YST	1 (17)[d]	0
Sem + YST	1 (29)	0
Germ cell tumors after chemo-therapy (tumors of indeterminate histologic type)	11 (11-41)	1 (41)[e]

[a]At National Cancer Center, Tokyo (1962~2003).
[b]MT = mature teratoma; IMT = immature teratoma; Ca = carcinoma; Sa = sarcoma; Sem = seminoma; Em = embryonal carcinoma; YST = yolk sac tumor (all YSTs were of adult type); Cho = choriocarcinoma; Ad = adenocarcinoma; CaSa = carcinosarcoma; NB = neuroblastoma.
[c]Five with IMT.
[d]Died of acute leukemia 9 months after surgery.
[e]MT with necrosis and history of elevated alpha-1-fetoprotein. During the same period, five patients treated without surgery were autopsied (two cases of YST, and one case each of Em, Sem, and IMT + Ca). All were males, aged 27 to 43 years. A case of IMT + Ca was complicated with malignant histiocytosis. One patient with YST + Sem diagnosed by biopsy died of tumor (no autopsy), and one patient with Sem diagnosed by biopsy is living and well.

than thymomas (87 versus 138) (Table 5-2); they accounted for 13 percent of all gonadal and extragonadal germ cell tumors resected. The remaining germ cell tumors were testicular (42 percent), ovarian (42 percent), and intracranial and sacrococcygeal (3 percent). This incidence depends upon the type of institution reporting.

Mature teratoma accounts for about 70 percent of germ cell tumors of the mediastinum. It is found in patients of all ages but most frequently in adolescents. In adult females, all tumors are mature teratomas, mostly cystic. Immature teratoma, the pure form of which accounts for about 1 percent and the mixed form for about 15 percent of all mediastinal germ cell tumors, is more frequent in children and adolescents. Teratoma with a secondary malignant component; malignant germ cell tumors such as seminoma, embryonal carcinoma, yolk sac tumor, and choriocarcinoma; and mixed germ cell tumors represent about 30 percent of all mediastinal germ cell tumors. They develop overwhelmingly in males, as is the case with immature teratoma, although there are a few reported cases of malignant germ cell tumor in female infants and young children, particularly yolk sac tumors (58).

Only one female patient had a malignant germ cell tumor at the National Cancer Center Hospital in Tokyo. She was 41 years of age and presented with an anterior mediastinal tumor of 8 cm in the greatest dimension and elevated alpha-fetoprotein (AFP) levels (4,210 ng/mL). She was treated with intensive chemotherapy followed by surgical resection. The resected tumor revealed foci of mature teratoma and areas of necrosis with ghost tumor cells. Mixed germ cell tumor with mature teratoma and either yolk sac tumor or embryonal carcinoma was suspected, but immunostaining of selected areas were negative for tumor markers including AFP, placental alkaline phosphatase, and beta-human chorionic gonadotropin (β-hCG).

Mature teratomas are often clinically silent and are frequently found by chest X-ray examination. Some patients complain of cough, dyspnea, and chest pain, which are due to compression of the airways and other structures by a large mediastinal teratoma. Rarely, patients cough up the contents of the tumor, including hair. This happens after destruction of the bronchi, probably as a result of friction and compression of the lung tissue by the tumor (fig. 5-1).

Most patients with immature teratoma, teratoma with a secondary malignant component, and other malignant germ cell tumors are symptomatic at the time of diagnosis. They present not only with cough, dyspnea, and chest pain due to compression of organs by the rapidly growing tumor, but also with fatigue and weight loss. Gynecomastia may be evident when the tumor contains choriocarcinoma.

Patients with Klinefelter syndrome are predisposed to develop germ cell tumors, particularly those of an extragonadal origin (22,23,38). Lachman et al. (30), in their review of the literature found 20 cases of primary mediastinal germ

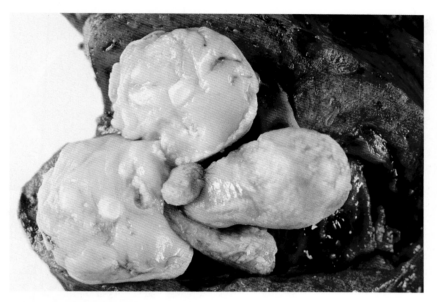

Figure 5-1

**MATURE TERATOMA
INVADING THE LUNG**

Polypoid tumors occlude and distend a bronchus. The tumor surface is opaque to semitranslucent. Mature fat and cartilage are apparent at the cut surface.

cell tumor associated with Klinefelter syndrome and 252 cases of primary mediastinal germ cell tumor in the normal male population. The incidence of Klinefelter syndrome among patients with mediastinal germ cell tumors is roughly 30 to 40 times that of Klinefelter syndrome among the general population. Almost all kinds of germ cell tumors, both benign and malignant, occur in patients with Klinefelter syndrome. Hasle et al. (22) reported a case of a 14-year-old boy with Klinefelter syndrome and a mediastinal malignant germ cell tumor showing features of mixed choriocarcinoma and teratoma. These investigators reviewed 40 cases of primary mediastinal germ cell tumor associated with Klinefelter syndrome, all of which were of nonseminomatous histology. At least 8 percent of the male patients with primary mediastinal germ cell tumors had the syndrome, 50 times the expected frequency. In another study, Hasle et al. (23) found a total of 39 neoplasms of various kinds (relative risk of 1.1) and 4 malignant mediastinal germ cell tumors (relative risk of 67) among a cohort of 696 men with Klinefelter syndrome. They concluded that there was no increase in overall cancer incidence but a considerably elevated risk of developing a mediastinal germ cell tumor in the period from early adolescence until the age of 30 years.

The association of hematologic malignancies with mediastinal germ cell tumors has been investigated (17,47a,53). de Ment (17) reviewed 16 cases with simultaneous presentation, and 19 cases of hematologic malignancies that developed 48 months or more after chemotherapy for mediastinal germ cell tumor. This incidence is greater than would be expected by chance alone. de Ment proposed two hypotheses: that hematopoietic malignancies arise from pluripotent germ cells and that alternatively, teratocarcinoma cells may elaborate factor S, which promotes the growth and differentiation of leukemic blast cells. The most frequent synchronous hematologic malignancy seen by de Ment was malignant histiocytosis, followed by acute myelomonocytic leukemia. Many cases of the former were reclassified recently as anaplastic large cell lymphoma. We have also seen one case each of acute leukemia and malignant histiocytosis associated with mediastinal germ cell tumors (Table 5-2). Hematologic malignancies that develop after chemotherapy for germ cell tumors include acute myelogenous leukemia, acute megakaryocytic leukemia, and acute myelomonocytic leukemia.

Nichols et al. (47a) described 16 cases of hematologic neoplasia associated with mediastinal germ cell tumors, all of which were nonseminomatous germ cell tumors, the most important of which were tumors with yolk sac elements. The two most common hematologic neoplasms were acute megakaryoblastic leukemia and malignant histiocytosis. Their review suggested that the hematologic neoplasia is not

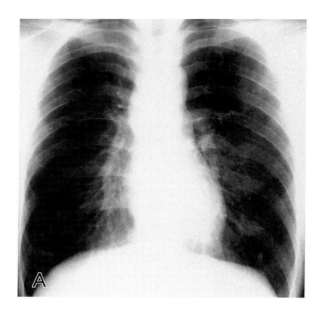

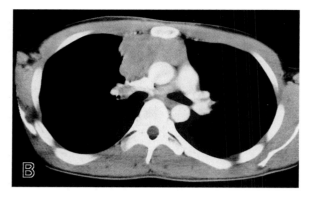

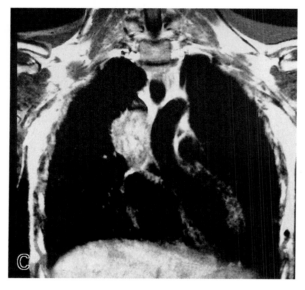

Figure 5-2

MEDIASTINAL SEMINOMA

A: A plain chest X ray reveals a tumorous density projecting toward the right lung from the right pulmonary hilum to the superior mediastinal region.

B: Enhanced computerized tomography (CT) with radiopaque material shows a retrosternal, well-defined tumorous density compressing the ascending aorta and superior vena cava posteriorly.

C: Thoracic magnetic resonance imaging (MRI) of a coronal section at the level of the ascending aorta reveals a nonhomogeneously enhanced tumor adjacent to the right border of the ascending aorta. (Fig. 3-170 from Fascicle 21, Third Series.)

the result of cisplatin-based chemotherapy for germ cell tumors. The finding of the marker chromosome isochromosome (12p) in both a germ cell tumor and leukemic blasts in one patient suggested that these tumors may arise from a common progenitor cell.

DIAGNOSTIC APPROACH

Posteroanterior and lateral chest roentgenograms frequently reveal a large, round or nodular mass in the anterior or anterosuperior mediastinum, in many instances displacing, and at times invading, the adjacent structures such as the trachea, lung, and major vessels (fig. 5-2). Areas of calcification may be seen in the tumor. Pleural effusion may be present in patients with malignant germ cell tumors. Air may accumulate within the tumor, if the tumor communicates with the trachea or bronchi (fig. 5-3). Roentgenologic

findings are not specific for germ cell tumors, and differentiation from other thymic tumors may be impossible. Computerized tomography (CT) is useful for detecting small tumors that are not seen on routine chest X rays.

Multilocular cyst formation is seen not only in mediastinal seminoma but also in a variety of conditions including thymoma, thymic carcinoma, and Hodgkin or other type of malignant lymphoma. Whenever an anterior (or superior) mediastinal tumor is detected in male patients, a serologic study for tumor markers should be done, including β-hCG for choriocarcinoma and AFP for yolk sac tumor.

For histologic confirmation of the nature of the tumor, a needle biopsy can be done either percutaneously or through a mediastinoscope (figs. 5-4–5-6). When the lung is invaded, transbronchial biopsy can also be attempted.

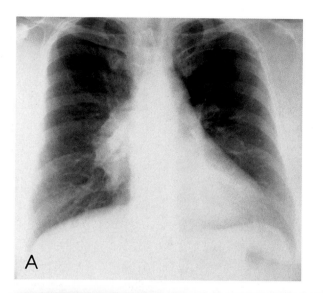

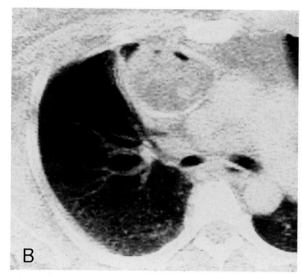

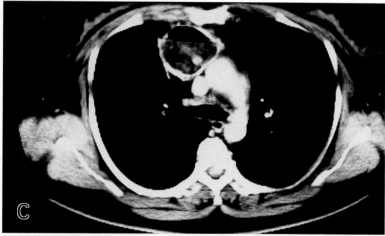

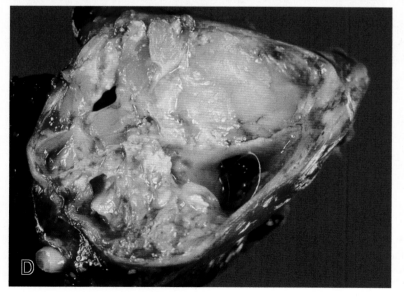

Figure 5-3

MEDIASTINAL MATURE TERATOMA

A: Plain chest X ray reveals a large tumor projecting toward the right lung from the right pulmonary hilar region, which overlaps the right cardiac border. A close look shows free air near the superior border of the tumor.

B: An enlarged CT view reveals engulfment of a B5 bronchus by the peripheral portion of the tumor. There are a few air spaces anteriorly and a ring-shaped calcification posteriorly on the right.

C: CT enhanced with radiopaque material at the level of the tracheal bifurcation shows a tumor anterior to the ascending aorta and superior vena cava compressing the right lung. The tumor is irregularly stained and has a fluid level.

D: A horizontal slice of the resected tumor shows fibrofatty tissue, calcified areas, and a few cystic spaces lined with a smooth membrane and containing a hair. In the left lower corner, the involved B5 bronchus is evident. (Fig. 3-171 from Fascicle 21, Third Series.)

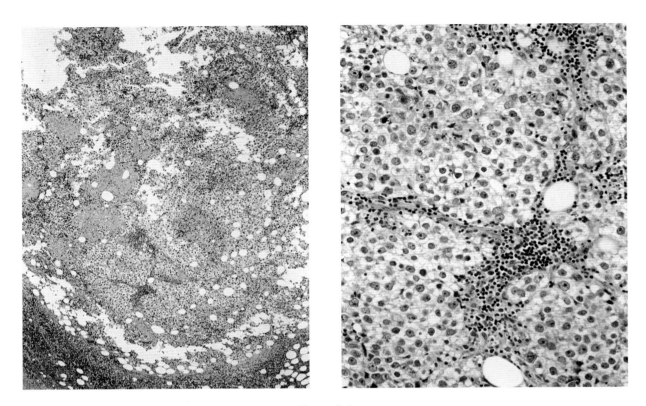

Figure 5-4

SEMINOMA DIAGNOSED BY PERCUTANEOUS NEEDLE BIOPSY

Left: Partly necrotic tumor tissue infiltrates fatty tissue. The tumor tissue consists of solid nests of moderately large polygonal cells with clear cytoplasm, round nuclei, and prominent nucleoli, supported by a fibrous stroma densely infiltrated by lymphoid cells, features characteristic of seminoma.

Right: High-power view.

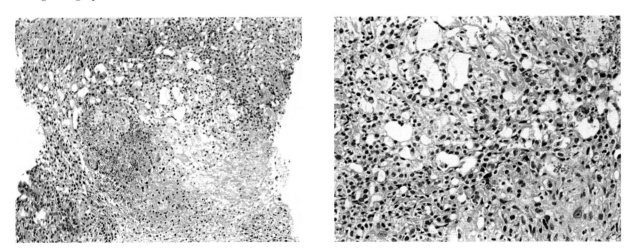

Figure 5-5

YOLK SAC TUMOR DIAGNOSED BY PERCUTANEOUS NEEDLE BIOPSY

Left: The tumor is necrotic and hemorrhagic in some areas, with a reticular pattern and solid growth. Intracellular and intercellular hyaline substances are also evident. These histologic features are characteristic of yolk sac tumor.

Right: High-power magnification. (Figs. 5-5 and 5-28 are from the same patient.)

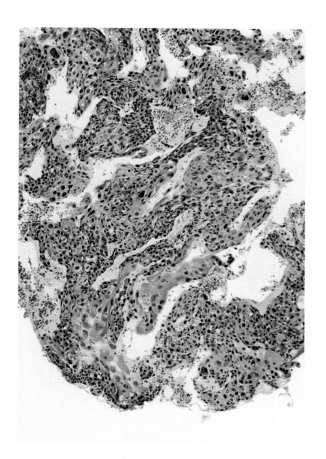 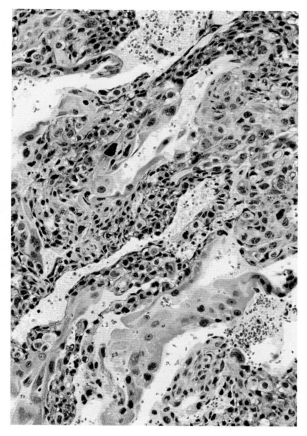

Figure 5-6

CHORIOCARCINOMA DIAGNOSED BY PERCUTANEOUS NEEDLE BIOPSY

Left: The viable tumor tissue is composed of round to polygonal mononuclear cells resembling cytotrophoblasts and multinucleated cells with deeply eosinophilic cytoplasm resembling syncytiotrophoblasts. A diagnosis of choriocarcinoma was confirmed by positive beta-human chorionic gonadotropin (β-hCG) immunostaining.

Right: Medium-power magnification.

Fine needle aspiration cytology has a high degree of accuracy in establishing a diagnosis of mediastinal germ cell tumors, particularly when serum levels and immunocytochemistry of tumor markers, such as AFP, β-hCG, and placental alkaline phosphatase, help confirm the diagnosis (11,14,16,44,54).

Mature cystic teratoma can easily be diagnosed by the recognition of normal cellular components and by the absence of atypical cells (fig. 5-7). Immature teratoma, on the contrary, may be difficult to diagnose, because cells may show some nuclear atypia with an increased nuclear to cytoplasmic ratio (fig. 5-8). The absence of obviously malignant cells, however, suggests immature teratoma.

Seminoma cells show characteristic features. They are large, with scant to moderately abundant cytoplasm, and round to slightly irregular, finely granular or vesicular nuclei, with either a central prominent nucleolus or two to three smaller nucleoli. Variable numbers of lymphocytes and plasma cells are present (fig. 5-9) (11,16). Cytochemical staining for placental alkaline phosphatase helps distinguish seminoma from poorly differentiated carcinoma (11,44). A characteristic "tigroid" background may be found in air-dried fine needle aspiration specimens that are stained by the Giemsa or Diff Quik stain, although this does not seem to be as well documented in mediastinal seminomas as with seminomas at other anatomic sites (11,16,38a)

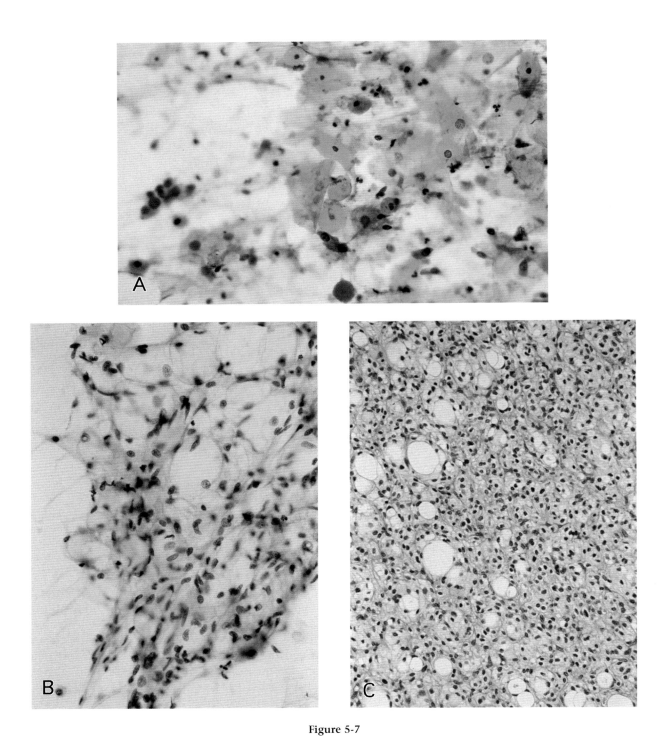

Figure 5-7

NEEDLE ASPIRATION CYTOLOGY OF MATURE CYSTIC TERATOMA

A: The smear consists largely of normal-appearing squamous epithelial cells and some inflammatory cells. No atypical cells are present.

B: A cell aggregate is composed of intact and degenerating fat cells with some foamy macrophages. Individual cells have bland nuclei.

C: Hematoxylin and eosin (H&E)-stained section of an area corresponding to the cellular aggregate shown in B. (Courtesy of Dr. Yoshiro Ebihara, Tokyo, Japan.)

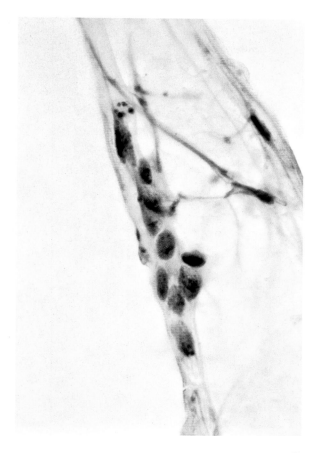
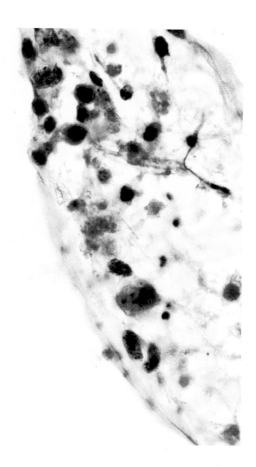

Figure 5-8

NEEDLE ASPIRATION CYTOLOGY OF IMMATURE TERATOMA

Left: Cells are cohesive, with distinct cytoplasm and mildly atypical nuclei, suggesting an epithelial nature.

Right: Dispersed cells in a mucinous background are not cohesive and are moderately pleomorphic, suggesting that they are mesenchymal in nature and probably immature cartilage cells. There are no cells that suggest malignant germ cell tumor. (Courtesy of Dr. Yoshiro Ebihara, Tokyo, Japan.)

Yolk sac tumor shows cohesive clusters of cells with large nuclei, vacuolated cytoplasm, and extracellular hyaline spheres or globules. Embryonal carcinoma has tumor cells with hyperchromatic nuclei and scanty cytoplasm arranged in tubules and papillae. Choriocarcinoma displays mononuclear cells with vesicular nuclei and distinct nucleoli, as well as multinucleated giant tumor cells (fig. 5-10) (16).

Distinction from thymoma can be made easily due to the cellular components. Occasional difficulty is encountered in distinguishing malignant germ cell tumors from either primary or metastatic poorly differentiated carcinoma with regard to cytologic diagnosis without any immunocytochemical staining (60,76).

TUMORS OF ONE HISTOLOGIC TYPE

Teratoma

Teratoma is either mature, immature, or with a secondary malignant component (either carcinoma or sarcoma). It accounts for more than half of all mediastinal germ cell tumors. Mature teratoma shows an equal gender distribution or slight female predominance, while immature teratoma occurs almost exclusively in males. In the second series Fascicle on Extragonadal Teratoma, Gonzalez-Crussi (20) classified teratoma as shown in Table 5-3 into broad categories of benign and malignant. While this may be useful in practice for better communication with clinicians, the

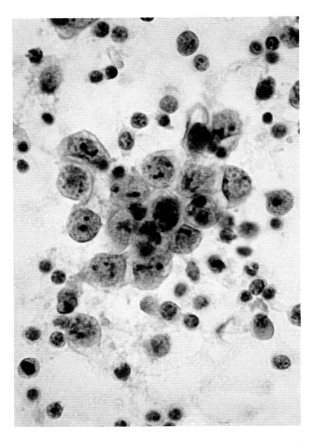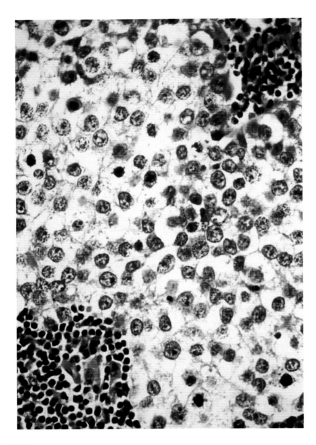

Figure 5-9

NEEDLE ASPIRATION CYTOLOGY OF MEDIASTINAL SEMINOMA

Left: Large round cells in an aggregate possess vesicular nuclei, varying sized distinct nucleoli, and a small amount of cytoplasm. They are surrounded by lymphoid cells.

Right: Histologically, the resected tumor has the typical features of seminoma. The patient was 29-year-old man in whom serum alpha-fetoprotein (AFP) and β-hCG were within the normal range.

classification may not correlate well with prognosis (see TNM classification and staging).

Grossly, mature teratomas are often cystic and are rarely predominantly solid (figs. 5-3, 5-11). They are encapsulated and occasionally adhere to the surrounding structures with fibrous tissue. The cut surface reveals a variegated appearance: unilocular or multilocular cavities containing brown fluid or oily or grumous material with or without hair. In the cyst walls or solid areas, fatty tissue, medullary soft tissue, and flecks of cartilaginous tissue can be identified. When the tumor invades the lung, mature teratoma tissue may become exposed in the bronchial lumen (fig. 5-1).

Immature teratomas are often large, at times weighing over 1 kg. They are solid and frequently adhere to adjacent structures. The cut surface varies in appearance, depending upon the constituent tissues (fig. 5-12). Areas of hemorrhage and necrosis, if present, suggest a mixed germ cell tumor, i.e., the presence of a malignant germ cell tumor component.

Microscopically, teratomas are composed of an abnormal mixture of several tissues derived from more than two, and often three, embryonic layers: ectoderm, entoderm, and mesoderm. In mature teratoma of the mediastinum, skin and its appendages are usually found, followed in order of frequency by bronchial tissue, gastrointestinal mucosa, smooth muscle, and fat (80 to 90 percent of cases). Bone, cartilage, and exocrine and endocrine pancreatic tissues occur in 50 to 60 percent of cases; salivary gland and central

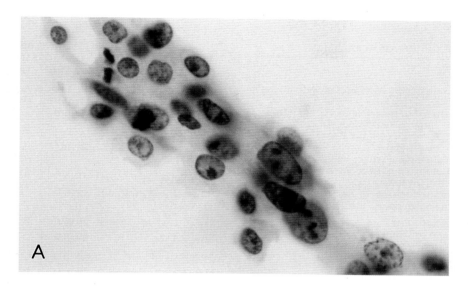

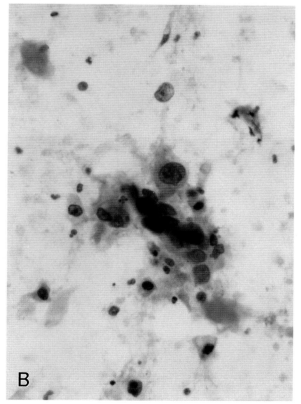

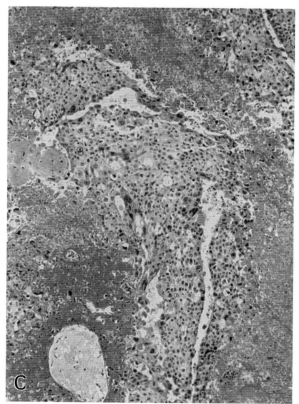

Figure 5-10

NEEDLE ASPIRATION CYTOLOGY OF MEDIASTINAL CHORIOCARCINOMA

A: Cells with vesicular nuclei, prominent nucleoli, and faintly stained cytoplasm are shown. These features are consistent with those of cytotrophoblasts.

B: A multinucleated giant tumor cell with hyperchromatic nuclei and without structural detail is considered to be a syncytial trophoblast.

C: The hemorrhagic tumor has nests of cytotrophoblasts bordered by syncytial trophoblasts. (Courtesy of Dr. Yoshiro Ebihara, Tokyo, Japan.)

Table 5-3

CLASSIFICATION OF TERATOMAS[a]

Benign Teratomas
  Mature teratoma
    Grade 0 (all component tissues appear well differentiated)
    Grade 1 (occasional microscopic foci contain incompletely differentiated tissue, not exceeding 10 percent of the sampled surface)
  Immature teratoma, benign
    Grade 2 (immature tissues make up between 10 and 50 percent of the sampled tumor surface)
    Grade 3 (over half the surface examined is composed of undifferentiated tissues of uncertain metastatic potential; a benign course is still possible)

Malignant Teratomas
  With areas of germ cell tumor
    Germinoma (seminoma, dysgerminoma)
    Embryonal carcinoma
    Choriocarcinoma
    Yolk sac tumor
    Mixed (any combination of the above)
  With nongerminal malignant tumor pattern
    Carcinoma
    Sarcoma
    Malignant embryonal tumor
    Mixed
  Immature teratoma, malignant: a teratoma that would otherwise be classified as benign immature teratoma, but which subsequently became metastatic

[a]Modified from Table 3-12 from Fascicle 21, Third Series.

Table 5-4

FREQUENCY OF THE ORGANS AND TISSUE PRESENT IN MATURE TERATOMA OF MEDIASTINUM AND GONADS[a,b]

	No. Cases Examined (%)		
	Media-stinum	Ovary	Infant Testis
Skin and adnexa	35 (100)	72 (100)	6 (100)
Bronchial mucosa and glands	30 (86)	45 (63)	6 (100)
Gastrointestinal mucosa	31 (89)	9 (13)	4 (67)
Pancreas (exocrine and endocrine)	19 (54)	0 (0)	0 (0)
Fat	28 (80)	39 (54)	6 (100)
Muscle	29 (83)	51 (71)	4 (67)
Salivary gland	11 (31)	15 (21)	4 (67)
Bone and cartilage	22 (63)	36 (50)	5 (83)
Nervous tissue	8 (23)	27 (38)	6 (100)
Melanin-containing cells	1 (3)	15 (21)	2 (33)
Hepatocytes	1 (3)	0 (0)	0 (0)
Thyroid	0 (0)	12 (17)	0 (0)

[a]National Cancer Center Hospital, Tokyo, 1962-1981.
[b]Modified from Table 3-14, Fascicle 21, Third Series.

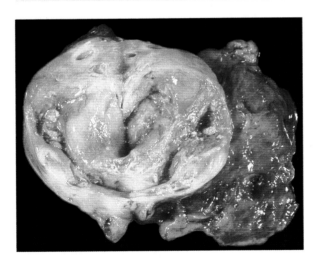

Figure 5-11

MATURE CYSTIC TERATOMA

The lining of the cyst is smooth in some areas and granular in others.

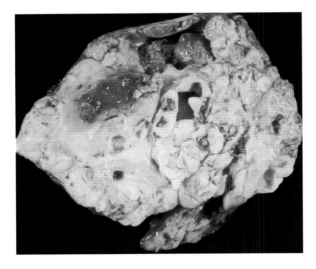

Figure 5-12

IMMATURE TERATOMA

A large immature teratoma has a variegated appearance on cut section, corresponding to its constituent tissues.

nervous tissue including ependyma in 20 to 30 percent of cases; and prostatic gland and hepatocytes in rare cases (Table 5-4; figs. 5-13–5-15).

The presence of pancreatic tissue in a teratoma is of interest, since it is not seen in teratomas of the gonads. Suda et al. (61) reported

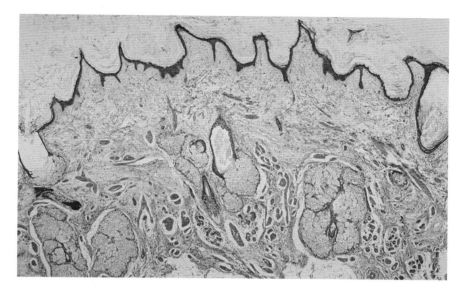

Figure 5-13

MATURE TERATOMA

Between the epidermis and subcutaneous fat are sebaceous and sweat glands, hair follicles, and smooth muscle, all of which are mature.

that among 17 teratomas with pancreatic tissue, 11 were located in the anterior mediastinum, 5 in the sacrococcygeal region, and 1 in the retroperitoneal space. A slightly lower blood glucose level was found in one case and a very high level of amylase in the fistulous discharge from a teratoma was found in another case. Bordi et al. (8). described a teratoma showing the precise topographic distribution of endocrine cells that is seen in normal islets. Gastrointestinal tissue has also frequently been found in mediastinal teratomas. The authors have not yet seen thyroid follicles in a mediastinal teratoma.

One mediastinal teratoma in a 25-year-old man contained lobules of mature glandular tissue which resembled prostatic or Skene glands, although the basal cells were inconspicuous in some acini. The acinar cells were strongly positive for prostatic acid phosphatase, and scattered cells were intensely positive for prostate-specific antigen (PSA). The Alcian blue–periodic acid–Schiff (PAS) stain revealed the presence of cytoplasmic mucus in some cells showing mucus cell metaplasia. Within the stroma, bundles of smooth muscle cells were found, as in the normal prostate, but in addition, a few spindle-shaped melanocytes were present (fig. 5-15). PSA was not demonstrated in the other components of this teratoma, but other glandular components in immature teratomas have immunostained with antibody against prostatic acid phosphatase. The presence of prostatic tissue has been occasionally reported in mature cystic teratoma of the ovary (37).

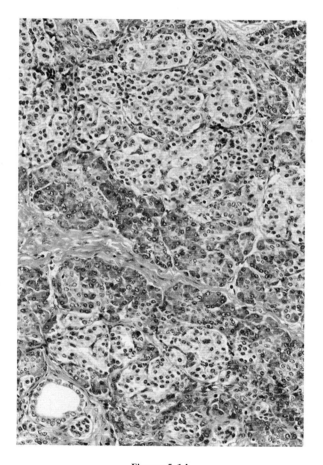

Figure 5-14

MATURE TERATOMA

Exocrine pancreatic acini and islets of Langerhans are evident.

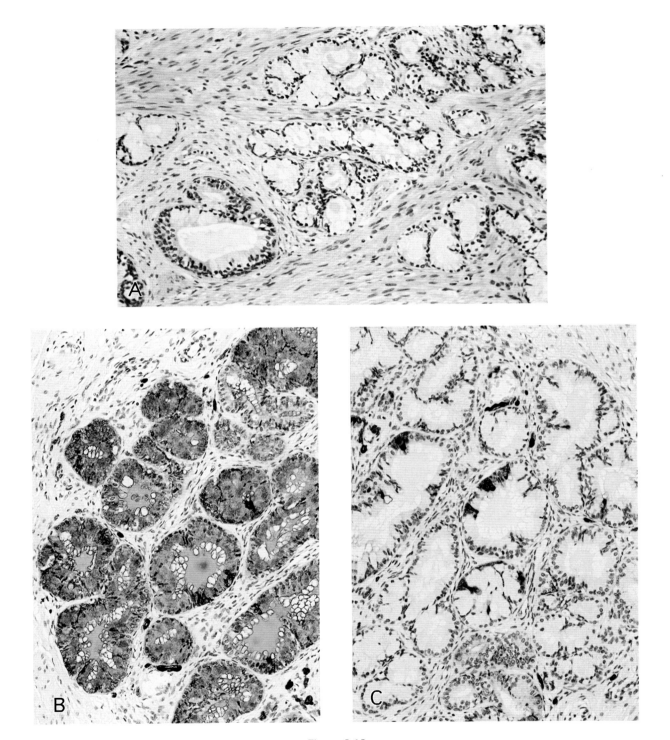

Figure 5-15

MATURE TERATOMA

A: Glandular tissue with interposing smooth muscle cells suggests differentiation toward prostatic tissue.

B: The glandular cells are strongly positive for prostatic acid phosphatase. Melanocytes are scattered within the smooth muscle.

C: A few cells are positive for prostate-specific antigen.

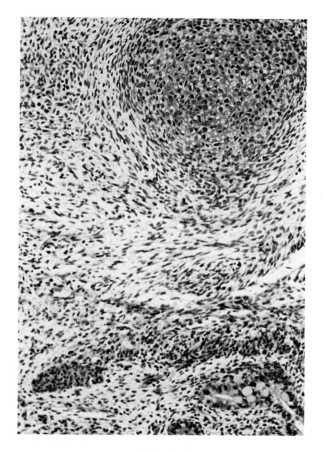

Figure 5-16

IMMATURE TERATOMA

Glands are lined by columnar cells with cytoplasmic mucus. A single lobule of immature cartilage is evident. The tissue between the glands and the cartilage consists of proliferating spindle-shaped cells. There is no evidence of malignancy, however.

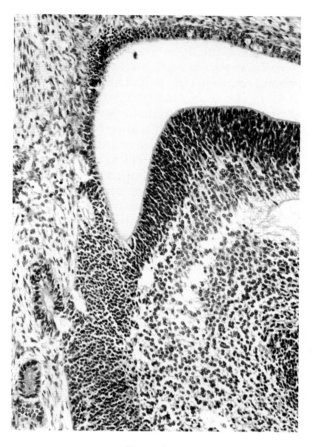

Figure 5-17

IMMATURE TERATOMA

Immature neural tissue with neuroepithelium-forming tubules is seen. Some cells contain melanin pigment. Spindle-shaped supporting cells are also immature but show no nuclear atypia.

Histologically, immature teratoma uncomplicated by obvious malignant germ cell tumor or carcinoma shows tissue derived from all three germinal layers in various stages of maturation, from embryonic to fetal. Immature tissue includes epithelia of ectodermal and entodermal derivatives, bone, cartilage, and muscle (fig. 5-16). In many immature teratomas, neural tissue occupies large areas, and consists of not only glial elements but also neuroepithelium with tubules, rosettes, and retinal anlage (fig. 5-17). Thurlbeck and Scully (63) graded immature teratoma of the ovary according to the amount of immature tissue present, particularly neuroepithelium, and the degree of differentiation, and found the grading

to have prognostic value. As yet, no such study has been conducted for mediastinal teratomas. The authors have seen three patients with immature teratoma, in whom the tumor consisted of large areas of mature tissues and small amounts of immature somatic tissue (mature teratoma, benign, grade 1 of Gonzalez-Crussi classification) (Table 5-3). All were alive and well after surgical resection of the tumor.

A 37-year-old man with a 10 x 12 cm solid tumor, which consisted of abundant immature neuroectodermal and epithelial tissues and a small amount of mature tissue (grade 3), died of metastasis to the lung 15 months after surgery (case of author). The metastatic immature teratoma contained microscopic foci of solid embryonal carcinoma and malignant nongerm cell tumor (fig. 5-18). In seven other patients, immature teratoma was complicated by malignant germ cell and nongerm cell components (Table 5-2).

As in the ovary, malignant transformation of mature cystic teratoma (dermoid) occurs in the mediastinum, with features of squamous cell carcinoma, adenocarcinoma, or poorly differentiated carcinoma (43,51). A goblet cell carcinoid with features of both adenocarcinoma and carcinoid tumor arose in a mature teratoma of the mediastinum (31), as in the ovary (15). Seminoma (germinoma), embryonal carcinoma, yolk sac tumor, and choriocarcinoma have been found in the mediastinum in pure form or in combination with each other and with immature teratoma. Indeed, the presence of a microscopic focus of malignant germ cell tumor in an immature teratoma suggests malignant transformation, and this appears to occur frequently (figs. 5-19, 5-21) (see Mixed Germ Cell Tumors).

Seminoma (Germinoma)

Mediastinal *seminomas (germinomas)* are rare tumors, occurring in male patients of the second, third, and fourth decades of life and very rarely in females. In the past, this entity was diagnosed erroneously as seminomatous thymoma. Patients with mediastinal seminoma may be asymptomatic, and the tumor may be found radiographically as a large anterior mediastinal mass (fig. 5-2). Alternatively, patients present with nonspecific symptoms and signs of a mediastinal tumor, including superior vena cava syndrome and cervical lymphadenopathy. In order to establish a diagnosis of mediastinal seminoma, it is necessary to exclude the presence of a primary tumor in the testis or retroperitoneum, at least clinically.

Grossly, the tumor is large, soft, and well circumscribed, and its cut surface is usually homogeneous. Large tumors show foci of hemorrhage and coagulation necrosis. Moran and Suster (39) found 10 seminomas with prominent cystic changes among 120 primary thymic seminomas.

Microscopically, the tumor is composed of sheets of large polygonal cells with distinct cell membranes, clear or finely granular cytoplasm, and centrally located round nuclei with prominent nucleoli. The tumor cells are supported by a loose stroma densely infiltrated by lymphocytes (figs. 5-4, 5-19). The tumor cell cytoplasm contains glycogen. Isolated giant tumor cells that resemble syncytiotrophoblasts, like those in testicular seminoma, may also be present. Individual cell necrosis or foci of coagulation necrosis provokes a granulomatous reaction. No cases of spermatocytic or anaplastic seminoma arising in the mediastinum have been reported (35).

In the multilocular thymic seminomas, the cystic spaces are lined by squamous or cuboidal epithelium showing severe chronic inflammatory changes with hyperplastic lymph follicles; the walls of the cysts contain residual thymic parenchyma. These features may represent a reactive change secondary to thymic epithelial hyperplasia, and are indistinguishable from acquired multilocular thymic cysts. Extensive sampling of the solid areas is necessary to find the neoplastic components to distinguish these seminomas from acquired multilocular thymic cysts (39). Similar cystic changes are also noted in thymoma, Hodgkin lymphoma, mucosa-associated lymphoid tissue (MALT) lymphoma, and certain types of thymic carcinoma, such as basaloid carcinoma.

The entities in the differential diagnosis include lymphoepithelioma-like carcinoma of the thymus and diffuse large cell lymphoma with sclerosis of the anterior mediastinum. Although hematoxylin and eosin (H&E)-stained sections are sufficient to establish a diagnosis in most cases, immunohistochemistry is helpful in difficult cases. Mediastinal seminomas are frequently positive for placental alkaline phosphatase (fig. 5-20) and vimentin. CD117 immunoreactivity is commonly seen in the cell membrane or in the paranuclear region (33,71). OCT4, a transcription factor expressed in embryonic stem cells and germ cells, has been found to be a useful marker in the identification of testicular seminoma of the usual type and embryonal carcinoma (4,64,71), as well as dysgerminoma and the germ cell component of gonadoblastoma of the ovary (13). The validity of OCT4 has been tested recently for mediastinal germ cell tumors and thymomas, and all of 10 seminomas, 1 embryonal carcinoma, and 1 mixed germ cell tumor containing seminoma were immunoreactive for OCT4 (27a). All of 22 thymomas and 34 nonseminomatous germ cell

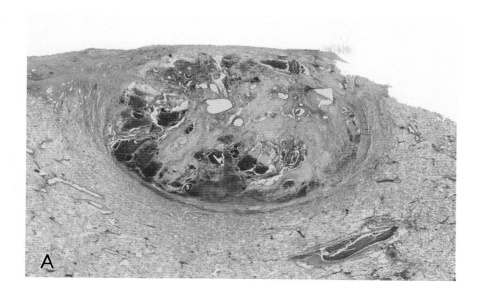

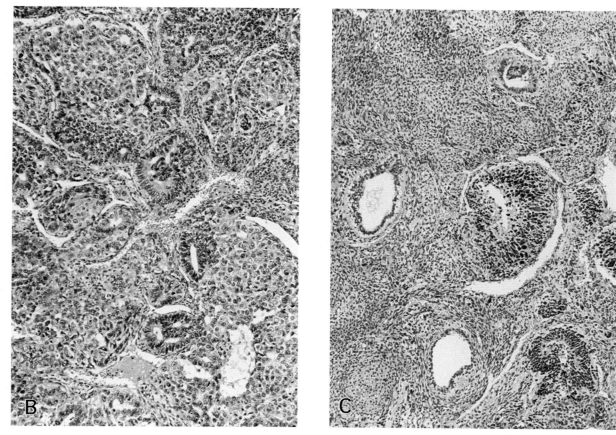

Figure 5-18

MALIGNANT IMMATURE TERATOMA WITH A NONGERM CELL COMPONENT

The primary tumor consisted largely of immature teratoma. The predominantly immature teratoma metastatic to the lung (A), however, contains adenocarcinoma and largely solid carcinoma, suggesting embryonal carcinoma in some areas (B) and microscopic foci of what appears to be neuroblastoma in others (C).

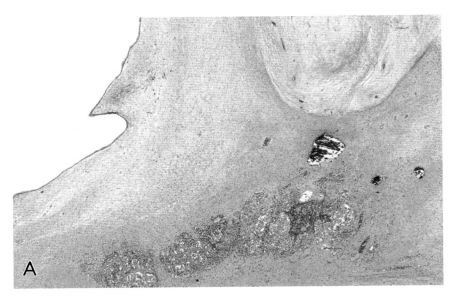

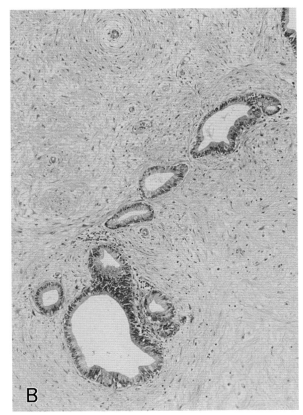

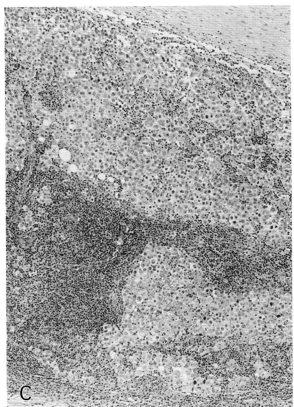

Figure 5-19

SMALL SEMINOMA IN THE WALL OF A MATURE CYSTIC TERATOMA

A: There is a small focus of seminoma within the wall of a cystic teratoma (lower portion of the figure).

B: Within a sclerotic wall of the cystic teratoma are several ductal structures with no nuclear atypia.

C: Medium-power view of the seminomatous focus shown in A reveals typical features of seminoma with variable numbers of lymphoid cells in the stroma.

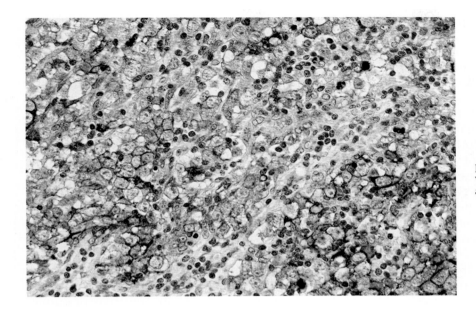

Figure 5-20

SEMINOMA

The cell membrane and cytoplasm of most tumor cells show variable staining for placental alkaline phosphatase.

tumors of various types were immunonegative for OCT4. Recently, transcription factors M2A (stainable with monoclonal antibody D2-40) and AP-2γ have been found to be sensitive markers for metastatic seminomas and pineal germinomas, although no primary seminomas have been tested (4a).

Focal and weak cytokeratin staining is noted in some mediastinal seminomas: 6 of 50 gonadal seminomas showed focal or diffuse cytokeratin reactivity (48). Epithelial membrane antigen (EMA) is negative in seminomas. Giant tumor cells resembling syncytiotrophoblasts are positive for β-hCG. In contrast, lymphoepithelioma-like undifferentiated carcinoma of the thymus is EMA positive and placental alkaline phosphatase negative. Diffuse large cell lymphomas are, of course, positive for leukocyte common antigen and frequently show a B-cell phenotype.

Embryonal Carcinoma

Embryonal carcinoma is a rare, highly malignant, anterior mediastinal tumor occurring predominantly in young males. It may be found in pure form or in association with other malignant germ cell tumors. When diagnosed, it is often large and invasive into the surrounding organs or structures, and is inoperable or only treated by tumor burden-reduction surgery. An elevated level of serum AFP is diagnostic for either embryonal carcinoma or yolk sac tumor. Patients with embryonal carcinoma and the clinical

and chromosomal abnormalities of Klinefelter syndrome have been reported (30,38).

Grossly, the cut surface of embryonal carcinoma is largely occupied by areas of coagulation necrosis and hemorrhage. Histologically, the tumor is composed of sheets, tubules, and papillary formations of large polygonal cells. These cells have round to oval nuclei, prominent nucleoli, often pale-stained cytoplasm, and indistinct cell borders. Mitotic figures are frequent.

Immunohistochemically, embryonal carcinomas are frequently positive for placental alkaline phosphatase and low molecular weight cytokeratin, and about one third are positive for AFP (48). The presence of AFP excludes the possibility of metastatic adenocarcinoma. As in seminoma, multinucleated giant tumor cells of the syncytiotrophoblastic type may be intermixed. These cells are positive immunohistochemically for β-hCG. Staining of the cell membrane and cytoplasm with CD30 (Ki-1) is frequently seen in embryonal carcinoma (18,32,33), but CD117 expression is usually absent (33). The validity of OCT4 as a marker of mediastinal embryonal carcinoma should be verified. Absence of Schiller-Duval bodies and a reticular pattern allows differentiation from yolk sac tumor.

Yolk Sac Tumor (Endodermal Sinus Tumor)

Although *yolk sac tumor* is a rare tumor in the mediastinum, it is the most frequent malignant mediastinal germ cell tumor treated at the

National Cancer Center Hospital in Tokyo. There are two distinct age groups, one in infants and young children and the other in postpubertal adolescents and adults. Only two of six children with mediastinal yolk sac tumor reported by Hawkins et al. (24) were girls aged 2 and 10 years, but another report indicated a female predominance with a female to male ratio of 4 to 1 (58). The vast majority of postpubertal patients are males, and they are frequently in their twenties and thirties (45,59,67). Of 76 cases collected by Marchevsky and Kaneko (35), only 1 occurred in a female patient (21). Yolk sac tumor is highly malignant, and often large and invasive when detected. The serum level of AFP is markedly elevated. The tumor occurs as a pure form or in combination with immature teratoma or other forms of malignant germ cell tumor (figs. 5-5, 5-21–5-23).

The tumor cells grow diffusely, forming tubular and papillary structures. Characteristic and diagnostic features are a reticular pattern with various-sized spaces lined by flattened cells, and the presence of Schiller-Duval bodies, which are papillae composed of a central vessel covered by columnar tumor cells lying in spaces (fig. 5-23, left). Ulbright et al. (73) studied yolk sac differentiation in germ cell tumors and found hepatic-like foci in 22 percent of cases, enteric-like glands in 34 percent, and parietal yolk sac structures in 92 percent. This last feature is characterized by the intercellular accumulation of basement membrane substance in generally thick and longitudinally arranged bands of eosinophilic material. Eosinophilic hyaline droplets may be seen within and outside the cells, which are PAS-positive and may contain immunoreactive AFP (fig. 5-23). Four cases of hepatoid yolk sac tumor of the anterior mediastinum were reported by Moran and Suster (40). Yolk sac tumors also contain immunoreactive alpha-1-antitrypsin and cytokeratin. Placental alkaline phosphatase is present in about half of the cases and carcinoembryonic antigen in 11 percent (48).

Choriocarcinoma

Choriocarcinoma is also a rare malignant germ cell tumor arising in the anterior mediastinum. It develops in predominantly male adults, most commonly in the third decade of life. Gyneco-mastia is a frequent finding, and an elevated serum level of β-hCG is diagnostic.

Grossly, the tumor is characteristically hemorrhagic. It becomes extensively necrotic after effective chemotherapy, with or without radiotherapy (figs. 5-24, 5-25).

Microscopically, choriocarcinoma consists of mononuclear cytotrophoblastic cells and giant syncytiotrophoblastic cells, frequently bordering extensive areas of hemorrhage. Choriocarcinoma is seen as a pure form or in combination with immature teratoma or other germ cell tumors such as embryonal carcinoma. Immunohistochemically, β-hCG is positive in the syncytiotrophoblastic cells and some cytotrophoblastic cells (fig. 5-26). Cytokeratin is positive in all cases and placental alkaline phosphatase and EMA in about half (48). Cytotrophoblasts are variably positive for human placental lactogen (39a).

Choriocarcinoma is a highly aggressive tumor with early hematogenous dissemination to lung, kidney, spleen, brain, heart, adrenal gland, and bone.

TUMORS OF MORE THAN ONE HISTOLOGIC TYPE: MIXED GERM CELL TUMORS

Any combination of germ cell tumors can be seen in adults. The incidence of mixed germ cell tumors is second only to teratoma, at around 20 percent of all mediastinal germ cell tumors, and almost equal to that of seminoma. Mixed germ cell tumors overwhelmingly affect males (41,42,66). The two most frequent components are teratoma, often immature teratoma, and embryonal carcinoma, followed by yolk sac tumor, seminoma, and choriocarcinoma. In children, however, most mixed germ cell tumors are yolk sac tumors combined with mature or immature teratoma, affecting both sexes of children younger than 8 years of age and occurring almost exclusively in boys older than 8 years (56,58).

Teratoma with Nongerminal Malignant Tumor

Multiple sections of immature teratoma occasionally disclose microscopic foci of nongerm cell malignant tumors, such as adenocarcinoma, undifferentiated carcinoma, or sarcoma (figs. 5-18, 5-27). Germ cell tumors in which nongerminal malignancy predominates are rare,

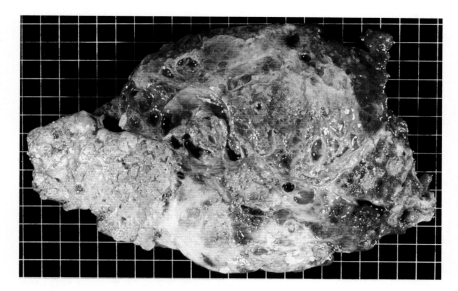

Figure 5-21

MIXED GERM CELL TUMOR COMPOSED OF IMMATURE TERATOMA AND YOLK SAC TUMOR: GROSS FEATURES

An irregular large tumor is composed of abundant immature cartilage (left), and extensive hemorrhagic and necrotic areas of yolk sac tumor (right).

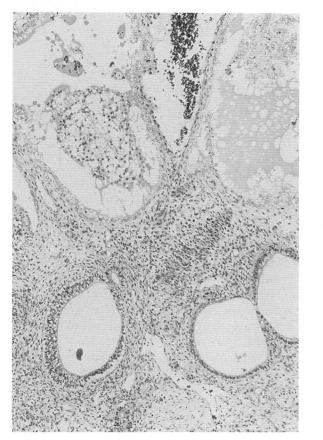

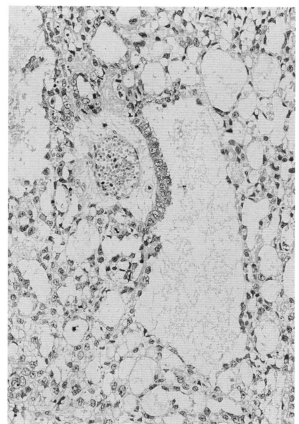

Figure 5-22

SMALL YOLK SAC TUMOR IN IMMATURE TERATOMA

Left: Within the immature teratoma containing glands and smooth muscle is a microscopic focus of tumor showing a reticular pattern.

Right: In another area there is a typical yolk sac tumor with a reticular pattern and an incomplete Schiller-Duval body.

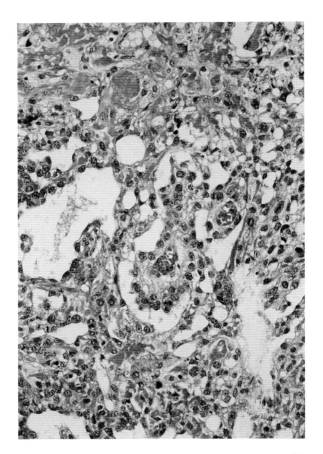 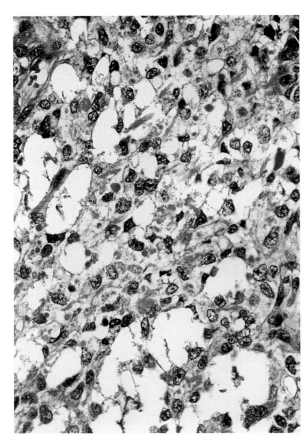

Figure 5-23

YOLK SAC TUMOR

Left: Typical Schiller-Duval bodies are shown. Also seen are intracytoplasmic eosinophilic droplets and extracellular irregularly shaped eosinophilic material.

Right: In this area showing a reticular pattern, eosinophilic hyaline droplets are evident both within and outside the tumor cells.

however, and mostly affect men. The occurrence of carcinoma in teratoma, either mature or immature, is much less frequent than mesenchymal tumors (19,43). These malignant tumors are believed to arise within teratomatous foci.

A variety of malignant tumors have been described in association with germ cell tumor: embryonal rhabdomyosarcoma, angiosarcoma, myxoid liposarcoma, osteosarcoma, chondrosarcoma, leiomyosarcoma, malignant fibrous histiocytoma, malignant nerve sheath tumor, glioblastoma multiforme, neuroblastoma, nephroblastoma, adenosquamous carcinoma, and more, either in a pure form or in combination (34,53,72). Some components may remain after complete disappearance of the germ cell tumor following intensive chemotherapy.

Remnants are considered the result of selective action of chemotherapy. Therefore, chemotherapy protocols may need to be altered to include sarcoma-oriented drugs for this particular group of patients, although the role of other forms of chemotherapy remains unclear (34,72).

Recently, Malagon et al. (33a) reported 46 cases of germ cell tumor with a sarcomatous component, of which 23 arose in the mediastinum. They concluded that the presence of a sarcomatous component is a factor that portends more aggressive behavior. The sarcomatous component may behave as an independent tumor that can metastasize autonomously, and appears to be highly resistant to the standard combination chemotherapy commonly employed for the treatment of germ cell tumors.

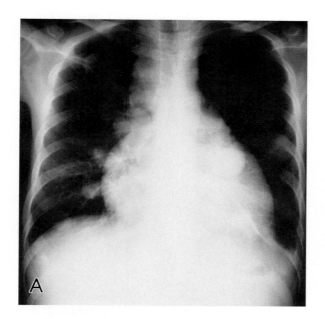
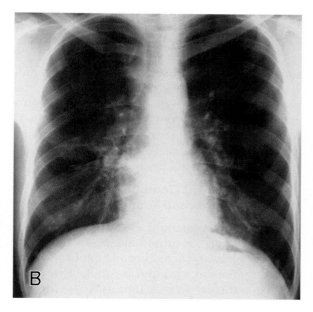
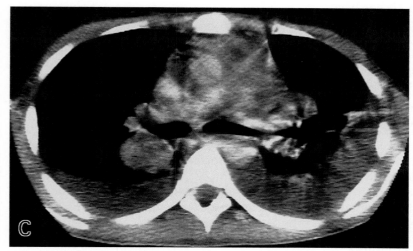
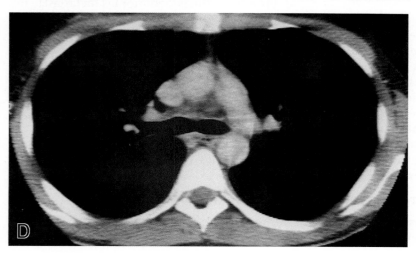

Figure 5-24

**CHORIOCARCINOMA AFTER
TREATMENT WITH
ANTITUMOR AGENTS**

A: Prior to chemotherapy, plain chest X ray shows widening of the mediastinal density, multiple metastases up to 3 cm in diameter in the lung field, enlargement of the cardiac density due to pericardial effusion, and bilateral pleural effusions.

B: After chemotherapy, a plain chest X ray reveals minimal widening of the superior mediastinum. The nodular tumorous densities in the lung field and the pleural effusion disappear, leaving only reticular densities in both lower lobes.

C: CT at the level of the tracheal bifurcation shows anterior mediastinal tumorous densities associated with the metastatic tumor in the lung and bilateral pleural effusions.

D: CT at the level of the tracheal bifurcation discloses some enlargement of the pretracheal lymph nodes and almost complete disappearance of the mediastinal tumor, lung metastases, and pleural effusion. (Fig. 3-189 from Fascicle 21, Third Series.) (Figs. 5-24–5-26 are from the same patient.)

MOLECULAR AND OTHER SPECIAL TECHNIQUES

Genetic abnormalities of mediastinal germ cell tumors parallel those of gonadal tumors. Depending on the setting of the tumor development, the genetic changes of mediastinal germ cell tumors can be divided into three categories (Table 5-5) (66,75): malignant germ cell tumors of infants and young children; malignant germ cell tumors of adolescents and adults; and pure teratoma.

Malignant Germ Cell Tumors of Infants and Young Children

These tumors are almost always yolk sac tumors. Prepubertal yolk sac tumors are mostly diploid or near tetraploid and are rarely aneuploid (49). The chromosomal abnormalities are similar to those of sacral or testicular yolk sac tumors. These include loss of chromosomes 1p and 6q and gain of 1q and 20q (26,50,58). Loss of distal 1p has been identified in 80 percent of infantile yolk sac tumors and is also common in another embryonal malignancy, neuroblastoma. It is probable that this location contains a tumor suppressor gene, but its identity has not been clarified.

Malignant Germ Cell Tumors of Adolescents and Adults

The genetic abnormalities of these tumors are similar to those of gonadal tumors. These tumors are aneuploid in most cases and consistently show gain of chromosome 12p, regardless of the histology (58). This finding correlates with the presence of an isochromosome 12p in these tumors.

Pure Teratoma (Immature and Mature)

Mediastinal teratomas in patients of all ages do not show genetic abnormalities (58). This is similar to mature teratomas of the ovary, the infant testis, and extragonadal sites. On the other hand, teratomas of the adult testis are different, carrying isochromosome 12p, which is common in malignant germ cell tumors. Mediastinal teratomas are similar to ovarian teratomas genetically; therefore, it is understandable that their malignant potential is also similar to the ovarian rather than the testicular counterpart.

TUMOR SPREAD AND STAGING

Mature teratomas do not metastasize and are considered benign, although they may locally

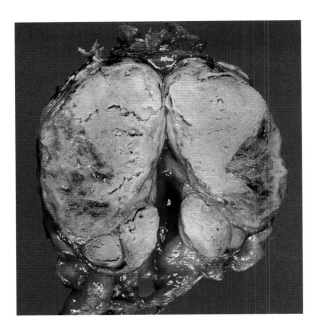

Figure 5-25

TREATED CHORIOCARCINOMA

The tumor is encapsulated and partly nodular. The cut surface shows extensive coagulation necrosis and hemorrhage. No viable tumor cells could be identified histologically.

destroy the lung by compression and friction (fig. 5-1) and may develop a secondary malignancy of nongerm cell or malignant germ cell type (19,43,56,62). Immature teratomas are often large and adhere to surrounding structures. They may metastasize to the lung, with or without secondary malignant components. Malignant germ cell tumors are usually divided into seminomas and nonseminomas. Seminomas metastasize frequently to lymph nodes and occasionally to the lung and elsewhere. Nonseminomas frequently reveal hematogenous metastases to the lung, which is followed by bone, liver, and brain.

The same TNM classification and staging system as proposed for thymic tumors by the International Union Against Cancer (UICC) (69), and by other investigators (2,68), and as proposed for thymic germ cell tumors by the WHO (66), may be used for staging (see Tables 2-11, 2-12, 5-6).

TREATMENT AND PROGNOSIS

Immature teratoma is frequently combined with malignant germ cell tumor (Table 5-2).

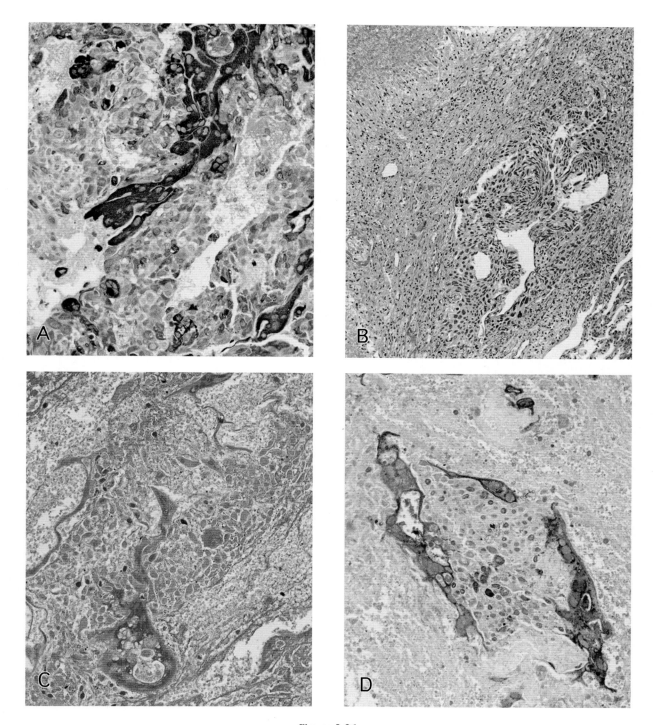

Figure 5-26

CHORIOCARCINOMA AFTER TREATMENT WITH ANTITUMOR AGENTS

A: The untreated mediastinal choriocarcinoma shown in figure 5-6 is stained for β-hCG as a control.

B: Several lung metastases removed surgically were almost entirely necrotic, and apparently viable tumor tissue remained in only one nodule between the lung tissue and the granulation tissue bordering the necrotic tissue.

C: Within the necrotic tissue, ghosts of cytotrophoblasts and syncytiotrophoblasts can be identified.

D: These cells show intense reactivity upon immunostaining with anti-β-hCG.

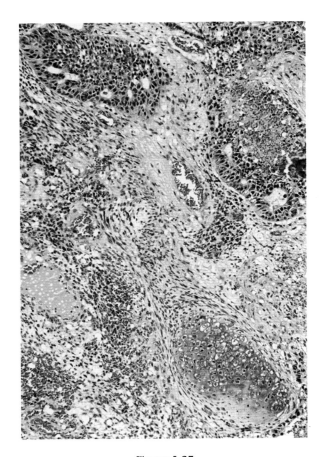

Figure 5-27

**IMMATURE TERATOMA WITH
NONGERMINAL MALIGNANT TUMOR**

Within this immature teratoma with a mesenchymal component are several nests of moderately differentiated adenocarcinoma.

Therefore, surgical removal is indicated whenever possible.

Encapsulated immature teratoma in infants and children younger than 15 years old seems to behave like mature teratoma (35), and complete surgical excision is effective treatment. A survival period of 3 years is obtained in over 80 percent of cases (36,56). Only 4 of 23 patients with gonadal and extragonadal immature teratomas with malignant foci, most commonly yolk sac tumors, developed recurrence after complete surgical excision (36). Resectable yolk sac tumors at earlier stages (stages I and II) are more often seen in the prepubertal age group, resulting in higher survival rates than for postpubertal patients. Therefore, grading by

Table 5-5

INTERRELATIONSHIP OF AGE, TUMOR TYPE, CLINICAL BEHAVIOR, AND GENETIC ALTERATIONS IN MEDIASTINAL GERM CELL TUMORS[a]

Age at Clinical Presentation	Histology	Clinical Behavior	Recurrent Genetic Aberrations
Prepubertal	Teratoma[b]	Benign if resectable	None
	Yolk sac tumor	Malignant (80% survival)	del(6q), del(1p), gain 20q, gain 1q, diploidy or tetraploidy
Adolescents and Adults	Teratoma Malignant GCT[c]	Benign Malignant (50% survival)	None i(12p), gain 21, loss 13, loss of Y, +Xc,[d] aneuploidy

[a]Modified from Table 3-10 from reference 75; data are derived from conventional cytogenetics, comparative genomic hybridization studies, and DNA ploidy analysis.
[b]Teratoma includes both mature and immature types.
[c]GCT = germ cell tumor; malignant GCT includes all histologic subtypes.
[d]+Xc = constitutional gain of the X-chromosome (Klinefelter syndrome).

the Gonzalez-Crussi classification (20) is of no prognostic significance.

Experience with pure immature teratoma in adults is limited. The patients must be watched carefully postoperatively for recurrence since a malignant germ cell component may have been overlooked at the time of histologic examination or because of sampling error of the specimen. If immature teratoma in postpubertal adolescents and adults is combined with malignant germ cell tumor, growth is aggressive and often only biopsy or tumor burden-reduction surgery can be performed. Cisplatin-based chemotherapy combined with radiotherapy and surgery may achieve cure in some patients.

By considering the malignant potential and responsiveness to treatment of the tumor, the International Germ Cell Cancer Collaborative Group (1,66) presented clinical risk groupings for malignant germ cell tumors in adults as follows: "good prognosis with a 5-year survival of 91 percent" for patients with seminoma displaying no nonpulmonary visceral metastases and normal AFP, regardless of β-hCG and lactate dehydrogenase (LDH) levels; "intermediate prognosis with a 5-year survival of 79 percent" for patients with seminoma displaying nonpulmonary visceral metastases and normal AFP, any β-hCG or

Table 5-6

TUMOR-NODE-METASTASIS (TNM) CLASSIFICATION (UICC) AND STAGING OF GERM CELL TUMORS[a,b]

T1	Tumor confined to the thymus and mediastinal fat
T1a	Tumor 5 cm or less in greatest dimension
T1b	Tumor larger than 5 cm
T2	Tumor infiltrating surrounding organs or tissues or accompanied by malignant effusion
T2a	Tumor 5 cm or less in greatest dimension
T2b	Tumor larger than 5 cm
T3	Tumor invades into neighboring structures, such as pericardium, mediastinal pleura, thoracic wall, great vessels, and lung
T4	Tumor with pleural or pericardial dissemination
N0	No regional lymph node metastasis
N1	Metastasis to regional lymph node
N2	Metastasis in other intrathoracic lymph nodes excluding anterior mediastinal lymph nodes
N3	Metastasis in scalene and/or supraclavicular lymph nodes
M0	No distant metastasis
M1	Distant metastasis
Stage I	Locoregional tumor, nonmetastatic, complete resection
Stage II	Locoregional tumor, nonmetastatic, macroscopic complete resection but microscopic residual tumor
Stage III	Locoregional tumor, regional lymph nodes negative or positive; no distant metastasis; biopsy only or gross residual tumor after primary resection
Stage IV	Tumor with distant metastasis

[a]Modified from reference 69.
[b]UICC = International Union Against Cancer.

LDH levels; and "poor prognosis with a 5-year survival of 48 percent" for patients with nonseminomatous malignant germ cell tumors.

The prognosis for patients with seminomas is excellent after surgical resection (62). Mediastinal seminoma is highly sensitive to radiotherapy, and therefore, not only total surgical removal of the tumor but also incomplete removal are followed by radiotherapy to the chest, neck, and at times retroperitoneum and other areas. This often cures the disease (27,55). Kersh et al. (29) reported a 100 percent actuarial 5-year survival rate in patients with mediastinal seminoma. Cisplatin-based combination chemotherapy, with or without secondary surgery, is preferred to initial radiotherapy for mediastinal seminoma, in which a long-term cure rate of almost 90 percent is obtained (7). Recurrence

after surgery or radiotherapy can also be treated by combination chemotherapy. Cisplatin-based chemotherapy for metastatic disease results in long-term survival in 80 percent or more of patients (46). Prognostic factors influencing survival negatively are liver metastases and more than one metastatic site (6).

Mediastinal nonseminomatous malignant germ cell tumors were invariably fatal until two decades ago. They are a clinically and biologically distinct subset of germ cell neoplasms, and patients have a poor prognosis, with the worst survival among patients with gonadal and extragonadal germ cell tumors (46,65). Nowadays, however, intensive chemotherapy using cisplatin, vinblastine, etoposide, and bleomycin for gonadal germ cell tumors is effective for extragonadal germ cell tumors including nonseminomatous malignant mediastinal germ cell tumors (figs. 5-24, 5-26, 5-28). An increasing incidence of successfully treated cases has been reported (9,24,59,62). An international analysis revealed that 45 percent of patients with mediastinal nonseminomatous malignant germ cell tumors were alive at 5 years after platinum-based induction chemotherapy, with or without secondary surgery (7). Preoperative intensive chemotherapy is frequently employed. When it is effective, the histology of the resected tumor may show extensive necrosis and markedly degenerating tumor cells, obscuring the histologic detail of the tumor, and making a definitive diagnosis impossible.

Moran and Suster (42) analyzed 64 mediastinal nonseminomatous malignant germ cell tumors and concluded that the clinical/pathologic staging of yolk sac tumor, embryonal carcinoma, and combined nonteratomatous germ cell tumor is an important parameter that helps predict the clinical outcome of patients. In contrast, mediastinal choriocarcinoma appears to follow a very aggressive clinical course, regardless of treatment modality or clinical stage. Poor-risk patients with extragonadal nonseminomatous germ cell tumors may be treated with high-dose etoposide and carboplatin followed by autologous bone marrow transplantation (47). There appears to be no significant difference in prognosis between patients with pure and mixed nonseminomatous germ cell tumors.

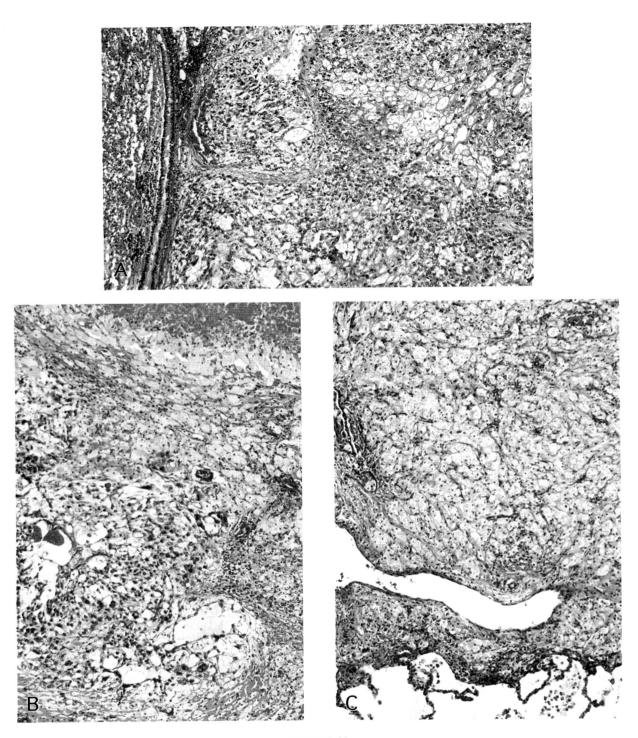

Figure 5-28

YOLK SAC TUMOR AFTER TREATMENT WITH ANTITUMOR AGENTS

A: Tumor metastatic to the right upper lobe of the lung shows only a mild degree of degenerative change.

B: Metastasis in the right lower lobe shows moderate therapeutic effects, as evidenced by large areas of necrosis bordered by foamy histiocytes and cytolytic changes in the remaining tumor cells.

C: The tumor in the left lower lobe has been completely replaced by foamy histiocytes.

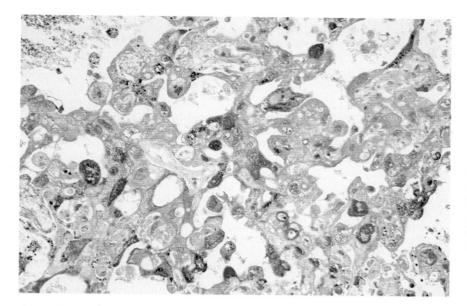

Figure 5-29

**YOLK SAC TUMOR
AFTER CHEMOTHERAPY**

The tumor cells are markedly enlarged and degenerative, and no definite histologic diagnosis was possible based on H&E-stained sections. However, a reticular pattern suggestive of yolk sac tumor was retained, and this was confirmed by immunostaining for AFP.

Therapeutic effectiveness can be monitored using chest X-ray films (fig. 5-24) and the serum level of markers such as AFP and β-hCG. Metastatic choriocarcinoma in the lung is extensively hemorrhagic, and abnormal densities remain even after β-hCG has been reduced to a normal level or even after complete disappearance of tumor cells. Also, surgical removal of multiple lung lesions following the return of the marker to a normal serum level has disclosed hemorrhagic and necrotic tissue surrounded by granulation or fibrous tissue in most nodules (fig. 5-25). Tumor cell ghosts may show β-hCG immunoreactivity. There may be microscopic remnants of viable tumor cells at the borders of the nodules (fig. 5-26B). Therefore, the timing of chemotherapy discontinuation is important, and at present, surgery is recommended even after effective chemotherapy, when abnormal densities remain on the imaging studies. The patient with an "entirely necrotic tumor" included in Table 5-2 had been treated in this manner, and is alive after more than 3 years without evidence of disease (3). Tumors remaining after such intensive treatment often show marked pleomorphism with frequent giant tumor cells (fig. 5-29), which may mimic the histology of choriocarcinoma. Immunohistochemistry should be done to establish a final diagnosis.

REFERENCES

1. International Germ Cell Consensus Classification: a prognostic factor-based staging system for metastatic germ cell tumours. International Germ Cell Cancer Collaborative Group. J Clin Oncol 1997;15: 594-603. (Comment in J Clin Oncol 1998;16:1244-7.)

2. Asamura H, Nakagawa K, Matsuno Y, Suzuki K, Watanabe S, Tsuchiya R. Thymoma needs a new staging system. Interactive Cardiovasc Thorac Surg 2004; 3:163-7.

3. Asamura H, Tsuchiya R, Goya T, et al. Malignant germ cell tumor of the mediastinum: a multimodality therapeutic approach. Surg Today 1994;24:137-41.

4. Berney DM. A practical approach to the reporting of germ cell tumours of the testis. Curr Diagn Pathol 2005;11:151-61.

4a. Biermann K, Klingmueller D, Koch A, et al. Diagnostic value of markers M2A, OCT3/4, AP-2gamma, PLAP, and c-KIT in the detection of extragonadal seminomas. Histopathology 2006;49:290-7.

5. Bitar FF, el-Zein C, Tawil A, Gharzuddine W, Obeid M. Intrapericardial teratoma in an adult: a rare presentation. Med Pediatr Oncol 1998;30:249-51.

6. Bokemeyer C, Droz JP, Horwich A, et al. Extragonadal seminoma: an international multicenter analysis of prognostic factors and long term treatment outcome. Cancer 2001;91:1394-401.

7. Bokemeyer C, Nichols CR, Droz JP, et al. Extragonadal germ cell tumors of the mediastinum and retroperitoneum: results from international analysis. J Clin Oncol 2002;20:1864-73.

8. Bordi C, De Vita O, Pollice L. Full pancreatic endocrine differentiation in a mediastinal teratoma. Hum Pathol 1985;16:961-3.

9. Bukowski RM, Wolf M, Kulander BG, Montie J, Crawford ED, Blumenstein B. Alternating combination chemotherapy in patients with extragonadal germ cell tumors. A Southwest Oncology Group study. Cancer 1993;71:2631-8.

10. Bussey KJ, Lawce HJ, Himoe E, et al. SNRPN methylation patterns in germ cell tumors as a reflection of primordial germ cell development. Genes Chromosomes Cancer 2001;32:342-52.

11. Caraway NP, Fanning CV, Amato RJ, Sneige N. Fine-needle aspiration cytology of seminoma: a review of 16 cases. Diagn Cytopathol 1995;12:327-33.

12. Chaganti RS, Rodriguez E, Mathew S. Origin of adult male mediastinal germ-cell tumours. Lancet 1994;343:1130-2.

13. Cheng L, Thomas A, Roth LM, Zheng W, Michael H, Karim FW. OCT4: a novel biomarker for dysgerminoma of the ovary. Am J Surg Pathol 2004;28:1341-1346.

14. Chhieng DC, Lin O, Moran CA, et al. Fine-needle aspiration biopsy of nonteratomatous germ cell tumors of the mediastinum. Am J Clin Pathol 2002;118:418-24.

15. Clement PB, Young RH. Germ cell tumours of the ovary, part I, Non-teratomatous germ cell tumours; part II, Teratomas excluding monodermal teratomas; part III, Monodermal teratomas. Current Diagn Pathol 1995;2:199-207, 208-213, 214-221.

16. Collins KA, Geisinger KR, Wakely PE Jr, Olympio G, Silverman JF. Extragonadal germ cell tumors: a fine-needle aspiration biopsy study. Diagn Cytopathol 1995;12:223-9.

17. de Ment SH. Association between mediastinal germ cell tumors and hematologic malignancies: an update. Hum Pathol 1990;21:699-703.

18. Ferreiro JA. Ber-H2 expression in testicular germ cell tumors. Hum Pathol 1994;25:522-4

19. Freilich RJ, Thompson SJ, Walker RW, Rosenblum MK. Adenocarcinomatous transformation of intracranial germ cell tumors. Am J Surg Pathol 1995;19:537-44.

20. Gonzalez-Crussi F. Extragonadal teratomas. Atlas of Tumor Pathology, 2nd Series, Fascicle 18, Washington, D.C: Armed Forces Institute of Pathology; 1982.

21. Gooneratne S, Keh P, Sreekanth S, Recant W, Talerman A. Anterior mediastinal endodermal sinus (yolk sac) tumor in a female infant Cancer 1985;56:1430-3.

22. Hasle H, Jacobsen BB, Asschenfeldt P, Andersen K. Mediastinal germ cell tumour associated with Klinefelter syndrome. A report of case and review of the literature. Eur J Pediatr 1992;151:735-9.

23. Hasle H, Mellemgaard A, Nielsen J, Hansen J. Cancer incidence in men with Klinefelter syndrome. Br J Cancer 1995;71:416-20.

24. Hawkins EP, Finegold MJ, Hawkins HK, Krischer JP, Starling KA, Weinberg A. Nongerminomatous malignant germ cell tumors in children. A review of 89 cases from the Pediatric Oncology Group, 1971-1984. Cancer 1986;58:2579-84.

25. Hoffner L, Deka R, Chakravarti A, Surti U. Cytogenetics and origins of pediatric germ cell tumors. Cancer Genet Cytogenet 1994;74:54-8.

26. Hu J, Schuster AE, Fritsch MK, Schneider DT, Lauer S, Perlman EJ. Deletion mapping of 6q21-26 and frequency of 1p36 deletion in childhood endodermal sinus tumors by microsatellite analysis. Oncogene 2001;20:8042-4.

27. Hurt RD, Bruckman JE, Farrow GM, Bernatz PE, Hahn RG, Earle JD. Primary anterior mediastinal seminoma. Cancer 1982;49:1658-63.

27a. Jung SM, Chu PH, Shin TF, et al. Expression of OCT4 in the primary germ cell tumors and thymoma in the mediastinum. Appl Immunohistochem Mol Morphol 2006;14:273-5.

28. Kaplan CG, Askin FB Benirschke K. Cytogenetics of extragonadal tumors. Teratology 1979;19:261-6.

29. Kersh CR, Constable WC, Hahn SS, et al. Primary malignant extragonadal germ cell tumors. An analysis of the effect of radiotherapy. Cancer 1990;65:2681-5.

30. Lachman MF, Kim K, Koo BC. Mediastinal teratoma associated with Klinefelter's syndrome. Arch Pathol Lab Med 1986;110:1067-71.

31. Lancaster KJ, Liang CY, Myers JC, McCabe KM. Goblet cell carcinoid arising in a mature teratoma of the mediastinum. Am J Surg Pathol 1997;21:109-13.

32. Latza U, Foss HD, Durkop H, et al. CD30 antigen in embryonal carcinoma and embryogenesis and release of the soluble molecule. Am J Pathol 1995;146:463-71.

33. Leroy X, Augusto D, Leteurtre E, Gosselin B. CD30 and CD117 (c-kit) used in combination are useful for distinguishing embryonal carcinoma and seminoma. J Histochem Cytochem 2002;50:283-5.

33a. Malagon HD, Valdez AM, Moran CA, Suster S. Germ cell tumor with sarcomatous components: a clinicopathologic and immunohistochemical study of 46 cases. Am J Surg Pathol 2007;31:1356-62.

34. Manivel C, Wick MR, Abenoza P, Rosai J. The occurrence of sarcomatous components in primary mediastinal germ cell tumors. Am J Surg Pathol 1986;10:711-7.

35. Marchevsky AM, Kaneko M. Surgical pathology of the mediastinum, 2nd ed. New York: Raven Press; 1992:155-79.

36. Marina NM, Cushing B, Giller R, et al. Complete surgical excision is effective treatment for children with immature teratomas with or without malignant elements: A Pediatric Oncology Group/Children's Cancer Group Intergroup Study. J Clin Oncol 1999;17:2137-43.

37. McLachlin CM, Srigley JR. Prostatic tissue in mature cystic teratomas of the ovary. Am J Surg Pathol 1992;16:780-4.

38. McNeil MM, Leong AS, Sage RE. Primary mediastinal embryonal carcinoma in association with Klinefelter's syndrome. Cancer 1981;47:343-5.

38a. Kwon MS. Aspiration cytology of mediastinal seminoma: report of a case with emphasis on the diagnostic role of aspiration cytology, cell block and immunohistochemistry. Acta Cytol 2005;49:669-72.

39. Moran CA, Suster S. Mediastinal seminomas with prominent cystic changes. A clinicopathologic study of 10 cases. Am J Surg Pathol 1995;19:1047-53.

39a. Moran CA, Suster S. Primary mediastinal choriocarcinomas: a clinicopathologic and immunohistochemical study of eight cases. Am J Surg Pathol 1997;21:1007-12.

40. Moran CA, Suster S. Hepatoid yolk sac tumors of the mediastinum: a clinicopathologic and immunohistochemical study of four cases. Am J Surg Pathol 1997;21:1210-4.

41. Moran CA, Suster S. Primary germ cell tumors of the mediastinum: I. Analysis of 322 cases with special emphasis on teratomatous lesions and a proposal for histopathologic classification and clinical staging. Cancer 1997;80:681-90.

42. Moran CA, Suster S, Koss MN. Primary germ cell tumors of the mediastinum III. Yolk sac tumor, embryonal carcinoma choriocarcinoma, and combined nonteratomatous germ cell tumors of the mediastinum---a clinicopathologic and immunohistochemical study of 64 cases. Cancer 1997;80:699-707.

43. Morinaga S, Nomori H, Kobayashi R, Atsumi Y. Well-differentiated adenocarcinoma arising from mature cystic teratoma of the mediastinum (teratoma with malignant transformation). Report of a surgical case. Am J Clin Pathol 1994;101:531-4.

44. Motoyama T, Yamamoto O, Iwamoto H, Watanabe H. Fine needle aspiration cytology of primary mediastinal germ cell tumors. Acta Cytol 1995;39:725-32.

45. Mukai K, Adams WR. Yolk sac tumor of the anterior mediastinum. Case report with light- and electron-microscopic examination and immunohistochemical study of alpha-fetoprotein. Am J Surg Pathol 1979;3:77-83.

46. Nichols CR. Mediastinal germ cell tumors. Clinical features and biologic correlates. Chest 1991;99:472-9.

47. Nichols CR, Andersen J, Lazarus HM, et al. High-dose carboplatin and etoposide with autologous bone marrow transplantation in refractory germ cell cancer: an Eastern Cooperative Oncology Group protocol. J Clin Oncol 1992;10:558-63.

47a. Nichols CR, Roth BJ, Heerema N, Griep J, Tricot G. Hematologic neoplasia associated with primary mediastinal germ-cell tumors. N Engl J Med 1990;322:1425-9.

48. Niehans GA, Manival JC, Copland GT, Scheithauer BW, Wick MR. Immunohistochemistry of germ cell and trophoblastic neoplasms. Cancer 1988;62:1113-23.

49. Oosterhuis JW, Rammeloo RH, Cornelisse CJ, De Jong B, Dam A, Sleijfer DT. Ploidy of malignant mediastinal germ-cell tumors. Hum Pathol 1990;21:729-32.

50. Perlman EJ, Hu J, Ho DM, Cushing B, Lauer S, Castleberry RP. Genetic analysis of childhood endodermal sinus tumors by comparative genomic hybridization. J Pediatr Hematol Oncol 2000;22:100-5.

51. Rosai J, Levine GD. Tumors of the thymus, Atlas of Tumor Pathology, 2nd Series, Fascicle 13. Washington, DC: Armed Forces Institute of Pathology; 1976.

52. Roy N, Blurton DJ, Azakie A, Karl TR. Immature intrapericardial teratoma in a newborn with elevated alpha-fetoprotein. Ann Thorac Surg 2004;78:e6-8.

53. Saito A, Watanabe K, Kusakabe T, Abe M, Suzuki T. Mediastinal mature teratoma with coexistence of angiosarcoma, granulocytic sarcoma and a hematopoietic region in the tumor. A rare case of association between hematological malignancy and mediastinal germ cell tumor. Pathol Int 1998;48:749-53.

54. Sangalli G, Livraghi T, Giordano F, Tavani E, Schiaffino E. Primary mediastinal embryonal carcinoma and choriocarcinoma. A case report. Act Cytol 1986;30:543-6.

55. Schantz A, Sewall W, Castleman B. Mediastinal germinoma. A study of 21 cases with an excellent prognosis. Cancer 1972;30:1189-94.

56. Schneider DT, Calaminus G, Reinhard H, et al. Primary mediastinal germ cell tumors in children and adolescents: results of German cooperative protocols MAKEI 83/86, 89, and 96. J Clin Oncol 2000;18:832-9.

57. Schneider DT, Schuster AE, Fritsch MK, et al. Multipoint imprinting analysis indicates a common precursor cell for gonadal and nongonadal pediatric germ cell tumors. Cancer Res 2001;61:7268-76.

58. Schneider DT, Schuster AE, Fritsch MK, et al. Genetic analysis of mediastinal nonseminomatous germ cell tumors in children and adolescents. Genes Chromosomes Cancer 2002;34:115-25.

59. Sham JS, Fu KH, Chiu CS, et al. Experience with the management of primary endodermal sinus tumor of the mediastinum. Cancer 1989;64:756-61.

60. Singh HK, Silverman JF, Powers CN, Geisinger KR, Frable WJ. Diagnostic pitfalls in fine-needle aspiration biopsy of the mediastinum. Diagn Cytopathol 1997;17:121-6.

61. Suda K, Mizuguchi K, Hebisawa A, Wakabayashi T, Saito S. Pancreatic tissue in teratoma. Arch Pathol Lab Med 1984;108:835-7.

62. Takeda S, Miyoshi S, Ohta M, Minami M, Masaoka A, Matsuda H. Primary germ cell tumors in the mediastinum: a 50-year experience at a single Japanese institution. Cancer 2003;97:367-76.

63. Thurlbeck WM, Scully RE. Solid teratoma of the ovary. A clinicopathological analysis of 9 cases. Cancer 1960;13:804-11.

64. Timothy DJ, Ulbright TM, Eble JN, Baldridge LA, Cheng, L. OCT4 staining in testicular tumors: a sensitive and specific marker for seminoma and embryonal carcinoma. Am J Surg Pathol 2004;28:935-40.

65. Toner GC, Geller NL, Lin SY, Bosl GJ. Extragonadal and poor risk nonseminomatous germ cell tumors. Survival and prognostic features. Cancer 1991;67:2049-57.

66. Travis WD, Brambilla E, Müller-Hermelink HK, Harris CC, eds. World Health Organization Classification of Tumours. Pathology and genetics of tumours of the lung, thymus and heart. Lyon: IARC Press; 2004.

67. Truong LD, Harris L, Mattioli C, et al. Endodermal sinus tumor of the mediastinum. A report of seven cases and review of the literature. Cancer 1986;58:730-9.

68. Tsuchiya R, Koga K, Matsuno Y, Mukai K, Shimosato Y. Thymic carcinoma: proposed pathological TNM and staging. Pathol Int 1994;44:505-12.

69. UICC. TNM Supplement 2001, A commentary on uniform use, 2nd ed. Wittekind Ch, Mensen DE, Hutter RV, Sobin LH, eds. New York: Wiley-Liss; 2001.

70. Ulbright TM. Testicular and paratesticular tumors. In Mills SE, Carter D, Greenson JK, Oberman HA, Reuter V, Stoler MH, eds. Sternberg's diagnostic surgical pathology, 4th ed. Philadelphia: Lippincott Williams and Wilkins; 2004: 2167-232.

71. Ulbright TM. Germ cell tumors of the gonads: a selective review emphasizing problems in differential diagnosis, newly appreciated, and controversial issues. Mod Pathol 2005;18:(Suppl 2):S61-79.

72. Ulbright TM, Loehrer PJ, Roth LM, Einhorn LH, Williams SD, Clark SA. The development of non-germ cell malignancies within germ cell tumors. A clinicopathologic study of 11 cases. Cancer 1984;54:1824-33.

73. Ulbright TM, Roth LM, Brodhecker CA. Yolk sac differentiation in germ cell tumor. A morphologic study of 50 cases with emphasis on hepatic, enteric, and parietal yolk sac features. Am J Surg Pathol 1986;10:151-64.

74. Weidner N. Germ-cell tumors of the mediastinum. Semin Diagn Pathol 1999;16:42-50.

75. Wick MR, Perlman EJ, Orazi A, et al. Germ cell tumours of the mediastinum. In Travis WD, Brambilla E, Müller-Hermelink HK, Harris CC, eds. World Health Organization Classification of Tumours. Pathology and genetics of tumours of the lung, pleura, thymus and heart. Lyon: IARC Press; 2004:198-201.

76. Yang GC, Hwang SJ, Yee HT. Fine-needle aspiration cytology of unusual germ cell tumors of the mediastinum: atypical seminoma and parietal yolk sac tumor. Diagn Cytopathol 2002;27:69-74.

6 MALIGNANT LYMPHOMAS AND HEMATOPOIETIC NEOPLASMS

Malignant lymphoma of the mediastinum may be primary in this location or secondary to generalized disease. Mediastinal lymphoma arises either in the mediastinal lymph nodes or in the thymus, and manifests as an anterior, superior, or middle mediastinal mass. A general description of various malignant lymphomas and hematopoietic neoplasms can be obtained in the Third and Fourth Series Atlas of Tumor Pathology Fascicles on the bone marrow and lymphoid tissues; the World Health Organization (WHO) Classification of Tumours of the Haematopoietic and Lymphoid Tissues, and of Tumours of the Lung, Thymus and Heart; as well as other major textbooks of hematopathology (5,26a,32,78,82). Discussion in this chapter is confined principally to malignant lymphomas and hematopoietic tumors that present as primary neoplasms in the mediastinum, both within the thymus and the lymph nodes. The classification used is the Revised European and American Lymphoma (REAL) classification (18), updated in the WHO classification (26a).

B-CELL LYMPHOMAS

Primary Mediastinal Large B-Cell Lymphoma

General Features. Non-Hodgkin large cell lymphomas (with a B-cell phenotype) have been known for more than two decades. They were formerly labeled mediastinal histiocytic lymphoma, mediastinal clear cell lymphoma of B-cell type, or mediastinal diffuse large cell lymphoma with sclerosis (1,13,37,39,47–49,52, 61). Prior to 1980, before lymphocyte marker study was available, and because of compartmentalization or nesting by hyaline connective tissue, mediastinal large B-cell lymphomas were often mistaken for seminoma, undifferentiated thymic carcinoma, and Hodgkin lymphoma (61). In fact, the initial diagnoses of the first two cases seen at the National Cancer Center Hospital in Tokyo were anaplastic germinoma and undifferentiated carcinoma. In the REAL and WHO classifications, primary mediastinal large cell lymphomas with B-cell phenotype, reported previously under a variety of terms, were categorized as *primary mediastinal large B-cell lymphoma*, disregarding individual cell morphology and the presence or absence of interstitial sclerosis (18,26a).

Clinical Features. Primary mediastinal large B-cell lymphoma is an uncommon tumor. It occurs predominantly in adults in the third and fourth decades of life, with a slight female predominance; diffuse large B-cell lymphomas of other locations occur in an older age group with a male predominance (7,11,18). According to Perrone et al. (61), 85 percent of patients (52 of 60 patients) are 35 years of age or younger at the time of initial diagnosis, with a male to female ratio of about 1.0 to 2.5. Of 28 Japanese patients of the National Cancer Center Hospital in Tokyo, the age range was 18 to 80 years (mean, 37 years) and the male to female ratio was 4 to 3 (71).

Patients often complain of dyspnea, cough, chest pain, malaise, and fever, and frequently present with superior vena cava syndrome. Chest X ray and computerized tomography (CT) examinations often disclose a large mass in the anterior mediastinum, frequently invading large vessels, pericardium, pleura, lungs, and chest wall (fig. 6-1). Pleural and pericardial effusions may be present. The lesion tends to remain within the thorax, but sometimes involves extrathoracic organs such as lymph nodes, kidney, liver, pancreas, gastrointestinal tract, central nervous system, and ovary.

Gross Findings. The tumor is usually larger than 10 cm in greatest dimension. The cut surface is ivory colored, with or without foci of coagulation necrosis (figs. 6-1, 6-2). Thymic tissue may be attached to the tumor. In small tumors, foci of necrosis are absent and there may be granularity due to lobulation (fig. 6-3).

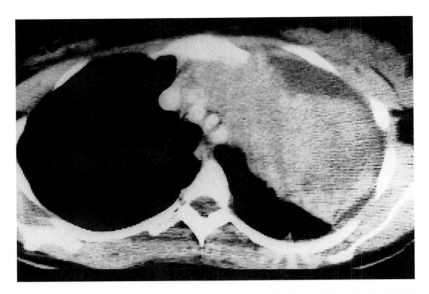

Figure 6-1

**PRIMARY MEDIASTINAL
LARGE B-CELL LYMPHOMA**

Top: Enhanced computerized tomography (CT) with radiopaque material at the level above the aortic arch reveals a huge tumor which extends from the anterior mediastinum to the left thoracic cavity, displacing the left lung posteriorly. The major vessels shown from the left to right are the superior vena cava and brachiocephalic, left common carotid, and left subclavian arteries. (Fig. 3-204 from Fascicle 21, Third Series.)

Bottom: A horizontal section of the gross specimen shows lobulation, conspicuous in the central portion. A small amount of the lung parenchyma (left) and a part of the chest wall (right) are attached. The hole appearing in the center is an artifact.

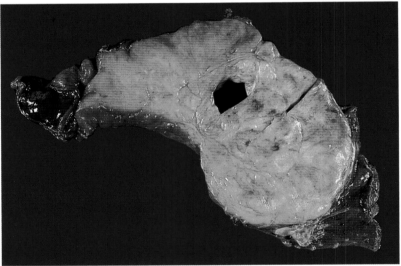

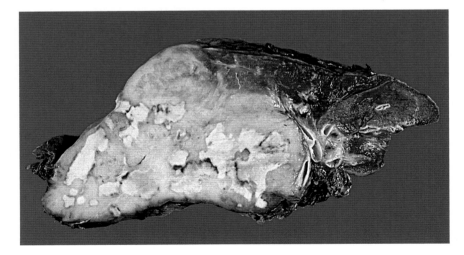

Figure 6-2

**PRIMARY MEDIASTINAL
LARGE B-CELL LYMPHOMA**

The horizontal cut surface of the large tumor shows invasive growth into the left upper lobe of the lung and irregular areas of coagulation necrosis. Lobulation is inconspicuous due to the high cellularity. (Fig. 3-205 from Fascicle 21, Third Series.)

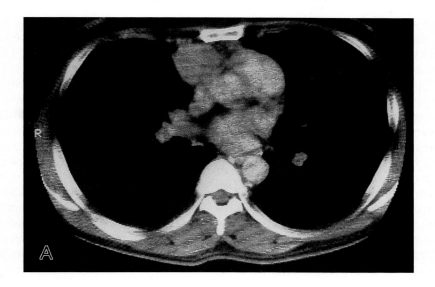

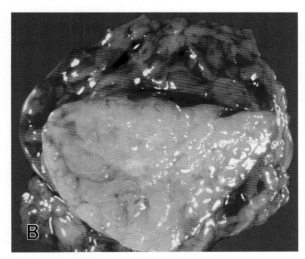

Figure 6-3

PRIMARY MEDIASTINAL LARGE B-CELL LYMPHOMA

A: Enhanced CT at the level below the tracheal carina discloses a homogeneous tumorous density with smooth borders anterior to the heart, and adjacent to the pericardium and right lung. (A&B, fig. 3-206A&B from Fascicle 21, Third Series.)

B: Horizontal cut surface of the tumor shows lobulation and nodularity without foci of coagulation necrosis.

C: Low-power view shows lobulation with fibrous bands resembling nodular sclerosis type Hodgkin lymphoma.

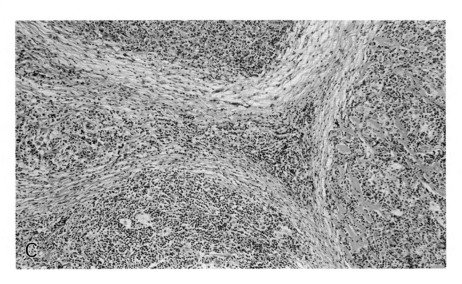

Microscopic Findings. The tumors reveal two common patterns: the presence of large cells with clear cytoplasm (38 percent of cases) and the presence of fibrosis (marked in 25 percent of cases) (7). The clear cell type is characterized by the diffuse growth of tumor cells with abundant clear cytoplasm. Tumor cells show a high S-phase component and rapid growth; the immunophenotype corresponds to the terminal stage of B-cell differentiation (48,49). Tumors with fibrosis are often compartmentalized into epithelial tumor–like solid nests by hyaline connective tissue of varying thickness (fig. 6-4), into lobules by broad fibrous bands (fig. 6-3C), and into a spindle cell sarcomatous pattern by thin sclerotic interstitium surrounding individual tumor cells and compressing them into spindle cells.

The histologic features vary. In a study of 29 tumors, 6 were immunoblastic, 14 were large cell not otherwise specified, 6 were large cell noncleaved, 1 was large cell cleaved, and 2 were not subclassifiable (37).

Tumor cells are medium-sized to large and possess abundant, pale, clear, and lightly acidophilic to basophilic cytoplasm. The nuclei are either large and vesicular with prominent nucleoli, or indented, reniform, or even multilobated (fig. 6-5). Small reactive lymphocytes and macrophages are seen in some areas (figs. 6-4, 6-5). Fixation artifacts, such as dense nuclei and apparently empty or vacuolated cytoplasm, may be seen. Mitotic figures are frequently observed.

Cytologic Findings. Features seen in fine needle aspiration cytology smears and imprint smears vary from case to case (fig. 6-6). In one study, azurophil granules were seen in the cytoplasm in imprint smears stained with the May-Giemsa stain. This finding is said to be rare in nodal B-cell tumors (52).

Immunohistochemical Findings. The tumor cells are CD19, CD20, CD22, and CD79a positive, and CD5, CD10, and CD21 negative (fig. 6-7) (28,52). CD30 is frequently positive but weak (78). Surface and cytoplasmic immunoglobulins are often negative, and when positive, are of immunoglobulin (Ig)G or IgA type, contrasting with the IgM or IgD type seen in large cell lymphoma of nodal origin (37,47). The discrepancy between the lack of immunoglobulin and the constitutive CD79a is charac-

teristic of this disease (28,78). Negative CD21 suggests an origin from the B cells present in the normal thymus (24). Although this hypothesis has been generally accepted, de Leval et al. (14) raised the possibility that mediastinal large B-cell lymphoma may arise from thymic B-cell follicles acquired in early adulthood, because of a phenotype with positive bcl-6 (19/19 cases) and CD10 (6/19 cases) in their series.

Molecular and Other Special Diagnostic Techniques. Southern blot analysis has disclosed unique heavy and kappa light chain immunoglobulin gene rearrangements, thereby genotypically establishing a B-cell origin and a germline T-cell receptor gene in all but one case (52,69). Clonal immunoglobulin gene rearrangements were demonstrated in two cases of mediastinal large B-cell lymphoma of clear cell type (4). C-*myc* gene alterations were found in three of six cases, none of which displayed a *bcl*-2 gene rearrangement or contained Epstein-Barr viral sequences (52,70). Analysis of molecular genetic patterns in 16 primary mediastinal large B-cell lymphomas revealed infrequent occurrence (6 percent) of *bcl*-6 gene rearrangement compared with other diffuse large B-cell lymphomas (up to 45 percent), suggesting that primary mediastinal large B-cell lymphomas represent a distinct subtype of diffuse large B-cell lymphoma (79). In another study, however, molecular analysis revealed *bcl*-6 gene mutations in more than half of the 45 cases (62). The data on the frequency of *bcl*-6 mutations in this disease are conflicting, ranging from 6 to 50 percent (78).

There are a few reports describing specific chromosomal alterations in primary mediastinal large B-cell lymphoma. Among these, gain of chromosomes 9, 19, or X, or loss of chromosome 4 has been described as characteristic, in contrast to diffuse large B-cell lymphoma of other primary sites (57). Gain of chromosome 9p and amplification of the *REL* gene have also been reported (27). The *MAL* gene is reportedly overexpressed in this type of malignant lymphoma, and it is suggested that its gene product may be useful as a molecular marker in the clinical setting (12).

Differential Diagnosis. Tumors to be distinguished from primary mediastinal large B-cell lymphoma are seminoma, undifferentiated thymic carcinoma, Hodgkin lymphoma, mediastinal

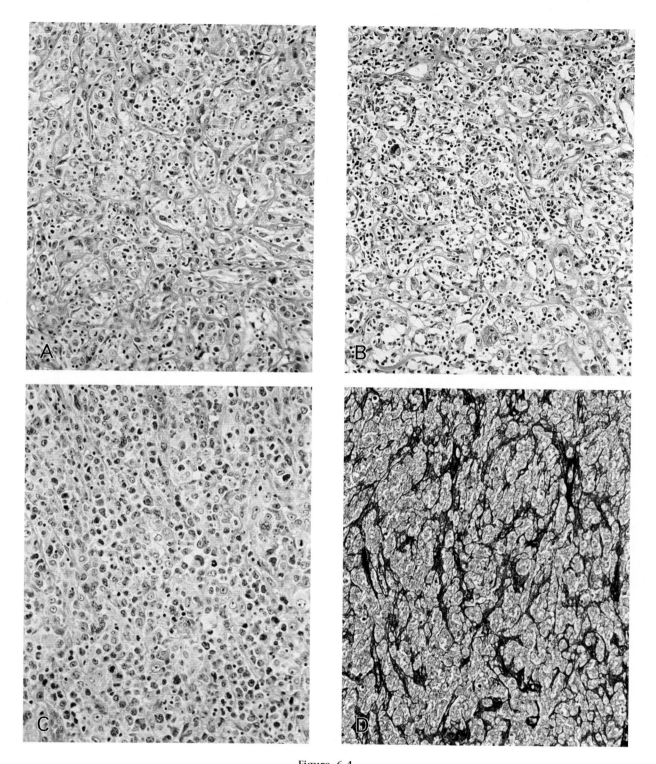

Figure 6-4

PRIMARY MEDIASTINAL LARGE B-CELL LYMPHOMA

A–C: The compartmentalization induced by interstitial sclerosis of various degrees is shown.
D: Silver impregnation shows both complete and incomplete compartmentalization.

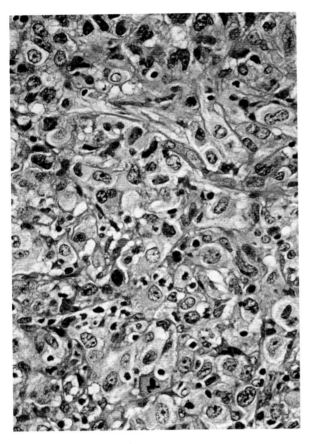

Figure 6-5

PRIMARY MEDIASTINAL LARGE B-CELL LYMPHOMA

High magnification shows large tumor cells with abundant pale cytoplasm, round to reniform vesicular nuclei, and prominent nucleoli. A mitotic figure is present. Most small lymphoid cells are of reactive T-cell phenotype.

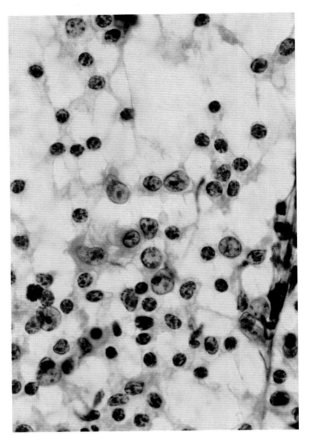

Figure 6-6

**PRIMARY MEDIASTINAL LARGE
B-CELL LYMPHOMA: CYTOLOGY**

The tumor cells are medium sized, with round vesicular or finely granular nuclei and distinct nucleoli. The pale staining cytoplasm is moderate in amount or lytic. There are scattered small reactive lymphocytes.

involvement of diffuse large cell and immunoblastic lymphoma of extrathoracic origin, metastatic undifferentiated carcinoma of extrathoracic origin, and metastatic amelanotic melanoma. The same differential diagnosis should be considered concerning fine-needle aspiration cytology of the mediastinum (74).

Rare pleomorphic large cell lymphomas of the mediastinum (nine cases reported) consist of three histologic growth patterns that can cause diagnostic difficulty: sarcomatoid, anaplastic carcinoma-like, and lymphocyte depleted Hodgkin lymphoma-like (75). Immunohistochemical studies show that the tumor cells stain for CD20 and CD45, and do not stain with a large panel of markers including keratin, carcinoembryonic antigen,

epithelial membrane antigen, vimentin, actin, desmin, HMB45, S-100 protein, CD3, CD15, CD30, and CD45RO, differentiating it from carcinoma, sarcoma, melanoma, or T-cell lymphoma.

Prognosis. Initially, the prognosis of patients with primary mediastinal large B-cell lymphoma was reported to be poor. Unfavorable prognostic factors were age less than 25 years at diagnosis, tumor outside the thoracic cavity, disease recurrence, and immunoblastic tumor histology. Favorable signs were good response to initial therapy and marked tumor sclerosis (61). In one study, performance status, pericardial effusion, bulky mediastinal tumor, and residual mediastinal abnormality after intensive treatment were additional poor prognostic factors

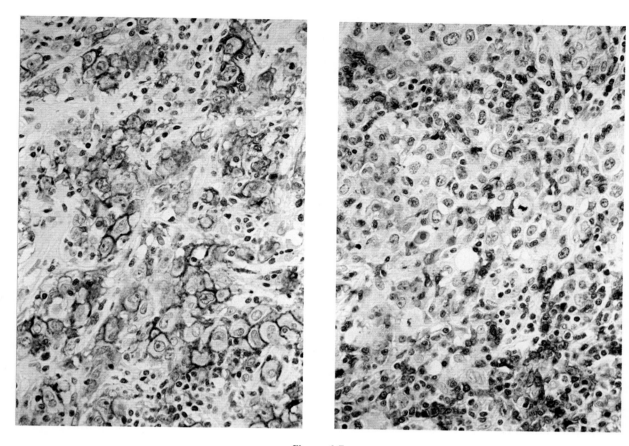

Figure 6-7

PRIMARY MEDIASTINAL LARGE B-CELL LYMPHOMA: IMMUNOHISTOCHEMISTRY

The tumor cells show marked membrane staining with CD20 antibody (left), and no reactivity with CD45RO antibody (right), indicating a B-cell phenotype. Small lymphocytes of a reactive nature are strongly positive for CD45RO (T cell).

(38). Lately, the prognosis has improved and a 5-year survival rate of about 50 percent is obtained with intense chemotherapy combined with radiotherapy (30,37,52). Tumors without bulky mass are found to be curable (26,37). Although confirmatory studies are needed, 28 cases encountered between 1982 and 2002 at the National Cancer Center Hospital in Tokyo indicated the relatively unfavorable prognosis for patients, with estimated 3-year overall and failure-free survival rates of 32 percent and 33 percent, respectively (71).

Thymic Extranodal Marginal Zone B-Cell Lymphoma of Mucosa-Associated Lymphoid Tissue

General Features. In 1987, Isaacson and Spencer (25) reviewed malignant lymphomas of

mucosa-associated lymphoid tissue (MALT) that involved the gastrointestinal tract, salivary gland, lung, and thyroid gland; most were of B-cell type and tended to remain localized for prolonged periods. In 1990, Isaacson et al. (23) reported two cases of low-grade B-cell lymphoma of MALT arising in the thymus. A report followed of a similar case but associated with Sjögren syndrome (76). The cases were characterized as "lymphoepithelial lesions," most closely resembling MALT lymphoma arising in myoepithelial sialadenitis. In the thymus, Hassall corpuscles were considered to correspond to a mucosal structure.

Thymic extranodal marginal zone B-cell lymphoma of MALT is a rare neoplasm. More than half of the cases reported are from Japan. Patients are of a mean age of 56.5 years at diagnosis and the male to female ratio is about 1 to 3. The disease

231

is frequently associated with autoimmune disease, particularly with Sjögren's syndrome, with a high frequency of IgA phenotype and clonal immunoglobulin heavy chain gene rearrangement, but not associated with Epstein-Barr virus (22,42,45,51,58,68,71a,84,85). Coexistence in the thymus and stomach of marginal zone B-cell lymphoma of MALT in a patient with Sjögren syndrome has been reported (51).

Gross Findings. The reported tumors are often encapsulated masses of 7.5 to 13.0 cm in greatest dimension. They are very soft, with a pale tan homogeneous cut surface. Some are studded with fluid-filled cysts of up to a few centimeters in diameter. Some tumors have ill-defined borders within thymic (or mediastinal) tissue without recognizable encapsulation, as opposed to thymoma.

Microscopic Findings. The normal architecture of the thymus is obscured by a lymphoid infiltrate, in which Hassall corpuscles are seen. The lymphoid infiltrate consists of reactive type follicles and diffuse growth of lymphoma cells showing a predominantly centrocyte-like or monocytoid appearance. The cells possess variably irregular nuclei; abundant clear, faintly granular cytoplasm; and sharp cell borders. Plasma cell differentiation may be present and larger blast forms are scattered throughout. Mitotic counts are less than 1 per 10 high-power fields. Thymic epithelial cell nests, including Hassall corpuscles, are obliterated or isolated at times, due to the lymphocytic infiltration. Prominent lymphoepithelial lesions may be a diagnostic clue for distinguishing this lymphoma from thymic hyperplasia or from lymphocyte-predominant thymoma. Cysts are lined by attenuated epithelium infiltrated by centrocyte-like lymphocytes and contain eosinophilic proteinaceous fluid.

Immunohistochemical Findings. The lymphoid infiltrates consist largely of B cells, which are CD20 and CD79a positive. Both of the cases of Isaacson et al. (23) showed kappa light chain restriction, expressing IgM in case 1 and IgA in case 2. In the case of Takagi et al. (76), the cells monotypically stained for IgA and kappa light chain. The phenotypes of the centrocyte-like lymphocytes are CD20, CD22, and CD79a positive, and CD3, CD5, CD10, and CD23 negative. Bcl-2 positivity is found in some cases (42,58).

Molecular and Other Special Diagnostic Techniques. The histopathologic diagnosis of thymic extranodal marginal zone B-cell lymphoma of MALT is not always easy. To obtain evidence for the presence of a neoplastic B-cell clone in the lesion, molecular analysis of immunoglobulin gene rearrangement by Southern blotting, or an equivalent alternative assay, is recommended. Usually the genes for both the heavy and light chains of immunoglobulin show clonal rearrangements. In a certain proportion of MALT lymphomas at other anatomic sites, especially the lung and stomach, t(11;18)(q21;q21), resulting from the fusion of the *API* and the *MALT1* genes, is frequently found in the tumor. The proportion of cases in which the fused gene is detectable is known to vary among the anatomic sites of the primary tumor. Among 15 Japanese cases of thymic MALT lymphoma studied by reverse transcriptase-polymerase chain reaction (RT-PCR) using formalin-fixed paraffin-embedded tissues, however, not a single case was positive for the *API-MALT1* fusion gene (22). A tumor reported by Takagi et al. (76) revealed rearrangements of the immunoglobulin heavy chain-joining region gene, kappa light chain-joining region gene, and the T-cell receptor beta-chain gene constant region.

Marginal zone B-cell lymphomas of MALT are often localized when diagnosed, are relatively benign, and may be cured by surgical resection. In case 1 of Isaacson et al. (23), the patient was alive and free of disease 4 years after surgery without further treatment. In case 2, the tumor involved a left axillary lymph node which was excised 2 months after resection of the thymic lymphoma. The patient reported by Takagi et al. (76) had total surgical resection of the mediastinal tumor, which was 13 cm in its greatest dimension and confined to within the thymus except in a small area that involved the pericardium. An adjacent lymph node was also involved. Resection was followed by radiotherapy and the patient was in complete remission 20 months later.

The first case encountered at the National Cancer Center Hospital in Tokyo was a 43-year-old Japanese housewife with an unusual asymptomatic anterior mediastinal tumor detected by routine chest X ray. It was multicystic on CT scan

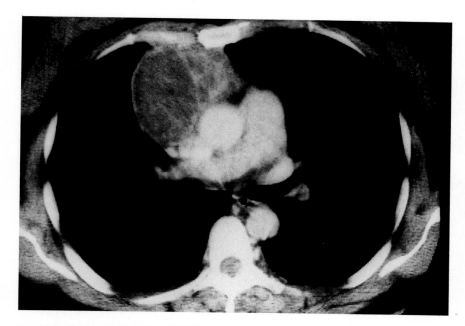

Figure 6-8

LOW-GRADE MARGINAL ZONE B-CELL LYMPHOMA OF MUCOSA-ASSOCIATED LYMPHOID TISSUE (MALT) OF THE THYMUS

CT at the level of the right pulmonary artery enhanced with radiopaque material reveals a roughly oval, clearly defined tumor with a smooth border in the anterior mediastinum. The tumor is lobulated and non-homogeneous, strongly suggestive of a multiloculated cystic lesion. The preoperative diagnosis was cystic teratoma. (Fig. 3-210 from Fascicle 21, Third Series.) (Figs. 6-8–6-11 are from the same patient.)

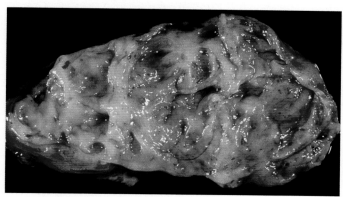
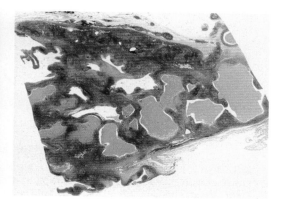

Figure 6-9

LOW-GRADE MARGINAL ZONE B-CELL LYMPHOMA OF MALT OF THE THYMUS

Left: The cut surface of the tumor shows variously sized, multiple cystic spaces with intervening medullary pale tan tissue.

Right: Low-power magnification reveals a partly and thinly encapsulated tumor, which is lobulated. A few fat cells lie between the lobules. Irregular cystic spaces containing serous fluid are present within or in association with lobules. Scanty thymic tissue is attached to the tumor at the top.

(fig. 6-8) and preoperatively suspected to be a teratoma. The thymic tumor was 10.0 x 8.5 x 2.0 cm and weighed 125 g. The cut surface of the mass revealed a thinly encapsulated tumor with multiple, irregular cystic spaces varying in size, and intervening pale tan medullary tissue (fig. 6-9, left). Histologically, scant thymic tissue of normal appearance for the patient's age was attached to the tumor. The tumor itself was lobulated, with cystic spaces within lobules and a few fat cells between lobules (fig. 6-9, right). Cortices and

medullae were indistinct but enlarged Hassall corpuscles could be recognized. Cystic spaces containing serous fluid, lymphoid cells, and degenerated Hassall corpuscles, with or without calcification, were bordered by atypical hyperplastic thymic tissue with squamoid epithelium infiltrated by lymphocytes. This area was considered to be a focus of a lymphoepithelial lesion (fig. 6-10, left). Some cystic spaces were devoid of lining epithelium and bordered by lymphoid tissue directly. No perivascular spaces or other

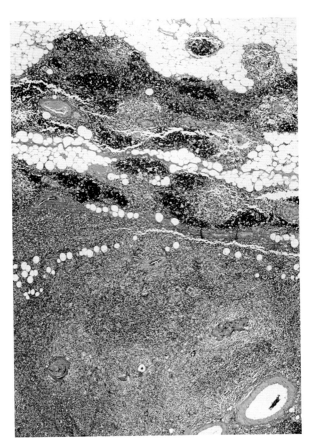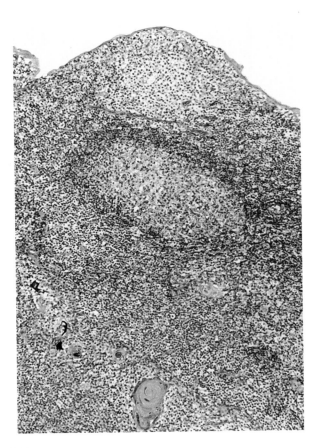

Figure 6-10

LOW-GRADE MARGINAL ZONE B-CELL LYMPHOMA OF MALT OF THE THYMUS

Left: Thymic tissue of normal appearance is shown on the top. The tumor, on the bottom, contains prominent Hassall corpuscles. Cortices and medulla are still recognizable, although blurred in some areas.

Right: A cyst is lined by attenuated squamoid epithelial cells, beneath which is a small monotonous area of uniform clear lymphoid cells facing a lymph follicle with a germinal center. In the lower left corner, a Hassall corpuscle is surrounded by atypical clear lymphoid cells.

structures characteristic of thymoma were seen. Lymph follicles with germinal centers were seen in some areas (fig. 6-10, right). There was diffuse growth of uniform, medium-sized lymphoid cells that had round granular nuclei, small nucleoli, and clear, faintly granular cytoplasm. Cell borders were not distinct (fig. 6-11, left). Mitotic figures were rare. There were scattered larger blast-like cells. This atypical lymphoid tissue infiltrated the thymic cortices and medullae and formed parts of the cyst walls.

Originally, because of lack of awareness of such a lesion in the thymus; clear delineation of the lesion from normal thymic tissue; the presence of thymic tissue components such as Hassall cor-

puscles, lymphoid cells, and fat; and no definite features suggestive of malignancy, we considered this lesion as a hamartoma or atypical lymphoid hyperplasia of the thymus, although no such entity had ever been reported. Later, the atypical lymphoid cells were found to show a B-cell phenotype (fig. 6-11, right), and the lesion was diagnosed as low-grade B-cell lymphoma of MALT primary in the thymus, although restriction of light chain expression could not be verified. The patient is alive with no evidence of recurrence more than 9 years after surgery.

The second case seen at the National Cancer Center Hospital (85) was a 55-year-old woman who had a history of rheumatoid arthritis, and

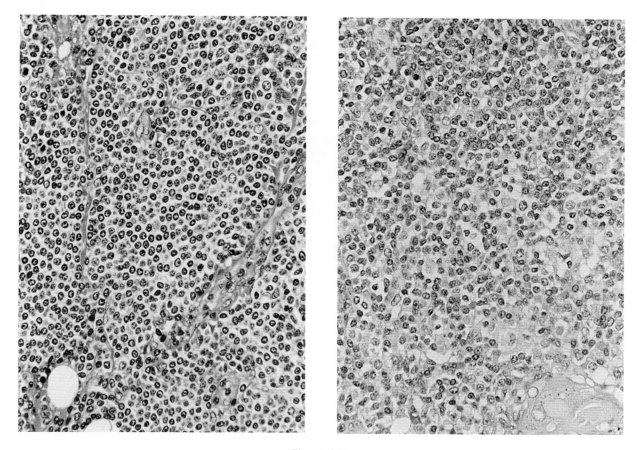

Figure 6-11

LOW-GRADE MARGINAL ZONE B-CELL LYMPHOMA OF MALT IN THE THYMUS

Left: High magnification of the tumor reveals diffuse monotonous growth of medium-sized lymphoid cells with round granular nuclei, small nucleoli, and clear or faintly granular cytoplasm. The cell border is indistinct. Mitotic figures are not seen.

Right: CD20 immunostaining reveals many positive cells and scattered large blast-like cells. A Hassall corpuscle is seen at the right upper corner.

complained of back pain. An anterior mediastinal tumor was found by CT scan. The tumor was solid, 7.5 x 6.2 x 2.0 cm in size, weighed 50 g, and was confined to within the thymus. This tumor was in continuity with the thymic parenchyma. Scattered within the tumor were lymph follicles with germinal centers. The medulla of the thymus was almost completely replaced by monotonous, small to medium-sized centrocyte-like or monocytoid cells, characterized by moderately abundant, clear or finely granular cytoplasm and round or indented nuclei. Mitotic figures were occasionally seen (fig. 6-12). However, follicular colonization was not evident on hematoxylin and eosin (H&E)-stained sections. Immunohistochemically, atypical

monocytoid cells were found to be of B-cell phenotype, showed kappa light chain restriction, and expressed IgA (fig. 6-13). The diagnosis was localized MALT lymphoma.

Imprint cytology of low-grade marginal zone B-cell lymphoma of MALT in the thymus was reported by Nakamura et al. (53). The imprint smears revealed small to medium-sized lymphocytes with round to slightly irregular, often eccentric nuclei; slightly condensed chromatin; and inconspicuous nucleoli. The cytoplasm varied in amount and staining quality, the larger cells displaying moderate amounts of a pale (amphophilic) to slightly basophilic cytoplasm. Plasmacytoid lymphocytes were admixed and a few epithelial cells were found (fig. 6-14).

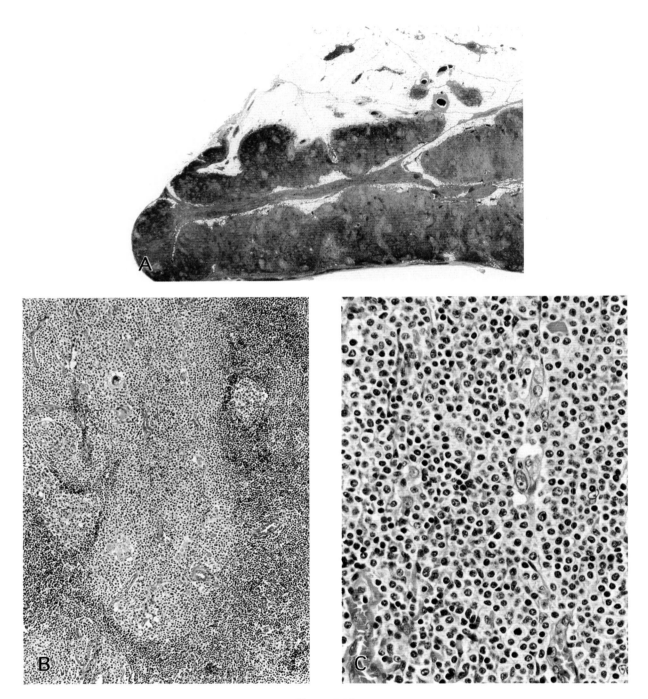

Figure 6-12

LOW-GRADE MARGINAL ZONE B-CELL LYMPHOMA OF MALT IN THE THYMUS

A: Low power reveals a nonencapsulated, in part lobulated, nodular tumor abutting the involuting thymus. The tumor is studded with multiple pale zones, but no cystic changes are seen.

B: The medullae of the thymus have been almost completely replaced by the monotonous growth of small round cells surrounding a well-formed Hassall corpuscle, adjacent to which is a lymph follicle with a germinal center.

C: Higher-power magnification reveals that the proliferating cells surrounding attenuated Hassall corpuscles are medium-sized monocytoid cells with clear cytoplasm and round or indented nuclei. A few mitotic figures are seen. (Figs. 6-12 and 6-13 are from the same patient.)

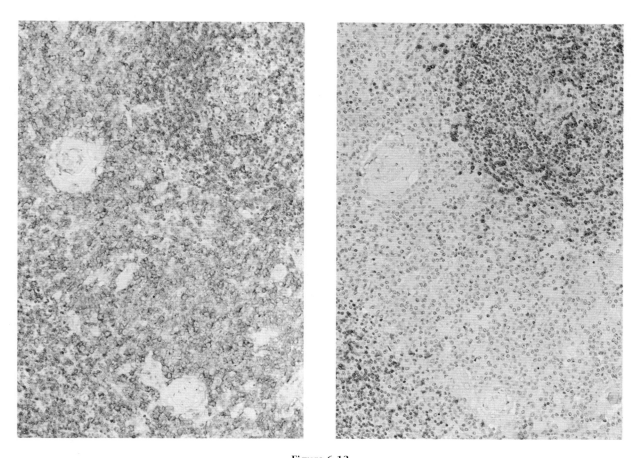

Figure 6-13

LOW-GRADE MARGINAL ZONE B-CELL LYMPHOMA OF MALT IN THE THYMUS

Left: A Hassall corpuscle is surrounded by the diffuse growth of atypical monocytoid B lymphocytes reactive with CD20 antibody.

Right: Almost no T lymphocytes reactive with CD45RO antibody remain in the zone with diffuse growth of atypical B lymphocytes.

Differential Diagnosis. The cytologic diagnosis of thymic disease is often difficult, as is the histologic diagnosis, because of the mixture of reactive lymphoid cells. The differential diagnosis includes thymic hyperplasia of both true and follicular types, Castleman disease, thymoma, Hodgkin lymphoma, diffuse large B-cell lymphoma, and seminoma. A diagnosis of lymphoma is favored in a patient with Sjögren syndrome (53).

Prognosis. Low-grade marginal zone B-cell lymphomas of MALT appear to have an indolent clinical course. They may transform to high-grade diffuse large B-cell lymphomas as in MALT lymphomas of other sites, but transformation to higher grade occurs rarely in primary mediastinal MALT lymphomas (42).

T-CELL LYMPHOMAS

T-cell lymphomas primary in the mediastinum include precursor T-lymphoblastic leukemia/lymphoma (precursor T-cell acute lymphoblastic leukemia/precursor T-cell lymphoblastic lymphoma), anaplastic large-cell lymphoma, and other rare mature T- and natural killer (NK)-cell lymphomas.

Precursor T-Lymphoblastic Leukemia/ Lymphoblastic Lymphoma (Precursor T-Cell Acute Lymphoblastic Leukemia/ Precursor T-Cell Lymphoblastic Lymphoma)

General Features. *Precursor T-lymphoblastic leukemia* (ALL)/*lymphoma* (LBL) is mainly a disease of late childhood, adolescence, and young

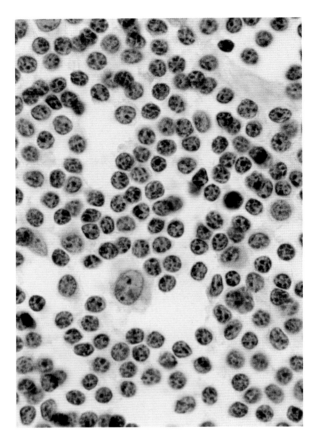 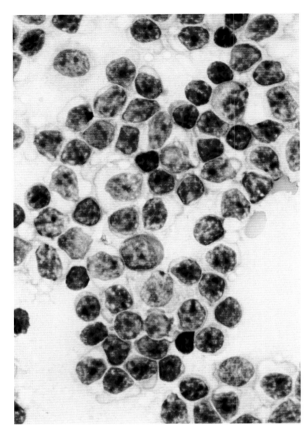

Figure 6-14

LOW-GRADE MARGINAL ZONE B-CELL LYMPHOMA OF MALT: CYTOLOGY

Left: In the background are small atypical lymphocytes of slightly irregular nuclear shape and chromatin aggregation, as well as scattered large lymphoid and plasma cells (Papanicolaou stain).

Right: Centrocyte-like cells and monocytoid cells with pale cytoplasm are seen (Giemsa stain).

adulthood. It has a peculiar predilection for the thymus. Although 20 percent of ALLs/LBLs are derived from precursor B-cells, most are derived from precursor T cells and express phenotypes corresponding to the various stages of the intrathymic differentiation of these cells (31).

ALL and LBL share overlapping clinical, pathologic, cytogenetic, and molecular features. For this reason, some investigators have suggested that ALL and LBL are simply different manifestations of the same disease. However, unlike those with ALL, patients with LBL have no or minimal peripheral blood or bone marrow involvement and normal or slightly decreased white blood cell and platelet counts at presentation. Twenty-five percent blast cells in the bone marrow is considered by some investigators as an arbitrary distinction between ALL and LBL.

Clinical Features. Patients with ALL/LBL typically present with acute respiratory distress due to the presence of a large mediastinal mass, with frequent pleural or pericardial effusions containing tumor cells (fig. 6-15) (67). Males are affected 2 to 4 times more frequently than females. Shortly after presentation, bone marrow, lymph node, and visceral involvement occur and leukemic spread follows. The central nervous system and gonads are often involved. An association with viral disease or decreased immune status has not been shown.

Microscopic Findings. ALL/LBL exhibits a diffuse, infiltrative pattern of growth. The infiltration involves the thymic parenchyma and can be confused with lymphocyte-predominant thymoma (type B1 or B2 thymoma) (fig. 6-16) (31,67). Proliferating tumor cells expand the

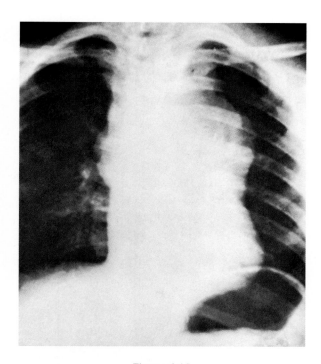

Figure 6-15

PRECURSOR T-LYMPHOBLASTIC LYMPHOMA

This chest X ray shows a large anterosuperior mediastinal mass. (Fig. 3-200 from Fascicle 21, Third Series.)

thymic lobules, surround persistent Hassall corpuscles, and infiltrate vessel walls, fibrous trabeculae, and the thymic capsule. In the periphery of the tumor, the tumor cells often split the collagen fibers and infiltrate between them in a single file arrangement (31).

The neoplastic cells of this lymphoma are medium sized, possessing round to oval or convoluted nuclei with finely dispersed and evenly distributed chromatin, inconspicuous or small nucleoli, thin but distinct nuclear membranes, and scanty cytoplasm with ill-defined cell borders (fig. 6-16). They resemble cortical thymocytes in terms of morphology, immunophenotype, and genotype. Nuclei are classified as convoluted when they possess one or more deep clefts or infoldings, resulting in a lobulated appearance. The mitotic index is high. A starry-sky appearance may be seen (fig. 6-16), which is less prominent than in Burkitt lymphoma. LBL is subdivided into convoluted and nonconvoluted subtypes according to the nuclear configuration of the neoplastic cells.

The presence of occasional convoluted nuclei qualifies an LBL as the convoluted subtype; about 80 percent of LBLs are classified as convoluted based on this criterion (31).

Cytologic Findings. Lymphoid cells seen in imprint smears of an enlarged cervical lymph node involved by LBL are either small with condensed chromatin, inconspicuous nucleoli, and scanty cytoplasm, or medium sized with finely granular chromatin, multiple small nucleoli, and a moderate amount of cytoplasm (fig. 6-17). Azurophil granules may be seen.

Immunohistochemical Findings. Confirmation of the histologic diagnosis can be made by the demonstration of terminal deoxynucleotidyltransferase (TdT) and immature immunophenotypes corresponding to different developmental stages of thymocytes: CD2, CD7, and cytoplasmic CD3 (early to pro-T); CD1a, sCD3, CD4, and CD8 (common thymocyte); and CD4 or CD8 (late thymocyte). During the past 10 years, 17 cases of T-ALL/LBL were seen at the National Cancer Center Hospital in Tokyo. They were divided into thymic type (8 cases) and nonthymic type (9 cases) depending on the distribution of tumor from the radiologic findings. Expression of CD8 was more frequent in the thymic type (6/7 versus 0/9), whereas expression of CD56 was more frequent in nonthymic, systemic type (0/7 versus 5/9) (55).

Genetic Alterations. Genetic studies of antigen receptor genes may be helpful in diagnosis if monoclonality is proven by the presence of rearrangements. Chromosomal translocations may be found in childhood cases. They usually involve T-cell receptor genes, and do not result in a chimeric transcript. Rare cases of thymic lymphoblastic lymphoma originating from a thymic precursor committed to NK cell differentiation was reported, of which the phenotype and genotype were different from the thymic T cells (21,33).

Differential Diagnosis. In adults, ALL/LBL should be distinguished from lymphocyte-rich thymoma (types B1 and B2 thymoma). This diagnostic dilemma most commonly occurs in small and often fragmented mediastinoscopic biopsies in which the characteristic features of thymoma, such as perivascular spaces, are absent. Careful observation of the cytologic and histologic manifestations usually prevents diagnostic confusion with type B1 or B2 thymoma (31). LBL destroys

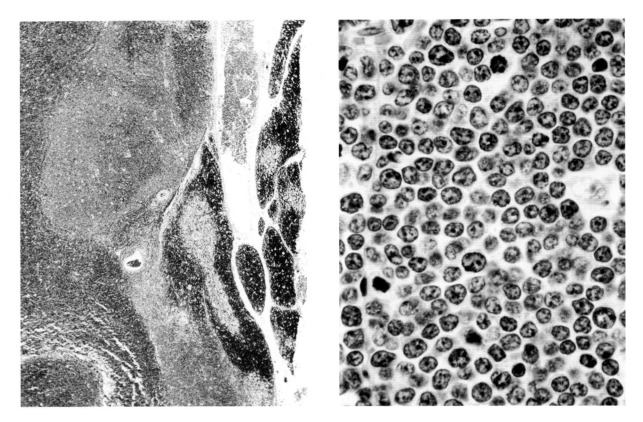

Figure 6-16

INVOLVEMENT OF THYMUS BY PRECURSOR T-LYMPHOBLASTIC LYMPHOMA

Left: Adjacent to the thymic tissue, a diffuse infiltrate of lymphoma cells is seen. A few Hassall corpuscles are trapped in the tumor. A starry sky appearance is also noted.

Right: At higher magnification, the neoplastic cells have an immature appearance. Scanty cytoplasm is difficult to recognize; some nuclei show clefts and infolding. Mitotic figures are frequent. (Courtesy of Dr. Koichi Shimizu, Tokyo, Japan.)

Figure 6-17

**PRECURSOR
T-LYMPHOBLASTIC LEUKEMIA
INVOLVING CERVICAL
LYMPH NODE**

In this imprint smear, tumor cells are uniform in appearance with granular, round to slightly irregular nuclei, distinct nucleoli, and scanty cytoplasm. Small reactive lymphocytes are scattered between tumor cells (Giemsa stain).

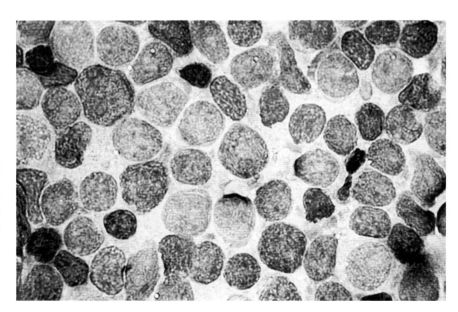

the normal thymic architecture, whereas the epithelial cell meshwork is maintained in type B1 or B2 thymoma. In contrast to neoplastic lymphoblasts, benign thymocytes in thymoma generally contain clumped chromatin and are mitotically inactive. Immunophenotyping is not usually helpful for the differential diagnosis because benign thymocytes express immunophenotypes similar to those of neoplastic T lymphoblasts.

Treatment and Prognosis. Adults with T-LBL have a more favorable outcome than those with B-LBL, with respective median disease-free survival periods of 28 and 14 months (3). The prognosis for children with LBL has improved remarkably through the use of recent multiagent chemotherapy, but nevertheless, approximately 20 to 25 percent of children do not respond to therapy (80).

Anaplastic Large Cell Lymphoma and Other Rare Mature T- and NK-Cell Lymphomas of the Mediastinum

Anaplastic large cell (Ki-1 positive) lymphoma (ALCL) is an uncommon non-Hodgkin lymphoma that mainly occurs in children and young adults. At times it involves the mediastinum and is characterized by marked nuclear pleomorphism (10,54). For details, readers are referred to the third series Fascicle on lymph nodes and the WHO classification of tumors of hematopoietic and lymphoid tissues (26a,82).

Grossly, ALCL may be cystic, and histologically, it may show cohesive growth mimicking cancer. Lymphoma cells are large with round or indented vesicular nuclei, often described as reniform, embryo-like, or horseshoe-shaped, with prominent nucleoli and abundant cytoplasm. Binucleated cells or multinucleated cells with individual nuclei dispersed in a wreath-like pattern may be present. Cells with embryo-like nuclei possess a characteristic paranuclear pale Golgi zone. In rare cases, numerous reactive histiocytes or neutrophils are present. A sarcomatoid variant is noted.

The tumor cells are positive for CD30 (Ki-1 antigen). It may be difficult to prove the phenotypic derivation of ALCL from the T-cell lineage, although CD2 and CD4 are most frequently positive, CD3 is often but not always positive, and other T-cell markers such as CD43 and CD45RO may be positive. Anaplastic lymphoma kinase (ALK) is expressed in the nuclei and cytoplasm or in the cytoplasm only in about half of the cases. ALK, which characterizes this tumor type, is a chimeric/fusion protein caused by t(2;5), specifically a translocation of the *ALK* gene located on chromosome 2, and *NPM* (nucleophosmin) on chromosome 5 (50,72). This constitutive overexpression of ALK is believed to be one of the factors in ALCL that drives cell growth. Positive expression of ALK is associated with an excellent prognosis (26a,78). Kaneko et al. (29) reported a specific chromosomal translocation, t(2;5)(p23;q35), in ALCL.

The differential diagnosis includes carcinoma, mediastinal large B-cell lymphoma, and Hodgkin lymphoma. Immunohistochemistry is essential for a definite diagnosis.

Other mature T- and NK-cell lymphomas of the mediastinum are so rare that the readers are referred to the Fascicle on tumors of the lymph nodes and hematopoietic system and the WHO classification of lymphomas (26a,78,82).

HODGKIN LYMPHOMA

General Features. *Hodgkin lymphoma* in the mediastinum may involve the thymus, mediastinal lymph nodes, or both, Of the major histologic subtypes, the nodular sclerosis type is by far the most common. Other types are exceedingly rare in the mediastinum, and the reader is referred to the third series Fascicle on tumors of hematopoietic tissue and lymph nodes and the WHO classification of lymphomas (26a,82).

Clinical Features. Most patients with nodular sclerosis type Hodgkin lymphoma are young women. Clinical symptoms related to local pressure (dyspnea, cough, or chest pain) may be present. Hodgkin lymphoma, however, is often detected by routine chest X ray, appearing as an anterior-superior mediastinal mass in an asymptomatic patient (67).

Gross Findings. A diagnosis of nodular sclerosis may be suspected at the time of macroscopic examination by the delineation of distinct nodules defined by retracted grayish white interconnecting bands on the cut surface of the gross specimen (fig. 6-18). When nodular sclerosis Hodgkin lymphoma involves the thymus, the tumor is sharply outlined and sometimes surrounded by a thick capsule. Unlike thymoma, the nodules may be multiple, and residual thymic remnants may be present (6).

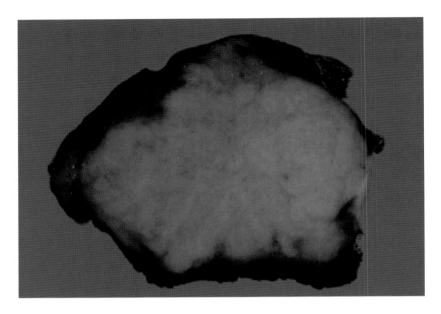

Figure 6-18

NODULAR SCLEROSIS TYPE HODGKIN LYMPHOMA

The distinct nodularity of the cut surface of this lymph node strongly suggests the diagnosis of Hodgkin lymphoma.

Microscopic Findings. Histologically, nodular sclerosis is characterized by orderly bands of interconnecting collagenous connective tissue that partially or entirely subdivide abnormal lymphoid tissue into isolated cellular nodules (fig. 6-19). In some cases, the entire lesion undergoes spontaneous sclerosis. At the opposite extreme, the lesion is predominantly cellular, with the formation of bands and isolation of nodules limited to only a small portion of the tumor.

The cellular proliferation within the nodules is polymorphic, with small and large lymphocytes, plasma cells, eosinophils, and histiocytes. The distinctive feature is the presence of Reed-Sternberg cells and their lacuna variants (fig. 6-20) (6). Reed-Sternberg cells (lacuna cells) occur in clusters and have abundant water-clear or slightly eosinophilic cytoplasm with sharply defined cellular borders situated in lacuna-like spaces. The lacuna-like spaces are artifacts of formalin fixation and are less obvious in tissues fixed in mercury-containing fixatives such as B5 (6). The nuclei of the lacuna cells are usually hyperlobated with delicate chromatin and small nucleoli.

Immunohistochemical Findings. Variants of nodular sclerosis Hodgkin disease occasionally present problems in diagnosis (6). These variants include a cellular phase without fibrous bands, as well as lymphocyte depleted, sarcomatous, and syncytial types. Immunohistochemistry is a great help in these cases. Reed-Sternberg cells and their lacuna variants are reactive frequently with CD15 antibody and consistently with CD30 antibody (fig. 6-21). The former is a granulocyte-associated antigen and the latter an activation marker (gp120). Leu-M1 is commonly used for CD15 and BerH2 and Ki-1 for CD30 (fig. 6-22). Leu-M1 and BerH2 are reactive with antigens in paraffin-embedded tissue. In a small proportion of cases, Reed-Sternberg cells and their variants express B-cell antigens such as CD20 but are negative for CD79a in the majority of cases (fig. 6-23) (6,78). Therefore, their precise phenotype is considered unclear, although occasional expression of CD20 and the presence of immunoglobulin gene rearrangements in almost all cases indicate a B-cell origin (36,86).

Molecular Findings. Molecular studies have revealed that the Reed-Sternberg cells originate from germinal center B cells of lymph follicles. This is supported by the findings that Reed-Sternberg cells frequently harbor somatic mutation of the *IgH* gene (43) and that molecular analysis of patients with composite Hodgkin and follicular lymphomas show these two tumor types to be monoclonal in origin (35). Thus, the *IgH* gene is clonally rearranged in Reed-Sternberg cells. However, these cells are not capable of producing immunoglobulin, probably because of the inherent abnormality of some of their transcription factors, which have not yet been clearly identified. Despite these genetic and functional abnormalities, Reed-Sternberg cells not only escape the apoptotic process, but also acquire

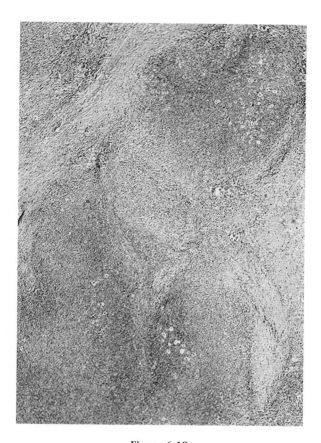

Figure 6-19

NODULAR SCLEROSIS TYPE HODGKIN LYMPHOMA

Bands of fibrous tissue subdivide the lymph node into multiple discrete nodules. Even at low magnification, scattered large tumor cells are seen.

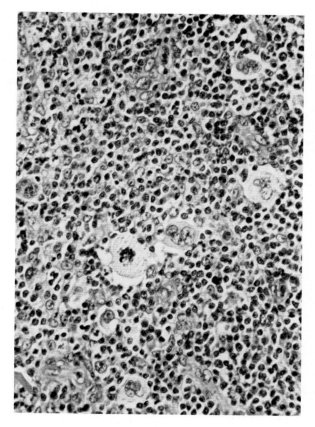

Figure 6-20

LACUNA CELLS WITH ABUNDANT CLEAR CYTOPLASM

The characteristic features of these cells are apparent in formalin-fixed tissue.

a growth advantage, as revealed by frequent expression of cell proliferation antigens such as Ki-67 and proliferating cell nuclear antigen (PCNA). Constitutive expression of transcription factor NFkB is believed to play a critical role in the growth of this tumor (34,83).

There have been 15 cases of composite or synchronous lymphoma with two distinct components of classic nodular sclerosis Hodgkin lymphoma and primary mediastinal large B-cell lymphoma reported (77). In this report, 21 mediastinal gray zone lymphomas with features transitional between these two tumors were analyzed for histologic features, immunophenotypes, and molecular changes. The results indicated the existence of gray zone lymphomas with transitional morphology and phenotype, further supporting accumulating evidence that classic nodular scle-

rosis Hodgkin lymphoma and mediastinal large B-cell lymphoma are related entities.

Differential Diagnosis. Nodular sclerosis type Hodgkin lymphoma has been misinterpreted as a form of thymoma (granulomatous thymoma), because the interlacing of fibrous bands and polymorphous inflammatory infiltration superficially resembles thymoma (67). In addition, thymic epithelial cells may react with a peculiar hyperplastic response to the presence of the lymphoma and resemble the spindle cell proliferation of thymoma (17). In Hodgkin lymphoma, fibrous bands are rounded and not angulated as in thymoma; epithelial hyperplasia is not present throughout the tumor; and diagnostic Reed-Sternberg cells or their lacunar variants are identifiable. Immunohistochemistry can clarify the situation.

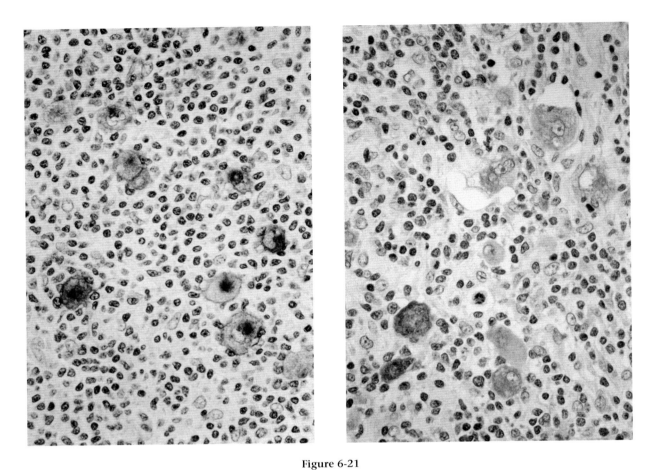

Figure 6-21

HODGKIN LYMPHOMA: IMMUNOHISTOCHEMISTRY

Left: The cell membrane and Golgi area are strongly positive for CD15.
Right: Cytoplasmic staining of lacuna cells by CD30.

Figure 6-22

**LACUNA CELLS
STAINED BY CD20**

The precise significance of positive staining is not known, although suggestive of tumor cells of B-cell lineage.

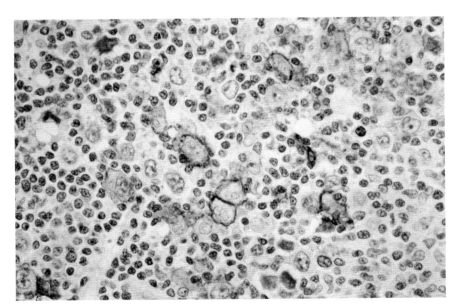

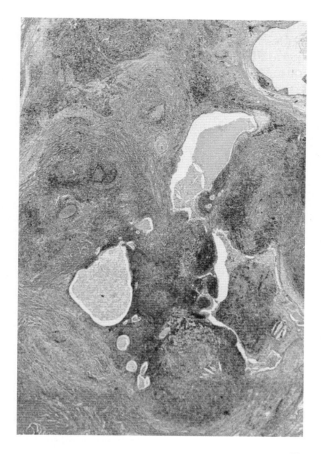 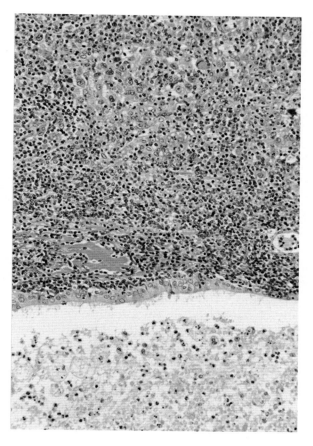

Figure 6-23

NODULAR SCLEROSIS TYPE HODGKIN LYMPHOMA

Left: A nodule of thymic Hodgkin lymphoma is in contact with an epithelium-lined cyst.

Right: Higher magnification reveals that part of the cyst is lined by non-neoplastic thymic epithelial cells. Mononuclear tumor cells infiltrated by lymphoid cells surround the cyst.

Another interesting feature frequently associated with Hodgkin lymphoma is the development of epithelium-lined cysts of various sizes (fig. 6-23) (67). They contain clear fluid or grumous material. This is the result of a peculiar reaction of the thymic epithelial cells. Occasionally, the entire lesion has a macroscopic appearance indistinguishable from that of benign thymic cysts. This cystic change may be seen in other disorders but is more common in Hodgkin lymphoma.

HISTIOCYTIC AND DENDRITIC CELL TUMORS

Histiocytic and dendritic cell tumors include Langerhans cell histiocytosis/sarcoma, follicular dendritic cell tumor/sarcoma, and interdigitat-

ing dendritic cell tumor/sarcoma. All occur in the mediastinum but are very rare. These tumors are dealt with briefly and readers are referred to monographs on hematopoietic and lymphoid tissues for details (26a,82).

The International Lymphoma Study Group (63) divided histiocytic and dendritic tumors into five groups (one histiocytic cell type, three dendritic cell types, and one unclassified) by analyzing 61 cases immunohistochemically. Six markers were utilized: CD68 and lysozyme (LYS) for histiocytes, CD1a for Langerhans cells, and CD21, CD35, and S-100 protein for follicular dendritic cells. This series of markers identified five groups: 1) histiocytic sarcoma with the phenotype of CD68 (100 percent), LYS (94 percent), CD1a (0 percent), S-100 protein (33 percent), CD21/35 (0 percent);

2) Langerhans cell tumor (Langerhans cell histiocytosis/sarcoma) with CD68 (96 percent), LYS (42 percent), CD1a (100 percent), S-100 protein (100 percent), CD21/35 (0 percent); 3) follicular dendritic cell tumor/sarcoma with CD68 (54 percent), LYS (8 percent), CD1a (0 percent), CD21/35 (100 percent); 4) interdigitating dendritic cell tumor/sarcoma with CD68 (50 percent), LYS (25 percent), CD1a (0 percent), S-100 protein (100 percent), CD21/35 (0 percent); and 5) unclassified tumors immunohistochemically, which were further classifiable into the above four groups using additional morphologic and ultrastructural features.

Langerhans Cell Histiocytosis and Sarcoma

Langerhans cell histiocytosis and sarcoma are neoplasms of Langerhans cells, which express CD1a and S-100 protein and are ultrastructurally characterized by the presence of Birbeck granules. Langerhans cell histiocytosis was previously called Langerhans cell granulomatosis. Even earlier, this lesion was designated as histiocytosis X, covering a spectrum of three entities: eosinophilic granuloma, Hand-Schuller-Christian disease, and Letterer-Siwe disease (40,73). It occurs primarily in the bone; commonly in the lung, skin, and lymph node; but rarely in the thymus and other sites.

Histologically, Langerhans cell histiocytosis shows diffuse infiltration of cells with grooved nuclei, fine chromatin, and eosinophilic cytoplasm, often admixed with multinucleated giant cells and eosinophils (fig. 6-24). Thymus involvement is either unifocal or multifocal. Langerhans cell histiocytosis in association with an asymptomatic multilocular thymic cyst was reported in a case discovered at the time of cardiac surgery (81). Langerhans cell sarcoma may be difficult to identify histologically but can be diagnosed by CD1a immunostaining (63).

Histiocytic Sarcoma

Histiocytic sarcoma is an extremely rare malignant tumor, consisting of cells with the morphologic and immunohistochemical features of histiocytes, such as large epithelioid cells with abundant eosinophilic cytoplasm, oval or irregular nuclei, vesicular chromatin, and large nucleoli. The neoplastic cells express the histiocytic markers CD68 and lysozyme, without follicular dendritic cell markers (CD21/35). Histiocytic sarcoma arises in lymph nodes, skin, and at extranodal sites including the gastrointestinal tract, nasal cavity, and lung (20). With systemic involvement, the disease is known as *malignant histiocytosis* (63,78).

Follicular Dendritic Cell Tumor/Sarcoma

This rare neoplasm shows follicular dendritic differentiation and involves lymph nodes of the neck, mediastinum, and axilla. Approximately 30 percent of the cases are located in extranodal sites, such as liver, tonsils, and intraabdominal soft tissues (60). Spindle to oval tumor cells possess eosinophilic cytoplasm and nuclei with clear or dispersed chromatin, inconspicuous or small nucleoli, and thin nuclear membranes. The neoplastic cells grow in a storiform pattern, whorls, fascicles, trabeculae, and even sheets (59,60). The diagnosis is confirmed immunohistochemically by positive CD21 and CD35 (2,8,9,15,41,59,60), or ultrastructurally by slender, complex, occasionally interdigitating cytoplasmic processes with desmosomes (59,60). Multinucleated tumor cells may be present. Necrosis, marked cellular atypia, a high mitotic rate, and abnormal mitoses may be seen in some cases, indicating aggressive behavior (59,60). About 30 percent of tumors recur and metastasize (60).

Some tumors are associated with hyaline-vascular type Castleman disease (8,9,41,60,82) and one tumor had a concomitant plasma cell variant of Castleman disease (2). Transformation of hyaline-vascular Castleman disease of the nasopharynx into a follicular dendritic cell sarcoma was documented by sequential biopsies (8).

Interdigitating Dendritic Cell Tumor/Sarcoma

Interdigitating dendritic cell tumor/sarcoma is a rare malignant neoplasm with the histologic and phenotypic features of interdigitating reticulum cells, which are dendritic nonphagocytic histiocytes found in thymus-dependent areas of lymphoid tissue (64,66). Mediastinal involvement is even rarer. The histology is similar to that of follicular dendritic cell sarcoma, but individual cells with a complex nuclear outline and abundant, variably eosinophilic cytoplasm suggest histiocytic differentiation. Immunohistochemically, the tumor cells are positive for S-100 protein and often show weak

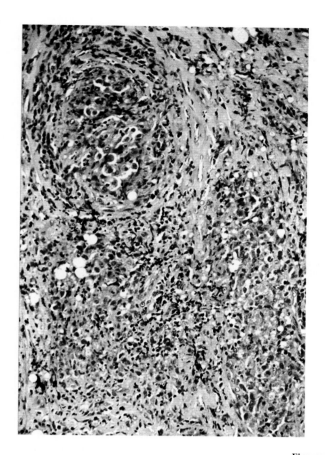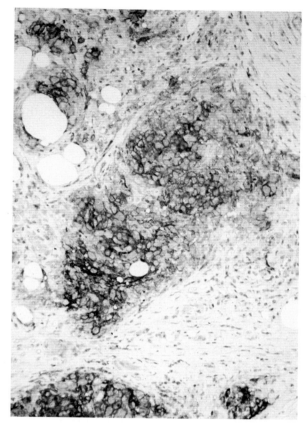

Figure 6-24

LANGERHANS CELL HISTIOCYTOSIS

Left: The biopsy was taken from an anterior mediastinal mass. Nodular aggregates of atypical polygonal cells with delicate nuclear membranes and eosinophilic cytoplasm are admixed with a few eosinophils and lymphocytes. Grooved or reniform nuclei were difficult to find at this magnification.

Right: Atypical cells stain for CD1a. The S-100 protein stain was also positive. (Courtesy of Dr. William D. Travis, New York, NY.)

staining for CD68, CD45, lysozyme, alpha-1-antichymotrypsin, and human leukocyte antigen (HLA)-DR. They are negative for CD1a, CD21, CD35, CD30, T-cell specific markers, B-cell specific markers, and myeloperoxidase (16,46, 64,66,78). Ultrastructurally, the tumor cells are devoid of Birbeck granules and well-formed desmosomes (78).

Most interdigitating dendritic cell tumors behave aggressively and are unresponsive to intensive chemotherapy regimens (64,66).

MYELOID SARCOMA AND EXTRAMEDULLARY ACUTE MYELOID LEUKEMIA

Myeloid (or *granulocytic*) *sarcoma* is a rare extramedullary tumor of immature myeloid cells.

It is frequently associated with hematologic disorders including acute myeloid leukemia, chronic myelogenous leukemia, and myelodysplastic syndrome. These hematologic disorders are often seen simultaneously or develop shortly after the tumor mass is detected. A case with superior vena cava syndrome has been reported (65). In patients with mediastinal germ cell tumors, hematopoietic precursor cells within the yolk sac tumor component are considered to be the source of the secondary hematologic malignancies (56).

Histologically, the tumor shows a diffuse infiltrate of immature round cells. If the tumor is composed of myeloid precursors or myeloblasts, it may be misdiagnosed as large cell lymphoma. Thus, a diagnosis of granulocytic

247

sarcoma should be considered when hematopoietic tumor cells do not stain with conventional antibodies against B- and T-lymphoid cells (44). Histochemical or immunohistochemical study is needed for confirmation of the diagnosis.

Commonly used myeloid-associated markers are lysozyme, myeloperoxidase, and naphthol AS-D chloroacetate esterase. In addition, a variety of markers are used for varying stages of myeloid cell development: CD34, CD43, CD117, and TdT for myeloid precursors in the thymus or immature myeloid cells, and CD13, CD15, and CD33 for a more committed myeloid lineage (19,78).

Mediastinal myeloid sarcoma is an aggressive disease. The prognosis is that of the underlying leukemia (26a,78).

REFERENCES

1. Addis BJ, Isaacson PG. Large cell lymphoma of the mediastinum: a B-cell tumour of probable thymic origin. Histopathology 1986;10:379-90.

2. Andriko JW, Kaldjian EP Tsokos M, Abbondanzo SL, Jaffe ES. Reticulum cell neoplasms of lymph nodes: a clinicopathologic study of 11 cases with recognition of a new subtype derived from fibroblastic reticular cells. Am J Surg Pathol 1998;22:1048-58.

3. Boucheix C, David B, Sebban C, et al. Immunophenotype of adult acute lymphoblastic leukemia, clinical parameters, and outcome: an analysis of a prospective trial including 562 tested patients (LALA87). French Group on Therapy for Adult Acute Lymphoblastic Leukemia. Blood 1994;84:1603-12.

4. Brandter LB, Smith CI, Hammerstrom L, Lindemalm C, Christensson B, Clonal immunoglobulin gene rearrangements in primary mediastinal clear cell lymphomas. Leukemia 1989;3:122-9.

5. Brunning RD, McKenna RW. Tumors of the bone marrow. Atlas of Tumor Pathology, 3rd Series, Fascicle 9, Washington DC: Armed Forces Institute of Pathology; 1994.

6. Burke JS. Hodgkin's disease. Histopathology and differential diagnosis. In Knowles DM, ed. Neoplastic hematopathology, 2nd ed. Philadelphia: Lippincott Williams & Wilkins; 2001:623-65.

7. Cazals-Hatem D, Lepage E, Brice P, et al. Primary mediastinal large B-cell lymphoma. A clinicopathologic study of 141 cases compared with 916 nonmediastinal large B-cell lymphoma, a GELA ("Groupe d'Etude des Lymphomes de L'Adulte") study. Am J Surg Pathol 1996;20:877-88.

8. Chan AC, Chan KW, Chan JK, Au WY, Ho WK, Ng WM. Development of follicular dendritic cell sarcoma in hyaline-vascular Castleman's disease of the nasopharynx. Histopathology 2001;38:510-8.

9. Chan JK, Fletcher CD, Nayler SJ, Cooper K. Follicular dendritic cell sarcoma. Clinicopathologic analysis of 17 cases suggesting a malignant potential higher than currently recognized. Cancer 1997;79:294-313

10. Chan JK, Ng CS, Hui PK, et al. Anaplastic large cell Ki-1 lymphoma. Delineation of two morphological types. Histopathology 1989;15:11-34.

11. A clinical evaluation of the International Lymphoma Study Group classification of non-Hodgkin's lymphoma. The Non-Hodgkin's Lymphoma Classification Project. Blood 1997;89:3909-18.

12. Copie-Bergman C, Plonquet A, Alonso MA, et al. MAL expression in lymphoid cells: further evidence for MAL as a distinct molecular marker of primary mediastinal large B-cell lymphomas. Mod Pathol 2002;15:1172-1180.

13. Davis RE, Dorfman RF, Warnke RA. Primary large-cell lymphoma of the thymus: a diffuse B-cell neoplasm presenting as primary mediastinal lymphoma. Hum Pathol 1990;21:1262-8

14. de Leval L, Ferry JA, Falini B, Shipp M, Harris NL. Expression of bcl-6 and CD10 in primary mediastinal large B-cell lymphoma. Evidence for derivation from germinal center B cells? Am J Surg Pathol 2001;25: 1277-82.

15. Dillon KM, Hill CM, Cameron CH, Attanoos RL, McCluggage WG. Mediastinal mixed dendritic cell sarcoma with hybrid features. J Clin Pathol 2002;55:791-4.

16. Fassina A, Marino F, Poletti A, Rea F, Pennelli N, Ninfo V. Follicular dendritic cell tumor of the mediastinum. Ann Diagn Pathol 2001;5:361-7.

17. Griffith RC. Thymus gland. In Kissane JM, ed. Anderson's pathology, 9th ed. St. Louis: CV Mosby; 1990:1493-516.

18. Harris NL, Jaffe ES, Stein H, et al. A revised European-American classification of lymphoid neoplasms: a proposal from the International Lymphoma Study Group. Blood 1994;84:1361-92.

19. Hishima T, Fukayama M, Hayashi Y, et al. Granulocytic sarcoma of the thymus in a nonleukemic patient. Virchows Arch 1999;435:447-51.

20. Hornick, JL, Jaffe ES, Fletcher CD. Extranodal histiocytic sarcoma: clinicopathologic analysis of 14 cases of a rare epithelioid malignancy. Am J Surg Pathol 2004;28:1133-44.

21. Ichinohasama R, Endoh K, Ishizawa K, et al. Thymic lymphoblastic lymphoma of committed natural killer cell precursor origin: a case report. Cancer 1996;77:2592-603.

22. Inagaki H, Chan JK, Ng JW, et al. Primary thymic extranodal marginal-zone B-cell lymphoma of mucosa-associated lymphoid tissue type exhibits distinctive clinicopathological and molecular features. Am J Pathol 2002;160:1435-43.

23. Isaacson PG, Chan JK, Tang C, Addis BJ. Low-grade B-cell lymphoma of mucosa-associated lymphoid tissue arising in the thymus. A thymic lymphoma mimicking myoepithelial sialadenitis. Am J Surg Pathol 1990;14:342-51.

24. Isaacson PG, Norton AJ, Addis BJ. The human thymus contains a novel population of B lymphocytes. Lancet 1987;2:1488-91.

25. Isaacson PG, Spencer J. Malignant lymphoma of mucosa-associated lymphoid tissue. Histopathology 1987;11:445-662.

26. Jacobson JO, Aisenberg AC, Lamarre L, et al. Mediastinal large cell lymphoma. An uncommon subset of adult lymphoma curable with combined modality therapy. Cancer 1988;62:1893-8.

26a. Jaffe ES, Harris NL, Stein H, Vardiman JV, eds. World Health Organization Classification of Tumours. Pathology and genetics of tumours of haematopoietic and lymphoid tissues. Lyon: IARC Press; 2001.

27. Joos S, Otano-Joos MI, Ziegler S, et al. Primary mediastinal (thymic) B-cell lymphoma is characterized by gains of chromosomal material including 9p and amplification of the REL gene. Blood 1996;87:1571-8.

28. Kanavaros P, Gaulard P, Charlotte F, et al. Discordant expression of immunoglobulin and its associated molecule mb-1/CD79a is frequently found in mediastinal large B cell lymphomas. Am J Pathol 1995;146:735-41.

29. Kaneko Y, Frizzera G, Edamura S, et al. A novel translocation, t(2;5)(p23;q35), in childhood phagocytic large T-cell lymphoma mimicking malignant histiocytosis. Blood 1989;73:806-13.

30. Kirn D, Mauch P, Shaffer K, et al. Large-cell and immunoblastic lymphoma of the mediastinum: prognostic features and treatment outcome in 57 patients. J Clin Oncol 1993;11:1336-43.

31. Knowles DM. Lymphoblastic lymphoma. In: Knowles DM, ed. Neoplastic hematopathology, 2nd ed. Philadelphia: Lippincott Williams & Wilkins; 2001:915-51.

32. Knowles DM, ed. Neoplastic hematopathology, 2nd ed. `Philadelphia: Lippincott Williams & Wilkins; 2001.

33. Koita H, Suzumiya J, Ohshima K, et al. Lymphoblastic lymphoma expressing natural killer cell phenotype with involvement of the mediastinum and nasal cavity. Am J Surg Pathol 1997;21:242-8

34. Krappmann D, Emmerich F, Kordes U, Scharschmidt E, Dorken B, Scheidereit C.. Molecular mechanisms of constitutive NF-kappaB/Rel activation in Hodgkin/Reed-Sternberg cells. Oncogene 1999;18:943-53.

35. Kuppers R, Sousa AB, Baur AS, Srickler JG, Rajewsky K, Hansmann ML. Common germinal-center B-cell origin of the malignant cells in two composite lymphomas, involving classical Hodgkin's disease and either follicular lymphoma or B-CLL. Mol Med 2001;7:285-92.

36. Kuppers R, Rajewsky K, Zhao M, et al. Hodgkin disease: Hodgkin and Reed-Sternberg cells picked from histological sections show clonal immunoglobulin gene rearrangements and appear to be derived from B cells at various stages of development. Proc Natl Acad Sci U S A 1994;91:10962-6.

37. Lamarre L, Jacobson JO, Aisenberg AC, Harris NL. Primary large cell lymphoma of the mediastinum. A histologic and immunophenotypic study of 29 cases. Am J Surg Pathol 1989;13:730-9.

38. Lazzarino M, Orlandi E, Paulli M, et al. Treatment outcome and prognostic factors for primary mediastinal (thymic) B-cell lymphoma: a multicenter study of 106 patients. J Clin Oncol 1997;15:1646-53.

39. Lichtenstein AK, Levine A, Taylor CR, et al. Primary mediastinal lymphoma in adults. Am J Med 1980;68:509-14.

40. Lieberman PH, Jones CR, Steinman RM, et al. Langerhans cell (eosinophilic) granulomatosis. A clinicopathologic study encompassing 50 years. Am J Surg Pathol 1996;20:519-52.

41. Lin O, Frizzera G. Angiomyoid and follicular dendritic cell proliferative lesions in Castleman's disease of hyaline-vascular type: a study of 10 cases. Am J Surg Pathol 1997;21:1295-306. (Erratum in: Am J Surg Pathol 1998;22:139)

42. Lorsbach RB, Pinkus GS, Shahsafaei A, Dorfman DM. Primary marginal zone lymphoma of the thymus. Am J Clin Pathol 2000;113:784-91.

43. Marafioti T, Hummel M, Anagnostopoulos I, et al. Origin of nodular lymphocyte-predominant Hodgkin's disease from a clonal expansion of highly mutated germinal–center B cells. N Engl J Med 1997;337:453-8.

44. McCluggage WG, Boyd HK, Jones FG, Mayne EE, Bharucha H. Mediastinal granulocytic sarcoma: a report of two cases. Arch Pathol Lab Med 1998;122:545-7.

45. McCluggage WG, McManus K, Qureshi R, McAleer S, Wotherspoon AC. Low-grade B-cell lymphoma of mucosa-associated lymphoid tissue (MALT) of thymus. Hum Pathol 2000;31:255-9.

46. Miettinen M, Fletcher CD, Lasota J. True histiocytic lymphoma of small intestine. Analysis of two S-100 protein-positive cases with features of interdigitating reticulum cell sarcoma. Am J Clin Pathol 1993;100:285-92.

47. Miller JB, Variakojis D, Bitran JD, et al. Diffuse histiocytic lymphoma with sclerosis: a clinicopathologic entity frequently causing superior vena caval obstruction. Cancer 1981;47:748-56.

48. Müller P, Lämmler B, Eberlein-Gonska M, et al. Primary mediastinal clear cell lymphoma of B-cell type. Virchows Arch A Pathol Anat Histopathol 1986;409:79-92.

49. Müller P, Moldenhauer B, Momburg F, et al. Mediastinal lymphoma of clear cell type is a tumor corresponding to terminal steps of B cell differentiation. Blood 1987;69:1087-95.

50. Morris SW, Kirstein MN, Valentine MB, et al. Fusion of a kinase gene, ALK, to a nucleolar protein gene, NPM, in non-Hodgkin's lymphoma. Science 1994;263:1281-1284. [Erratum appears in Science 1995;267:316-7].

51. Nagasaka T, Lai R, Harada T, et al. Coexisting thymic and gastric lymphomas of mucosa-associated lymphoid tissue in a patient with Sjögren syndrome. Arch Pathol Lab Med 2000;124:770-3.

52. Nakagawa A, Nakamura S, Koshikawa T, et al. Clinicopathologic study of primary mediastinal non-lymphoblastic non-Hodgkin's lymphomas among the Japanese. Acta Pathol Jpn 1993;43:44-54.

53. Nakamura S, Koshikawa T, Kaba S, Tokoro Y, Suchi T, Kurita S. Imprint cytology of low-grade B-cell lymphoma of mucosa-associated lymphoid tissue arising in the thymus. A case report. Diagn Cytopathol 1993;9:665-7.

54. Nakamura S, Takagi N, Kojima M, et al. Clinicopathologic study of large cell anaplastic lymphoma (Ki-1-positive large cell lymphoma) among the Japanese. Cancer 1991;68:118-29.

55. Onishi Y, Matsuno Y, Tateishi U, et al. Two entities of precursor T-cell lymphoblastic leukemia/lymphoma based on radiologic and immunophenotypic findings. Int J Hematol 2004;80:43-51.

56. Orazi A, Neiman RS, Ulbright TM, Heerema NA, John K, Nichols CR. Hematopoietic precursor cells within the yolk sac tumor component are the source of secondary hematopoietic malignancies in patients with mediastinal germ cell tumors. Cancer 1993;71:3873-81

57. Palanisamy N, Abou-Elella AA, Chaganti SR et al. Similar patterns of genomic alterations characterize primary mediastinal large-B-cell lymphoma and diffuse large-B-cell lymphoma. Genes Chromosomes Cancer 2002;33:114-122.

58. Parrens M, Dubus P, Danjoux M, et al. Mucosa-associated lymphoid tissue of the thymus hyperplasia vs lymphoma. Am J Clin Pathol 2002;117:51-6.

59. Perez-Ordonez B, Erlandson RA, Rosai J. Follicular dendritic cell tumor: report of 13 additional cases of a distinctive entity. Am J Surg Pathol 1996;20:944-55.

60. Perez-Ordonez B, Rosai J. Follicular dendritic cell tumor: review of the entity. Semin Diagn Pathol 1998;15:144-54.

61. Perrone T, Frizzera G, Rosai J. Mediastinal diffuse large-cell lymphoma with sclerosis. A clinicopathologic study of 60 cases. Am J Surg Pathol 1986;10:176-91.

62. Pileri SA, Gaidana G, Zinzani PL, et al. Primary mediastinal B-cell lymphoma: high frequency of BCL-6 mutations and consistent expression of the transcription factors OCT-2, BOB.1, and PU.1 in the absence of immunoglobulins. Am J Pathol 2003;162:243-53.

63. Pileri SA, Grogan TM, Harris NL, et al. Tumours of histiocytes and accessory dendritic cells: an immunohistochemical approach to classification from the International Lymphoma Study Group based on 61 cases. Histopathology 2002; 41:1-29.

64. Rabkin MS, Kjeldsberg CR, Hammond ME, Wittwer CT, Nathwani B. Clinical, ultrastructural immunohistochemical and DNA content analysis of lymphomas having features of interdigitating reticulum cells. Cancer 1988;61:1594-601.

65. Ravandi-Kashani F, Cortes J, Giles FJ. Myelodysplasia presenting as granulocytic sarcoma of mediastinum causing superior vena cava syndrome. Leuk Lymphoma 2000;36:631-7.

66. Rousselet MC, Francois S, Croue A, Maigre M, Saint-Andre JP, Ifrah N. A lymph node interdigitating reticulum cell sarcoma. Arch Pathol Lab Med. 1994;118:183-8.

67. Rosai J, Levine GD. Tumors of the thymus. Atlas of Tumor Pathology, 2nd Series, Fascicle 13, Washington, DC: Armed Forces Institute of Pathology; 1976;191-205.

68. Royer B, Cazals-Hatem D, Sibilia J, et al. Lymphomas in patients with Sjögren's syndrome are marginal zone B-cell neoplasms, arise in diverse extranodal and nodal sites, and are not associated with viruses. Blood 1997;90:766-75.

69. Scarpa A, Bonetti F, Menestrina F, et al. Mediastinal large-cell lymphoma with sclerosis. Genotypic analysis establishes its B nature. Virchows Arch A Pathol Anat Histopathol 1987;412:17-21.

70. Scarpa A, Borgato L, Chilosi M, et al. Evidence of c-myc gene abnormalities in mediastinal large B-cell lymphoma of young adult age. Blood 1991;78:780-8.

71. Sekiguchi N, Nishimoto J, Tanimoto K, et al. Primary mediastinal large B-cell lymphoma: a single-institution clinical study in Japan. Int J Hematol 2004;79:465-71.

71a. Shimizu K, Ishii G, Nagai K, et al. Extranodal marginal zone B-cell lymphoma of mucosa-associated lymphoid tissue (MALT) lymphoma in the thymus: report of four cases. Jpn J Clin Oncol 2005;35:412-6.

72. Shiota M, Nakamura S, Ichinohasama R, et al. Anaplastic large cell lymphomas expressing the novel chimeric protein p80NPM/ALK: a distinct clinicopathologic entity. Blood 1995;86:1954-60.

73. Siegal GP, Dehner LP, Rosai J. Histiocytosis X (Langerhans' cell granulomatosis) of the thymus. A clinicopathologic study of four childhood cases. Am J Surg Pathol 1985;9:117-24.

74. Singh HK, Silverman JF, Powers CN, Geisinger KR, Frable WJ. Diagnostic pitfalls in fine-needle aspiration biopsy of the mediastinum. Diagn Cytopathol 1997;17:121-6.

75. Suster S, Moran CA. Pleomorphic large cell lymphomas of the mediastinum. Am J Surg Pathol 1996;20:224-32.

76. Takagi N, Nakamura S, Yamamoto K, et al. Malignant lymphoma of mucosa-associated lymphoid tissue arising in the thymus of a patient with Sjogren's syndrome. A morphologic, phenotypic, and genotypic study. Cancer 1992;69:1347-55.

77. Traverse-Glehen A, Pittaluga S, Gaulard P, et al. Mediastinal gray zone lymphoma: the missing link between classic Hodgkin's lymphoma and mediastinal large B-cell lymphoma. Am J Surg Pathol 2005;29:1411-21.

78. Travis WB, Brambilla E, Müller-Hermelink HK, Harris CC, eds. World Health Organization Classification of Tumours. Pathology and genetics of tumours of the lung, thymus and heart. Lyon: IARC Press; 2004.

79. Tsang P, Cesarman E, Chadburn A, Liu YF, Knowles DM. Molecular characterization of primary mediastinal B cell lymphoma. Am J Pathol 1996;148:2017-25.

80. Uckun FM, Sensel MG, Sun L, et al. Biology and treatment of childhood T-lineage acute lymphoblastic leukemia. Blood 1998;91:735-46.

81. Wakely P Jr, Suster S. Langerhans' cell histiocytosis of the thymus associated with multilocular thymic cyst. Hum Pathol 2000;31:1532-5.

82. Warnke RA, Weiss LM, Chan JK, Cleary ML, Dorfman RF. Tumors of the lymph nodes and spleen. Atlas of Tumor Pathology, 3rd Series, Fascicle 14, Washington, DC: Armed Forces Institute of Pathology; 1995,.

83. Wood KM, Roff M, Hay RT. Defective IkappaB-alpha in Hodgkin cell lines with constitutively active NF-kappaB. Oncogene 1998;16:2131-9.

84. Yamasaki S, Matsushita H, Tanimura S, et al. B-cell lymphoma of mucosa-associated lymphoid tissue of the thymus: a report of two cases with a background of Sjögren's syndrome and monoclonal gammopathy. Hum Pathol 1998;29:1021-4.

85. Yokose T, Kodama T, Matsuno Y, Shimosato Y, Mukai K. Low-grade B-cell lymphoma of mucosa-associated lymphoid tissue in the thymus of a patient with rheumatoid arthritis. Pathol Int 1998;48:74-81.

86. Zukerberg LR, Collins AB, Ferry JA, Harris NL. Coexpression of CD15 and CD20 by Reed-Sternberg cells in Hodgkin's disease. Am J Pathol 1991;139:475-83.

7 SECONDARY INVOLVEMENT OF THE THYMUS BY CARCINOMA AND MESOTHELIOMA

SECONDARY CARCINOMA INVOLVING THE THYMUS

The mediastinum, particularly the anterior mediastinum, is frequently involved by carcinoma of various organs, either by direct extension from the neighboring organs or via mediastinal lymph node metastasis. Hematogenous metastasis to the thymus is rare.

Carcinoma of the lung involves the thymus more frequently than carcinoma of other organs (fig. 7-1), usually by direct invasion by both hilar and peripheral tumors. All the major histologic types of lung cancer can involve the thymus. Other routes of cancer spread include downward growth of thyroid cancer and cancers of the head and neck region, anterolateral extension of tracheal carcinoma, and extension through the chest wall by breast carcinoma. Involvement of the thymus through lymph node metastasis to the anterosuperior mediastinum occurs in cancer of various organs, not only from the lung and breast but also from abdominal organs

(stomach), the pelvis (prostate gland), and head and neck region (tongue).

Unless the primary tumor is clinically latent, the source of the metastasis to the thymus is easily recognized because of the generally advanced stage of the primary tumor. Even when the primary is clinically latent, the histology of the tumor suggests the primary site in many cases.

Moran et al. (11) reported three cases of low-grade serous carcinoma of the ovary metastatic to the anterior mediastinum, 3, 5, and 20 years after the initial diagnosis of a serous borderline tumor of the ovary. The tumors simulated a multilocular thymic cyst, and papillary tumors were found within and in continuity with the cystic structures. The authors interpreted the findings as metastatic from the ovarian borderline tumor because of the past history of an ovarian neoplasm and their histologic similarities. They also raised the possibility of a primary malignancy associated with multilocular thymic cysts. This possibility should be considered, since papillary

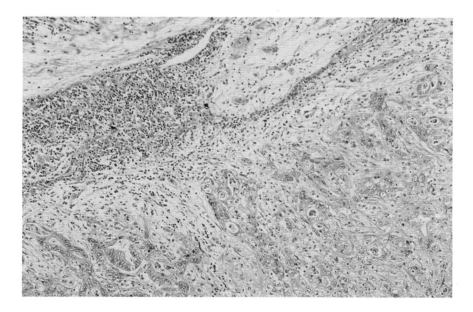

Figure 7-1

METASTATIC CARCINOMA IN THE THYMUS

Nests of moderately differentiated adenocarcinoma cells metastatic from the lung invade a lobule of atrophic thymus.

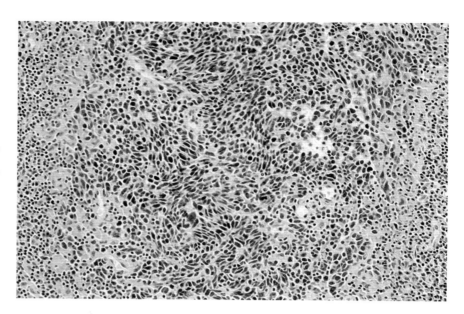

Figure 7-2

SMALL (OAT) CELL CARCINOMA IN A PULMONARY HILAR LYMPH NODE

Small tumor cells, typical of oat cell type small cell carcinoma, grow within a lymph node of the left pulmonary hilum. No primary tumor was found in the resected left upper lobe of the lung. The patient survived over 10 years without recurrence.

carcinoma with psammomatous bodies similar to ovarian serous carcinoma is known to arise in the thymus (10).

Distinction between Thymic and Pulmonary Carcinomas

As described in the chapter on thymic carcinoma, there are many identical and similarly named tumors in the thymus and lung: squamous cell carcinoma, mucoepidermoid carcinoma, adenosquamous carcinoma, undifferentiated large cell carcinoma, small cell/neuroendocrine carcinoma, sarcomatoid carcinoma, and carcinoid tumors. If the tumor is confined to one organ, the diagnosis can be made with ease. If the tumor involves both organs in continuity, the primary site may be difficult to determine.

The chapter on thymic carcinoma details the characteristic features of well-differentiated thymic squamous cell carcinoma that distinguish it from bronchial squamous cell carcinoma, such as nuclear features and broad sclerotic stroma (see figs. 3-9–3-11). No distinctive histologic differences are present in poorly differentiated squamous cell carcinoma, small cell carcinoma, and carcinoid tumors. In those cases, the gross topographic relationship of the tumor with the two organs and the location of the areas with the most abundant stroma or coagulation necrosis, which suggests the site of origin of the

tumor, help identify the primary site. Small cell carcinoma of the lung frequently forms a large mass in the anterior and middle mediastinum, and had even been designated mediastinal sarcoma until 1926 (2).

While extremely rare, carcinoma may originate in an epithelial inclusion in a lymph node or extrathymic mediastinal soft tissue (7). We encountered a case of small cell (typical oat cell) carcinoma in the middle mediastinum involving a lymph node of the left pulmonary hilum in a 65-year-old male. No primary tumor was found in the resected but otherwise unremarkable left upper lobe of the lung. The patient survived for more than 10 years without recurrence (fig. 7-2). This could well be a case of spontaneous regression of the primary lung cancer but the possibility of small cell carcinoma originating in a lymph node cannot be ruled out.

Immunohistochemically, squamous cell carcinomas of the thymus are often positive for CD5 and CD70, but those originating in other organs are negative for these markers (8,9). Thyroid transcription factor (TTF)-1, a transcriptional protein expressed by thyroid and pulmonary epithelia, is an excellent marker for their neoplastic counterparts, and is present in about 75 percent of pulmonary adenocarcinomas and in a smaller percentage of large cell carcinomas (25 percent) and squamous cell carcinomas (10 percent). TTF-1 is absent in cancers other than pulmonary and thyroid cancer (12,13). A variety of cytokeratins, such as cytokeratin (CK) 7 and CK20, may also be useful for determining the primary site, but a study of their use in thymic cancer is needed. Squamous cell carcinomas immunoreactive for both CD5 and kit (CD117) are best interpreted as thymic carcinoma, whereas neoplasms negative for both are more likely pulmonary squamous cell carcinoma involving the mediastinum, when the clinical setting is compatible (11a).

MESOTHELIOMA INVOLVING THE THYMUS

Malignant pleural mesothelioma of the diffuse type may invade the thymus in continuity, but involvement is almost always superficial. Mixed polygonal and spindle cell thymoma and sarcomatoid carcinoma of the thymus may mimic biphasic fibrous and epithelial mesothelioma. The modes of local growth, extension, and spread, together with some difference in cytologic appearance, can assist in the differential diagnosis. For a discussion of mesothelioma in detail, readers are referred to monographs published by the Armed Forces Institute of Pathology and American Registry of Pathology (1,3a) and the World Health Organization (WHO) (15).

The former designation of localized fibrous mesothelioma was divided into three types by Carter and Otis (3): 1) a localized, histologically benign, keratin-negative spindle cell tumor; 2) a diffuse, histologically malignant keratin-positive tumor; and 3) a histologically malignant, keratin-negative, spindle cell tumor. Fibrous tumors of types 1 and 3 are considered immunohistochemically and ultrastructurally to be derived from submesothelial connective tissue cells rather than from mesothelial cells, and are now termed solitary (localized) fibrous tumors of the pleura (5,16). This neoplasm is dealt with separately in chapter 11. The tumor of type 2 is a sarcomatoid mesothelioma.

Crotty et al (4) described a case of desmoplastic malignant mesothelioma of the mediastinum, which had been diagnosed as sclerosing mediastinitis by biopsy. In this case, immunostaining for keratin showed strong cytoplasmic positivity in both the sarcomatous cells and the cytologically bland cells within fibrous areas. Flint and Weiss (6) reported that CD34 and keratin expression distinguishes solitary fibrous tumor from desmoplastic mesothelioma. These studies indicate the importance of immunohistochemical staining in the differential diagnosis of fibrous tumors of the pleura, especially for malignant tumors. An extremely rare case of cystic adenomatoid tumor presenting as a mass in the anterior mediastinum with immunohistochemical and ultrastructural features characteristic of mesothelial cells has been reported (14).

REFERENCES

1. Battifora H, McCaughey WT. Tumors of the serosal membranes. Atlas of Tumor Pathology, 3rd Series, Fascicle 15, Washington DC: Armed Forces Institute of Pathology; 1995.
2. Bernard WG. The nature of the "oat celled sarcoma" of the mediastinum. J Pathol Bacteriol 1926;29:241-4.
3. Carter D, Otis CN. Three types of spindle cell tumors of the pleura. Fibroma, sarcoma, and sarcomatoid mesothelioma. Am J Surg Pathol 1988;12:747-53.
3a. Churg A, Cagle PT, Roggli VL. Tumors of the serosal membranes. Atlas of Tumor Pathology, 4th Series, Fascicle 3, Washington DC: American Registry of Pathology; 2006.
4. Crotty TB, Colby TV, Gay PC, Pisani RJ. Desmoplastic malignant mesothelioma masquerading as sclerosing mediastinitis: a diagnostic dilemma. Hum Pathol 1992;23:79-82.
5. England DM, Hochholzer L, McCarthy MJ. Localized benign and malignant fibrous tumors of the pleura. A clinicopathologic review of 223 cases. Am J Surg Pathol 1989;13:640-58.
6. Flint A, Weiss SW. CD-34 and keratin expression distinguishes solitary fibrous tumor (fibrous mesothelioma) of pleura from desmoplastic mesothelioma. Hum Pathol 1995;26:428-31.
7. Gould VE, Warren WH, Faber LP, Kuhn C, Franke WW. Malignant cells of epithelial phenotype limited to thoracic lymph nodes. Eur J Cancer 1990;26:1121-6.

8. Hishima T, Fukayama M, Fujisawa M, et al. CD5 expression in thymic carcinoma. Am J Pathol 1994;145:268-75.

9. Hishima T, Fukayama M, Hayashi Y, et al. CD70 expression in thymic carcinoma. Am J Surg Pathol 2000,24:742-6.

10. Matsuno Y, Morozumi N, Hirohashi S, Shimosato Y, Rosai J. Papillary carcinoma of the thymus: report of four cases of a new microscopic type of thymic carcinoma. Am J Surg Pathol 1998;22:873-80.

11. Moran CA, Suster S, Silva EG. Low-grade serous carcinoma of the ovary metastatic to the anterior mediastinum simulating multilocular thymic cysts: a clinicopathologic and immunohistochemical study of 3 cases. Am J Surg Pathol 2005;29:496-9.

11a. Nakagawa K, Matsuno Y, Kunitoh H, Maeshima A, Asamura H, Tsuchiya R. Immunohistochemical KIT (CD117) expression in thymic epithelial tumors. Chest 2005;128:140-4.

12. Ordonez NG. Value of thyroid transcription factor-1, E-cadherin, BG8, WT1, and CD44S immunostaining in distinguishing epithelial pleural mesothelioma from pulmonary and nonpulmonary adenocarcinoma. Am J Surg Pathol 2000;24:598-606.

13. Pecciarini M, Cangi G, Doglioni C. Immunohistochemistry in diagnostic pathology. Identifying the primary site of metastatic carcinoma: the increasing role of immunohistochemistry. Curr Diagn Pathol 2001;7:168-75.

14. Plaza JA, Dominguez F, Suster S. Cystic adenomatoid tumor of the mediastinum. Am J Surg Pathol 2004;28:132-8.

15. Travis WD, Brambilla E, M ller-Hermelink HK, Harris CC, eds. World Health Organization Classification of Tumours. Pathology and genetics of tumours of the lung, pleura, thymus and heart. Lyon: LARC Press; 2004:125-44.

16. Witkin GB, Rosai J. Solitary fibrous tumor of the mediastinum. A report of 14 cases. Am J Surg Pathol 1989;13:547-57.

8 OTHER TUMORS AND TUMOR-LIKE LESIONS OF THE THYMUS

THYMOLIPOMA

Definition. *Thymolipoma* is placed under the category of mesenchymal (or soft tissue) tumors of the thymus and mediastinum. It is defined as "a well-circumscribed thymic mass composed of mature adipose tissue and islands of microscopically unremarkable and non-neoplastic thymic parenchyma" in the original and revised World Health Organization (WHO) classifications (21,24).

Thymolipoma should be distinguished from lipoma and thymic lymphoid hyperplasia. Lipoma is one of the most common benign mesenchymal tumors of the mediastinum. It is often as large as thymolipoma. It can be located anywhere in the mediastinum and is made up of mature fat cells.

Clinical Features. Thymolipoma (or *lipothymoma*) often presents as a large asymptomatic mass in the anterior mediastinum. It can occur in both sexes at any age, but the mean age of patients is relatively young (20 to 30 years). It is a rare tumor. Patients may complain of symptoms attributable to the tumor mass, such as respiratory or cardiac problems (16).

Thymolipoma is radiolucent, therefore, the differential diagnosis includes cardiomegaly, pericardial cyst, and effusion. The combination of computerized tomography (CT) with location and attenuation values approaching those of fat; ultrasonography, with high echo due to the fat content; and magnetic resonance imaging (MRI), with strong signal intensity on T1-weighted spin-echo images should suggest thymolipoma (3,16,25).

Gross Findings. Most tumors weigh over 500 g and often exceed 2,000 g (range, 10 to 6,000 g). Grossly, the tumor diffusely enlarges the thymus, which often retains its normal configuration. The cut surface is yellow and is lobulated due to fibrous strands, resembling lipoma (figs. 8-1A, 8-2A). A close look, however, discloses milky white streaks and small nodules of thymic parenchyma (18).

Microscopic Findings. Histologically, thymolipoma is composed of mature fat and thymic parenchyma. The latter appears normal, although the medullary compartment may be reduced, with a scarcity of Hassall corpuscles (fig. 8-1B,C). A proportional increase of both thymic parenchyma (epithelial and lymphocytic) and mature fat indicates true hyperplasia of the thymus. The hamartomatous nature of the thymolipoma is illustrated by a tumor in a 6-year-old male child that showed the prominence of epithelial cells bordering nests of thymic parenchyma consisting of well-defined cortices and medullae and well-developed Hassall corpuscles (fig. 8-2B,C). Thymolipoma with clusters of polygonal myoid cells with eosinophilic cytoplasm in the medulla has been reported (9). The cells were positive for myoglobin and had a Z-band structure ultrastructurally.

An association with Graves disease, Hodgkin lymphoma, chronic lymphoid leukemia, hypogammaglobulinemia, and aplastic anemia has been reported (1,2). Thymolipoma associated with myasthenia gravis has also been reported (9,10,12,14,15). This association occurs more often in patients older than those presenting with thymolipoma alone. Thymectomy improves the symptoms of myasthenia gravis, although symptoms may recur postoperatively. Tumor weight is less than 200 g (average, 100 g), which is lower than the weight of thymolipoma unassociated with myasthenia gravis (average, 1,095 g). The presence of germinal centers has never been mentioned in either thymolipoma or the surrounding normal thymic tissue in cases complicated by myasthenia gravis. The prognosis is excellent after removal of the tumor, unless a paraneoplastic syndrome is present.

There is controversy as to the nature of thymolipoma. Some consider it abnormal hyperplasia of fat tissue, others a mixed tumor of mesenchymal and entodermal origin or hamartoma, and still others a thymoma with fatty changes (adipose involution). Moran et al.

257

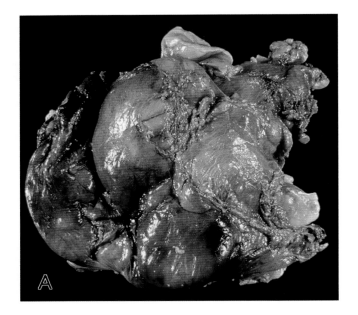

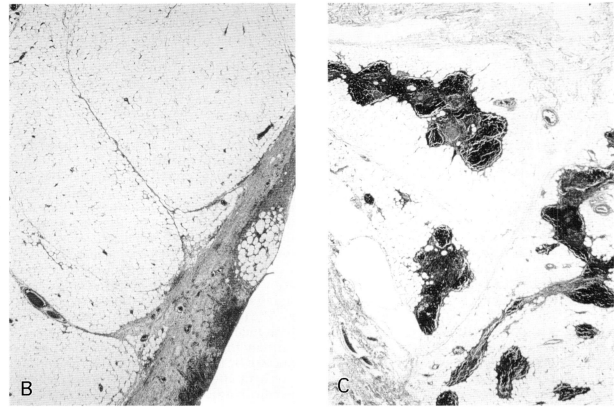

Figure 8-1

THYMOLIPOMA

A: Tumor in a 27-year-old woman is large, yellowish tan, and lobulated. It weighs 600 g.
B: The subcapsular portion of the tumor is composed of mature fat.
C: Thymic tissue is present. (Courtesy of Dr. Norikazu Tamaoki, Isehara, Japan.)

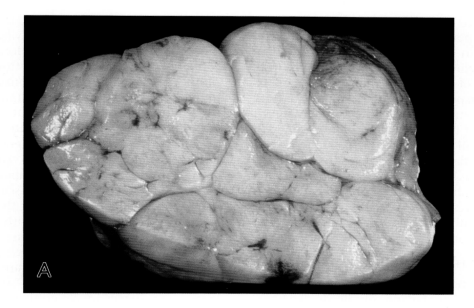

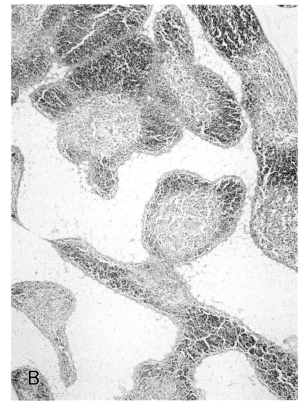
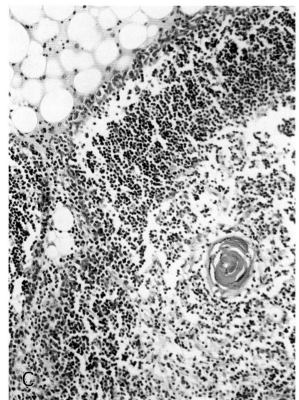

Figure 8-2

THYMOLIPOMA

A: The surgically resected tumor is thinly encapsulated and measures 12 x 11 x 7 cm.

B: The tumor is composed of irregular interconnecting nests of thymic parenchyma and mature fat. The former consists of well-defined cortices and medullae with well-developed Hassall corpuscles. Prominent epithelial cells border the nests.

C: Higher magnification. (Courtesy of Dr. Koichi Shimizu, Tokyo, Japan.)

(13) reported two cases of a histologic variant of thymolipoma, one in a 9-year-old girl and the other in a 32-year-old man, which they named thymofibrolipoma. The tumors were composed of "extensive areas of collagenous tissue interspersed with lakes of mature fatty tissue and strands of thymic parenchyma or remnants of normal thymic parenchyma with many Hassall corpuscles."

Differential Diagnosis. One thymolipoma was diagnosed erroneously as well-differentiated liposarcoma because of the presence of "atypical adipocytes" in the needle aspiration smear (17). The authors emphasized the necessity of differentiation from lipomatous tumors.

ECTOPIC HAMARTOMATOUS THYMOMA

Definition. A rare benign tumor of the lower neck consisting of fat and spindle-shaped fibroblastic and epithelial cells was described at about the same time by Smith and McClure (23) and Rosai et al. (19). This tumor was named 2 years later by Rosai et al. (20) as *ectopic hamartomatous thymoma*. Some additional cases have been reported and reviewed (4,8,22,26).

Clinical Features. This entity occurs in adults of a mean age of 52.5 years (26 to 79 years), and exhibits a marked male predominance (23 to 3). The tumors are located in the supraclavicular or suprasternal region, not attached to skin or bone, and are often present for many years (up to 30 years). This is not a mediastinal tumor, but it is described here since it is considered to originate in the thymic anlage associated with branchial pouches (8,20). Only one case of a carcinoma developing from an ectopic hamartomatous thymoma has been reported; the tumor did not metastasize. No cases of recurrence or metastasis have been reported after excision of this neoplasm (26).

Gross Findings. Grossly, the tumor is oval and well circumscribed, reaching as large as 19 cm in greatest dimension. The cut surface is solid, gray-white, and occasionally fasciculated.

Microscopic Findings. Histologically, ectopic hamartomatous thymoma is well circumscribed but may merge into surrounding adipose tissue. It is composed of several elements including spindle-shaped cells, fat cells, and squamous or glandular epithelial cell nests. The most conspicuous element is the spindle-shaped fibroblast-like cells, which are arranged in interlacing bundles. A storiform pattern may be seen. The nuclei are regular and oval to elongated, and contain fine chromatin and indistinct nucleoli. Although the spindle cells appear mesenchymal in nature, cytokeratin immunostains are positive, indicating their epithelial nature (figs. 8-3, 8-4). Epithelial islands with bland nuclei are present within the spindle cell element; they take the form of solid squamous cell nests, trabeculae, anastomosing cords, tubules, glands, and cysts. Groups of fat cells are scattered, and may occupy a major portion of the tumor or are inconspicuous. Myoid cells with myoglobin resembling fetal-type skeletal muscle have also been described (22). In one case, myoid cells simultaneously expressed cytokeratin, epithelial membrane antigen, myoglobin, and creatine kinase-mm, suggesting an epithelial cell origin (26). CD1a- and CD99-positive immature T cells, specific for thymic origin, were not found in several tumors studied (5,11a,26).

Histogenesis. Ectopic hamartomatous thymoma is considered to arise from the thymic anlage associated with branchial pouches (8). However, tumors identical to ectopic hamartomatous thymoma have not been seen in the normally located mediastinal thymus.

In 1991, Chan and Rosai (4) proposed a unifying concept for tumors of the neck showing thymic or related branchial pouch differentiation. On the benign end of the spectrum is the above-described ectopic hamartomatous thymoma; in the middle of the spectrum is the ectopic cervical thymoma, which is considered to arise from the cervical thymus and is histologically and biologically identical to mediastinal thymoma. On the malignant end are spindle epithelial tumor with thymus-like differentiation (SETTLE) and carcinoma showing thymus-like differentiation (CASTLE). In SETTLE, the spindle cell component may predominate and shows diffuse and strong immunoreactivity for cytokeratin using AE1/3 and CAM5.2 antibodies and vimentin (6). CASTLE resembles thymic lymphoepithelioma-like carcinoma or squamous cell carcinoma, and shows positive immunostaining for p63, high molecular weight cytokeratin, carcinoembryonic antigen, and CD5, providing evidence of thymic differentiation and thyroid solid cell nest origin (16a).

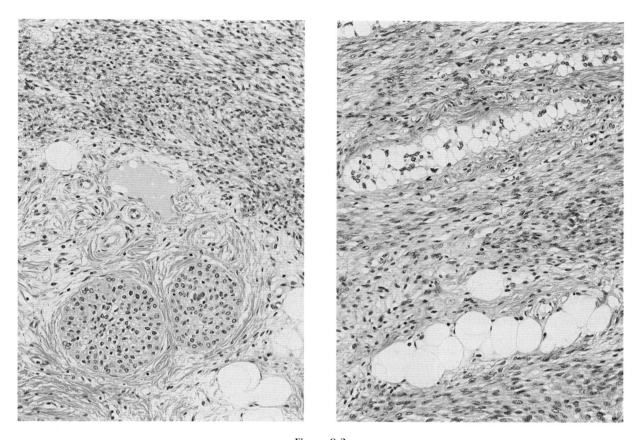

Figure 8-3

ECTOPIC HAMARTOMATOUS THYMOMA

Left: The tumor is composed of a mixture of fat cells, elongated fibroblast-like cells, and a few solid nests of squamous cells.

Right: Individual cells of a few nests seen on the top are markedly vacuolated, resembling fat cells, but they are much smaller than the fat cells seen on the bottom. (Courtesy of Dr. Tamotsu Sugai, Morioka, Japan.)

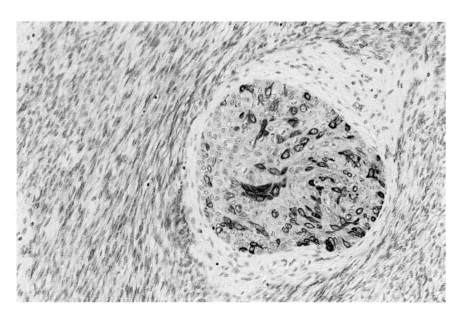

Figure 8-4

ECTOPIC HAMARTOMATOUS THYMOMA

Some squamous cells are strongly positive for cytokeratin. Fibrous tissue surrounding a squamous cell nest is negative but spindle-shaped tumor cells are weakly positive for cytokeratin. (Courtesy of Dr. Tamotsu Sugai, Morioka, Japan.)

After analyzing 21 cases of "ectopic hamartomatous thymoma" clinicopathologically and immunohistochemically, Fetsch et al. (7) found no compelling evidence of a thymic derivation and, therefore, regard the current designation as inaccurate. They believe that the designation "branchial anlage mixed tumor" reflects the nature of this unusual neoplasm. If this interpretation is correct, the description of this neoplasm should be deleted from this chapter. Another paper by Kazakov et al. (11) described a case of "ectopic" ectopic hamartomatous thymoma situated deep on the interface of the posterior axillary region and back, in which spindle cells were positive for CD34 and muscle-specific actin immunohistochemically. The authors stated that the dorsal location of the tumor calls into question all of the so far suggested origins of ectopic hamartomatous thymoma.

Differential Diagnosis. Histologic distinction between ectopic hamartomatous thymoma and ectopic cervical thymoma is simple, since these two tumors are entirely different in nature. The characteristic findings of the former are described here and those of the latter were described in chapter 2. The differential diagnosis of ectopic hamartomatous thymoma includes pleomorphic adenoma of salivary or sweat gland origin, spindle cell carcinoma, and synovial sarcoma. The general histologic features of relatively low cellularity, and nuclear normochromasia, and the absent or minimal mitotic activity enable the establishment of a correct diagnosis.

MALIGNANT MELANOMA

Malignant melanoma arising in the thymus is extremely rare and only a few cases have been reported in the literature, presenting either as a primary intrathymic tumor or as an anterior mediastinal neoplasm involving the thymus (27,28,30). One case of the latter was in an 11-year-old boy, in whom incomplete resection was performed (30). A 26-year-old woman had a giant pigmented nevus without malignant change and multiple foci of pigmented nevus cell nests throughout the thymus with foci of malignant melanoma (28). The occurrence of primary malignant melanoma in the thymus in these cases is suggested by no detectable primary melanoma in organs other than the thymus together with the presence of benign nevus cell aggregates in the thymus (28,29), and the presence of melanocytes in carcinoid tumors and thymoma (see figs. 2-64, 2-85B).

THYMIC CYST

Congenital Thymic Cyst

General Features. *Thymic cysts* are rare lesions. They are most likely congenital and developmental in origin, and are found along the anatomic course of embryologic descent of the thymus from the third pharyngeal pouch; that is, from the lateral aspect of the neck at the mandibular angle to the sternal manubrium (31). Thymic cysts derived from an acquired reactive process are rarer than those congenitally formed (40). At the National Cancer Center Hospital, Tokyo, congenital thymic cysts comprise about 5 percent of surgically removed mediastinal space-occupying lesions (see Table 2-4) (38).

Clinical Features. There is no gender difference in incidence. Thymic cysts have been seen in the lateral aspect of the neck of children. In adults, the cyst is often asymptomatic, and found incidentally by chest X-ray examination. Occasionally, symptoms result from compression of surrounding organs or tissue.

Mediastinal cyst is diagnosed by its smooth and sharp contour on chest X ray, and the CT and echographic findings. Needle aspiration of the cyst content is also useful for diagnosis.

Gross Findings. Thymic cysts in the neck are tubular and those in the thymus are round or oval. They are uniloculated or multiloculated and thin walled; fatty thymic tissue is attached (fig. 8-5). The content is watery clear to straw colored, or chocolate colored due to previous hemorrhage. The lining of an uncomplicated cyst is smooth.

Microscopic Findings. Histologically, the cyst lining consists of flattened, cuboidal, columnar, ciliated columnar, or stratified squamous epithelium, and may be composed of, or continuous with, thymic tissue (figs. 8-6, 8-7). The epithelial lining may be destroyed by pressure and is replaced by granulation tissue, with or without cholesterol clefts or fibrous tissue (fig. 8-7, bottom). It is essential to find thymic tissue in the wall of the cyst in order to establish a diagnosis of thymic cyst, and it may be necessary to examine multiple sections of the cyst wall.

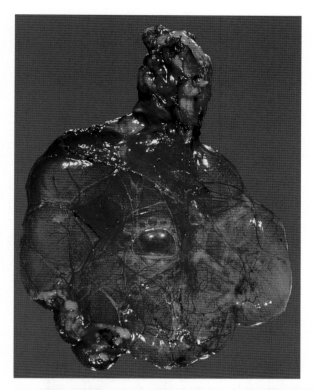

Figure 8-5

THYMIC CYST

Left: A large, thin-walled cyst of the thymus appears multiloculated from the outside.

Below: On sectioning, however, it was found to be unilocular.

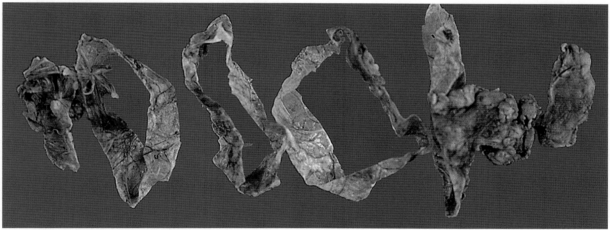

Malignant transformation of the epithelial cells of the thymic cyst is rare. Basaloid carcinoma of the thymus may show features suggestive of thymic cyst origin (see chapter 3, fig. 3-20). Well-differentiated papillary squamous cell carcinoma arising from the lining epithelium of a thymic cyst has been reported by Leong and Brown (34). A case of basaloid-squamous cell carcinoma arising in a multiloculated thymic cyst, which progressed to become undifferenti-ated carcinoma, is described in chapter 3 (see fig. 3-16).

Acquired Multilocular Thymic Cyst

In 1991, Suster and Rosai (40) reported 18 cases of multilocular thymic cysts that were related to an acquired reactive process. According to these authors, this was most likely the result of cystic transformation of medullary duct epithelium-derived structures (including

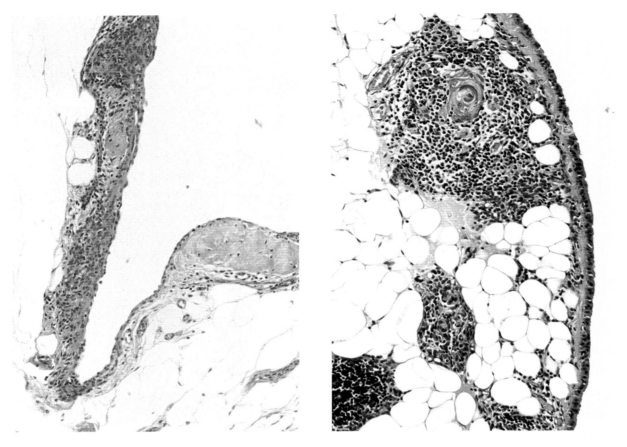

Figure 8-6

THYMIC CYST

Left: The cyst is lined in part by a single layer of flat cells, which are continuous with atrophic thymic tissue. The wall is partly collagenous.

Right: In other areas, the cyst is lined by a single layer of low columnar cells. Thymic tissue with a Hassall corpuscle is attached to the thin-walled cyst. Ciliated columnar cells were found in a small area.

Hassall corpuscles) induced by an acquired inflammatory process.

The lesions vary from 3 to 17 cm in greatest dimension. In most cases, they can be enucleated easily, but in some cases they adhere to the surrounding structures, making removal difficult. The cut surface shows multiloculated cavities of variegated appearance, filled with dark red blood or brown fluid and areas of recent hemorrhage and fibrosis (fig. 8-8).

Multilocular cysts are lined in part by squamous, columnar, or cuboidal epithelial cells, often continuous with the islands of non-neoplastic thymic tissue present in the cyst walls. They are associated with severe acute and chronic inflammation accompanied by fibrovascular proliferation, necrosis, hemorrhage, cholesterol granuloma formation, and reactive lymphoid hyperplasia with prominent germinal centers (fig. 8-8BC). The pseudoepitheliomatous hyperplasia in the lining of acquired multilocular thymic cysts noted in some cases is thought to be due to the inflammatory, hemorrhagic, and necrotizing changes that are often present in these lesions (36,39). Incidental thymoma and thymic carcinoma were found in two cases each.

Similar multilocular cysts were seen in association with thymic Hodgkin lymphoma and thymic seminoma (40). Marginal zone B-cell lymphoma (mucosa-associated lymphoid tissue [MALT] lymphoma) is also often multicystic (see fig. 6-9) (33). Prior to the recognition of this

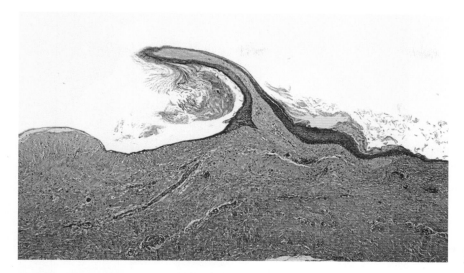

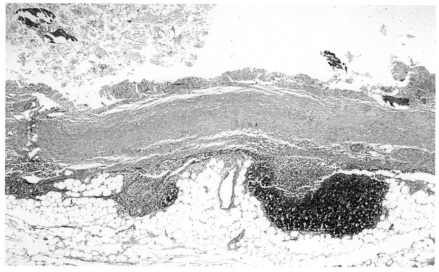

Figure 8-7

THYMIC CYST

Top: The cyst is partly lined by keratotic squamous epithelium. The cyst wall is collagenous.

Bottom: In another area, the lining epithelium has been denuded and replaced by histiocytes. The contents consist of keratotic debris and calcified material. Thymic tissue with Hassall corpuscles is present outside the cyst.

entity, some cases reported as acquired multiloculated thymic cyst were probably examples of lymphoid hyperplasia of MALT type, or low-grade marginal zone B-cell lymphoma. A multilocular thymic cyst associated with atypical lymphoid hyperplasia of MALT type in a patient with Sjögren's syndrome and suspicious for low-grade marginal zone B-cell lymphoma is shown in figure 8-9. This case was originally reported as acquired multilocular thymic cyst (32). It may be difficult to determine whether multilocular thymic cysts are congenital or acquired, if the inflammatory reaction is mild (fig. 8-10).

Differential Diagnosis. The differential diagnosis includes cystic thymoma, cystic teratoma, lymphangioma, and other mediastinal cysts or cystic lesions. Although the above are cystic and may be in the anterior mediastinum, as is thymic cyst, histologic distinction is easy. Even in difficult cases, multiple sectioning of cystic lesions usually leads to a correct diagnosis by examination of the characteristic findings for each lesion (35).

OTHER TUMOR-LIKE LESIONS

Inflammatory or non-neoplastic lesions, both cystic and solid, are rare in the anterior mediastinum. They include tuberculosis, hydatidosis (hydatid cyst) in endemic areas, and inflammatory pseudotumor of unknown etiology, as well as spontaneous thymic hemorrhage and choristoma of the thymus (35,37).

265

Figure 8-8

**ACQUIRED MULTILOCULAR
THYMIC CYST**

A: This multilocular thymic cyst has a fibrous wall of varying thickness.(Fig. 2 from Suster S, Rosai J. Multilocular thymic cyst: an acquired reactive process. Study of 18 cases. Am J Surg Pathol 1991;15:390.)

B: The cyst lining is continuous with the thymic lobules in the wall.

C: Thymic tissue around the cyst shows elongated, branching strands of epithelium surrounded by fibrous stroma and abundant lymphocytes.

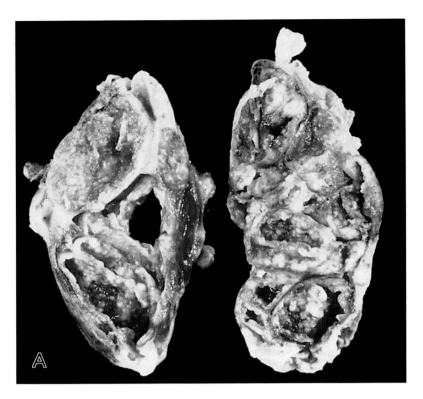

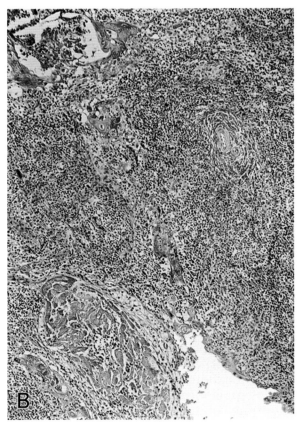

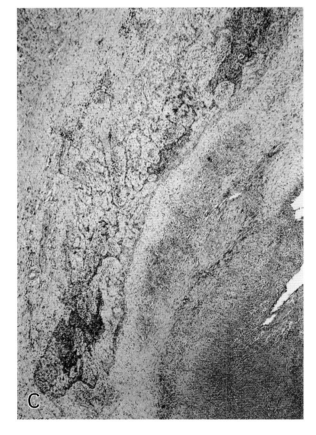

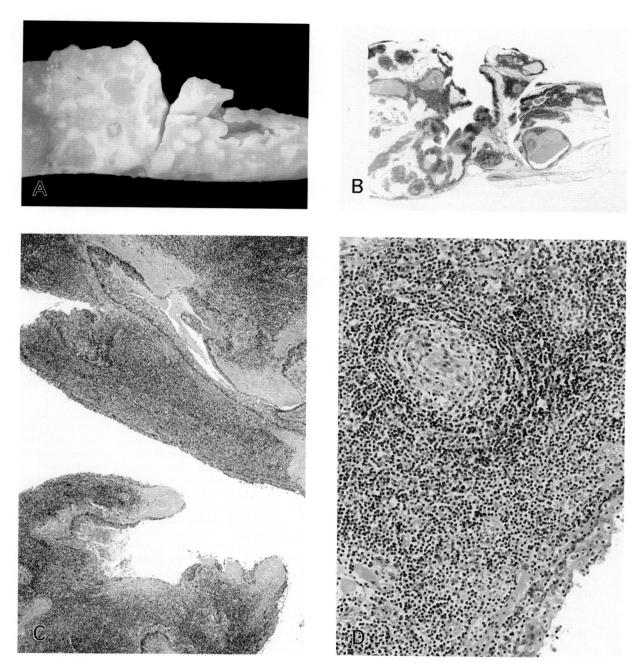

Figure 8-9

**MULTILOCULAR THYMIC CYST WITH ATYPICAL LYMPHOID
HYPERPLASIA OF MUCOSA-ASSOCIATED LYMPHOID TISSUE (MALT) TYPE**

A: The cut surface of the lesion, after formalin fixation, reveals multiple cysts containing gelatinous material and varying sized, milky white solid nodules.

B: Low-power view shows multilocular thymic cysts supported by lymphoid tissue.

C: Medium-power view discloses a cyst lined with stratified epithelium supported by abundant lymphoid tissue. Occasional lymph follicles contain germinal centers.

D: High-power view shows a lymphoepithelial lesion with a lymph follicle containing a germinal center. No areas with monocytoid clear lymphoid cells suggestive of low-grade marginal zone B-cell lymphoma are evident. (Courtesy of Dr. Kazuya Kondo, Tokushima, Japan.)

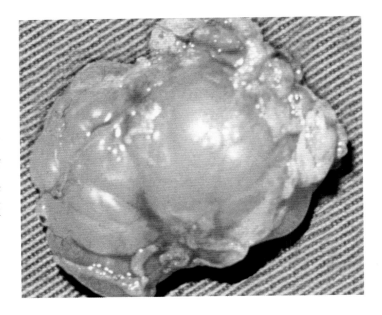

Figure 8-10

MULTILOCULAR THYMIC CYST OF EITHER CONGENITAL OR ACQUIRED TYPE

This thin-walled, clear fluid-filled multilocular thymic cyst was found incidentally in a 63-year-old woman. The cyst was lined by a single layer of flat or cuboidal cells or stratified squamous cells. There was involuted thymic tissue and chronic inflammatory cell infiltration of a mild degree in the cyst walls. (Courtesy of Drs. Yoshitaka Fujii and Tadaaki Eimoto, Nagoya, Japan.)

REFERENCES

Thymolipoma and Ectopic Hamartomatous Thymoma

1. Barnes RD, O'Gorman P. Two cases of aplastic anemia associated with tumours of the thymus. J Clin Pathol 1962;15:264-8.
2. Benton C, Gerard P. Thymolipoma in a patient with Graves' disease. Case report and review of the literature. J Thoracic Cardiovasc Surg 1966;51:428-33.
3. Brown LR, Aughenbaugh GL. Masses of the anterior mediastinum: CT and MR imaging. AJR Am J Roentgenol 1991;157:1171-80.
4. Chan JK, Rosai J. Tumors of the neck showing thymic or related branchial pouch differentiation: a unifying concept. Hum Pathol 1991;22:349-67.
5. Chan JK, Tsang WY, Seneviratne S, Pau MY. The MIC2 antibody 013. Practical application for the study of thymic epithelial tumors. Am J Surg Pathol 1995;19:1115-23.
6. Chetty R, Goetsch S, Nayler S, Cooper K. Spindle epithelial tumour with thymus-like element (SETTLE): the predominantly monophasic variant. Histopathology 1998;33:71-4.
7. Fetsch JF, Laskin WB, Michal M, et al. Ectopic hamartomatous thymoma: a clinicopathologic and immunohistochemical analysis of 21 cases with data supporting reclassification as a branchial anlage mixed tumor. Am J Surg Pathol 2004;28:1360-70.
8. Fetsch JF, Weiss SW. Ectopic hamartomatous thymoma: clinicopathologic, immunohistochemical, and histogenetic considerations in four new cases. Hum Pathol 1990;21:662-8.
9. Iseki M, Tsuda N, Kishikawa M, et al. Thymolipoma with striated myoid cells. Histological, immunohistochemical and ultrastructural study. Am J Surg Pathol 1990;14:395-8.
10. Jagadha V, Ramaswamy G. An unusual case of thymolipoma with hamartomatous changes. Arch Pathol Lab Med 1984;108:611-2.
11. Kazakov DV, Mukensnable P, Hes O, Michal M. 'Ectopic' ectopic hamartomatous thymoma. Histopathology 2004;45:202-4.
11a. Kushida Y, Haba R, Kobayashi S, Ishikawa M, Doi T, Kadota K. Ectopic hamartomatous thymoma: a case report with immunohistochemical study and review of the literature. J Cutan Pathol 2006;33:369-72.
12. Le Marc'hadour F, Pinel N, Pasquier B, Dieny A, Stoebner P, Couderc P. Thymolipoma in association with myasthenia gravis. Am J Surg Pathol 1991;15:802-9.
13. Moran CA, Zeren H, Koss MN. Thymofibrolipoma. A histologic variant of thymolipoma. Arch Pathol Lab Med 1994;118:281-2.
14. Otto HF, Loning T, Lachenmayer L, Janzen RW, Gurtler KF, Fischer K. Thymolipoma in association with myasthenia gravis. Cancer 1982;50:1623-8.

15. Reintgen D, Fetter BF, Roses A, McCarty KS Jr. Thymolipoma in association with myasthenia gravis. Arch Pathol Lab Med 1978;102:463-6.

16. Rasado-de-Christenson ML, Putgatch RD, Moran CA, Galobardes J. Thymolipoma: analysis of 27 cases. Radiology 1994;193:121-6.

16a. Reimann JD, Dorfman DM, Nose V. Carcinoma showing thymus-like differentiation of the thyroid (CASTLE): a comparative study: Evidence of thymic differentiation and solid cell nest origin. Am J Surg Pathol 2006;30:994-1001.

17. Romero-Guadarrama MB, Duran-Padilla MA, Cruz-Ortiz H, et al. Diagnosis of thymolipoma with fine needle aspiration biopsy. Report of a case initially misdiagnosed as liposarcoma. Acta Cytol 2004;48:441-6.

18. Rosai J, Levine GD. Tumors of the thymus. Atlas of Tumor Pathology, 2nd Series, Fascicle 13, Washington DC: Armed Forces Institute of Pathology; 1976.

19. Rosai J, Levine GD, Limas C. Spindle cell thymic anlage tumor: four cases of a previously undescribed benign neoplasm of lower neck [Abstract], Lab Invest 1982;46:70A.

20. Rosai J, Limas C, Husband EM. Ectopic hamartomatous thymoma. A distinctive benign lesion of lower neck. Am J Surg Pathol 1984;8:501-13.

21. Rosai J, Sobin LH, eds. Histological typing of tumours of the thymus. World Health Organization international histological classification of tumours, 2nd ed. New York: Springer; 1999

22. Saeed IT, Fletcher CD. Ectopic hamartomatous thymoma containing myoid cells. Histopathology 1990;17:572-4.

23. Smith PS, McClure J. Unusual subcutaneous mixed tumour exhibiting adipose, fibroblastic, and epithelial components. J Clin Pathol 1982;35:1074-7.

24. Travis WD, Brambilla E, Muller-Hermelink HK, Harris CC, eds. World Health Organization Classification of Tumours. Pathology and genetics of tumours of the lung, pleura, thymus and heart. Lyon: IARC Press; 2004.

25. Yeh HC, Gordon A, Kirschner PA, Cohen BA. Computed tomography and sonography of thymolipoma. AJR Am J Roentgenol 1983;140:1131-3.

26. Zhao C, Yamada T, Kuramochi S, et al. Two cases of ectopic hamartomatous thymoma. Virchow Arch 2000; 437:643-7.

Malignant Melanoma

27. Alli PM, Crain BJ, Heitmiller R, Argani P. Malignant melanoma presenting as an intrathymic tumor: a primary thymic melanoma? Arch Pathol Lab Med 2000;124:130-4.

28. Fushimi H, Kotoh K, Watanabe D, Tanio Y, Ogawa T, Miyoshi S. Malignant melanoma in the thymus. Am J Surg Pathol 2000;24:1305-8.

29. Parker JR, Ro JY, Ordonez NG. Benign nevus cell aggregates in the thymus: a case report. Mod Pathol 1999;12:329-32.

30. Vlodavsky E, Ben-Izhak O, Best LA, Kerner H. Primary malignant melanoma of the anterior mediastinum in a child. Am J Surg Pathol 2000;24:747-9

Thymic Cysts

31. Bieger RC, McAdams AJ. Thymic cysts. Arch Pathol 1966;82:535-41.

32. Kondo K, Miyoshi T, Sakiyama S, Shimosato Y, Monden Y. Multilocular thymic cyst associated with Sjögren's syndrome. Ann Thorac Surg 2001;72:1367-9.

33. Isaacson PG Chan JK, Tang C, Addis BJ. Low-grade B-cell lymphoma of mucosa-associated lymphoid tissue arising in the thymus. A thymic lymphoma mimicking myoepithelial sialadenitis. Am J Surg Pathol 1990;14:342-51.

34. Leong AS, Brown JH. Malignant transformation in a thymic cyst. Am J Surg Pathol 1984;8:471-5.

35. Marchevsky AM, Kaneko M. Surgical pathology of the mediastinum, 2nd ed. New York: Raven Press; 1992.

36. Michal M, Havlicek F. Pseudo-epitheliomatous hyperplasia in thymic cysts. Histopathology 1991;19:281-2.

37. Rosai J, Levine GD. Tumors of the thymus. Atlas of Tumor Pathology, 2nd Series, Fascicle 13, Washington, DC: Armed Forces Institute of Pathology; 1976.

38. Shimosato Y, Mukai K. Tumors of the mediastinum. Atlas of Tumor Pathology, 3rd Series, Fascicle 21, Washington, DC: Armed Forces Institute of Pathology; 1997.

39. Suster S, Barbuto D, Carlson G, Rosai J. Multilocular thymic cysts with pseudoepitheliomatous hyperplasia. Hum Pathol 1991;22:455-60.

40. Suster S, Rosai J. Multilocular thymic cyst: an acquired reactive process. Study of 18 cases. Am J Surg Pathol 1991;15:388-98.

9 NON-NEOPLASTIC CONDITIONS OF THE THYMUS

THYMUS IN IMMUNODEFICIENCY

Since the thymus is an important organ in the development and maintenance of the immune system, it is not surprising to find that morphologic changes in this organ are associated with various immunodeficiency disorders (2,3,6). The thymus is unique in several aspects when compared with other lymphoid organs. These characteristics also contribute to the distinct histologic changes associated with immunodeficiency disorders.

The morphologic features in the thymus that affect the immune system are divided into congenital (*thymic dysplasia*) and acquired (*thymic atrophy*) (Table 9-1) (6). Morphologically, the dysplastic thymus shows a depletion of lymphoid cells and a lack of maturation of the epithelial cells, which appear primitive and fail to differentiate into Hassall corpuscles. Thymic dysplasia is present at birth and is thought to

express a failure or arrest in the embryologic development of the organ. The terms "thymic hypoplasia" and "thymic alymphoplasia" are outdated designations and should be regarded as equivalent to, or variants of, dysplasia. The term "thymic aplasia," as observed in Di George syndrome, should be restricted to those cases with complete absence of a eutopic thymus gland, possibly with tiny remnants of normal mature tissue.

Thymic atrophy designates all regressive changes that are postnatally acquired. It is characterized by shrinkage of the thymus, depletion of the lymphoid populations, and varying alternations in the epithelial network (figs. 9-1–9-3) (6,7).

The thymus responds dramatically to episodes of severe stress by active lympholysis, resulting in a loss in size and weight. This stress-related involution, which may also be accidental, results

Table 9-1

A COMPARISON OF THE FEATURES OF INHERITED THYMIC DYSPLASIA (ITD) AND SEVERE THYMIC ATROPHY (STA)[a]

	ITD	STA
Weight of the gland	<5g	>5g
Foliated architecture	Well preserved	Blurred
Interlobular and perilobular tissue	Fatty	Fibroadipose with inflammatory cells
Size of the vessels	Small	Enlarged for the size of the lobules
Perivascular spaces	Empty	Fibrohyaline deposits
Thymic epithelial network	Maintained	Collapsed and disorganized
Epithelial maturation	Totally defective	Partially defective
Hassall corpuscles	Absent	Absent or necrotic and calcified
Cytokeratin expression	Present	Often reduced
Class II MHC expression	Present	Present
Lymphoid cells		
CD1	Absent	Absent
CD2	Absent or rare	Some present
CD4	Absent	Some present
CD8	Absent	Some present
Plasma cells	Absent	Present, sometimes numerous

[a]Table 1 from Nezelof C. Thymic pathology in primary and secondary immunodeficiencies. Histopathology 1992;21:506.

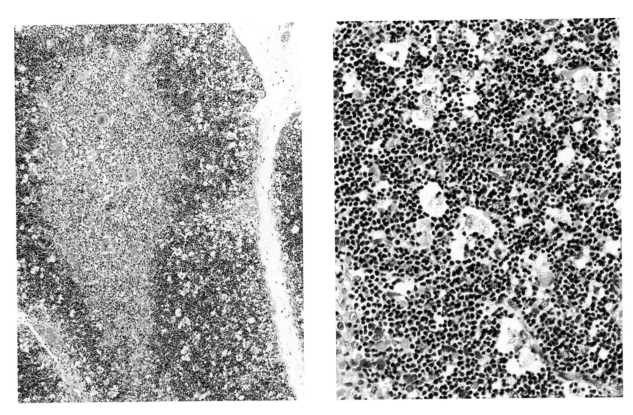

Figure 9-1

ACUTE THYMIC INVOLUTION WITH STARRY SKY APPEARANCE

Left: An abundance of macrophages containing degenerating lymphocytes and nuclear debris in the cortex of the thymus of an infant.

Right: High-power view. (Courtesy of Dr. Junichi Hata, Tokyo, Japan.)

from a sudden release of corticosteroids from the adrenal cortex causing rapid lympholysis of the cortical thymocytes. There are prominent karyorrhexis of thymocytes and active phagocytosis by macrophages, which create a prominent starry sky appearance, characteristically confined to the cortex (fig. 9-1) (10,11). Continuing stress results in extensive lympholysis with a loss of corticomedullary distinction, accentuation of the epithelial cells, and cystic dilation of Hassall corpuscles (fig. 9-2). With further loss of thymocytes, the lobular architecture progressively collapses and fibrosis ensues. Clinically significant immunosuppression due to extensive loss of cortical thymocytes may be seen in children undergoing major stress, such as with extensive thermal injury. Radiotherapy and intensive antitumor chemotherapy induce morphologic changes similar to those of stress involution (fig. 9-3) (10).

Thymus in Primary Immunodeficiencies

The primary immunodeficiency disorders are a heterogeneous group of genetic or acquired cellular defects that result in the faulty maturation, regulation, or function of antigen-specific lymphocytes (8). Several classifications of immunodeficiency have been proposed, but none is fully satisfactory. One of the classifications of these disorders is based on criteria that define the altered function of B or T lymphocytes, or both (8). As a group, these disorders are rarely encountered in clinical medicine, and their frequency is less than 1/50,000 to 100,000 population (3).

Dysplasia of the thymus is the most frequently and thoroughly described histologic lesion of the thymus associated with primary immunodeficiency disorders. Nezelof et al. (6) described four subtypes of thymic dysplasia: simple thymic dysplasia, pseudoglandular thymic

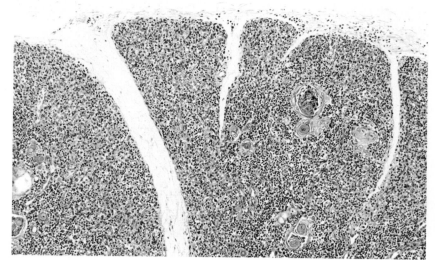

Figure 9-2

CHRONIC THYMIC INVOLUTION

The thymus in a 6-month-old female infant with Ebstein anomaly weighed 3 g. Lobulation is distinct. Loss of corticomedullary demarcation and marked reduction in the number of lymphocytes are the prominent features. (Courtesy of Dr. Junichi Hata, Tokyo, Japan.)

Figure 9-3

INVOLUTED THYMUS IN MEDIASTINAL CHORIOCARCINOMA TREATED BY CHEMOTHERAPY

The thymus lobule is reduced in size and fibrotic, and there is marked reduction in the number of lymphocytes. Calcified Hassall corpuscles are surrounded by nests of epithelial cells.

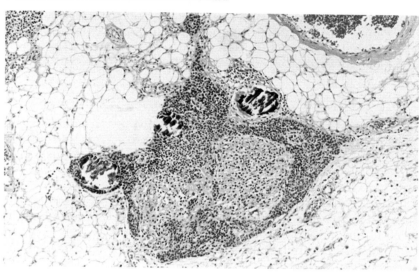

dysplasia, thymic dysplasia with corticomedullary differentiation, and thymic pseudoatrophy. In all subtypes, the thymus shows the following common features: loss of lymphoid cells, lack of a distinct corticomedullary junction, and lobular structures with an embryonal appearance. Pseudoglandular dysplasia is the most primitive form, whereas thymic dysplasia with corticomedullary differentiation and thymic pseudoatrophy are the better-differentiated forms.

These histologic patterns do not necessarily correlate with a precise inherited disease or a specific enzyme deficiency. They seem instead to reflect the severity of the disorder (6). The pseudoglandular pattern, the most primitive, is usually associated with complete agammaglobulinemia, early death, and, frequently, a total absence of peripheral lymph nodes. In contrast, the pseudoatrophic pattern correlates with normal or low levels of serum immunoglobulins, prolonged survival, and, occasionally, adenosine deaminase (7) or nucleoside phosphorylase enzymatic deficiency (fig. 9-4).

Well-established inherited T-cell deficiencies, such as the bare lymphocytes syndrome (lack of expression of major histocompatibility complex [MHC] class II), Wiskott-Aldrich disease, and a defect in the production of interleukin-2 are not associated with dysplastic thymus but with an otherwise normal atrophic gland (6). The thymus of patients with Down syndrome, who have a marked and definite defect in the

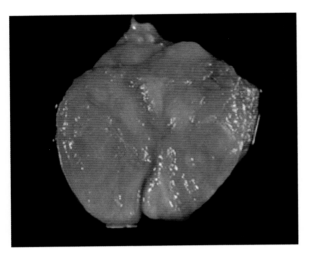
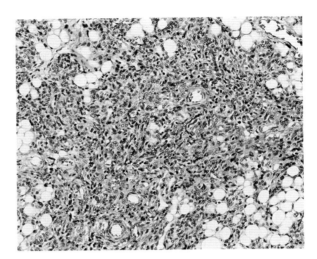

Figure 9-4

THYMIC DYSPLASIA

Left: The thymus in a 2-month-old male infant with adenosine deaminase-deficient severe combined immunodeficiency weighed only 0.8 g and consisted of loose fibrotic tissue with scattered fat lobules.

Right: Histologically, the thymus shows a vaguely foliated architecture with irregular borders. It was composed of spindle-shaped epithelial cells, rare lymphoid cells, absence of Hassall corpuscles, and scattered fat cells. (Courtesy of Dr. Junichi Hata, Tokyo, Japan.)

thymus-dependent immune system, shows morphologic changes resembling involution (1), that is, a small thymus with severe lymphocyte depletion, diminution of the cortex, and loss of corticomedullary demarcation. In addition, Hassall corpuscles are giant and cystic, with increased cellularity around them (fig. 9-5) (5). Although the distribution of epithelial cells positive for different subtypes of cytokeratins is similar to that in the thymus of normal children, the number of interdigitating cells is reduced or absent (4). It is postulated that alterations in the thymic microenvironment may correlate with the imbalances of immunity in patients with Down syndrome.

Thymus in Secondary Immunodeficiencies

Unlike inherited immunodeficiencies, acquired immunodeficiencies appear less delineated. In addition to the acquired immunodeficiency syndrome (AIDS), acquired immunodeficiency may be seen in patients with severe graft versus host disease (GVHD), chronic viral infections including late onset rubella syndrome, prolonged administration of glucocorticoid and cytotoxic drugs, severe and early protein malnutrition, and total body

irradiation (figs. 9-3, 9-6) (6,9). In all these circumstances, the thymus is assumed to have previously been normal, and the morphologic changes are therefore regarded as acquired, i.e., of atrophic and degenerative nature. Nezelof (6) uses the term severe thymic atrophy for these morphologic changes (Table 9-2).

THYMIC HYPERPLASIA

The term thymic hyperplasia embraces two distinct morphologic forms (12,15,17). The first, *true thymic hyperplasia*, indicates enlargement of the thymus through an increase in thymic tissue, which remains normally organized. The second form, *lymphoid hyperplasia*, is characterized by the presence of lymphoid follicles with germinal centers in a thymus gland that may be enlarged, atrophied, or involved by a neoplasm.

True Thymic Hyperplasia

True thymic hyperplasia is defined as enlargement of the thymus gland (as determined by weight and volume) beyond the upper limit of normal for that particular age (fig. 9-7). A histologically normal thymus can weigh in excess of 200 g (12). In order to establish the diagnosis of true thymic hyperplasia, reference

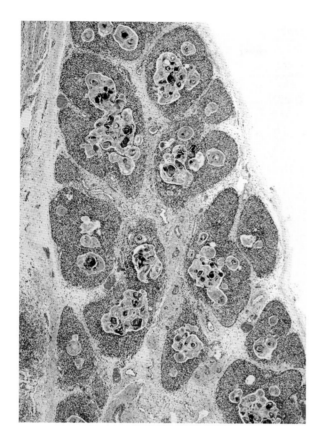 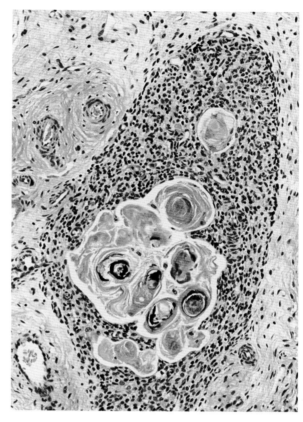

Figure 9-5

SMALL ABNORMAL THYMUS RESEMBLING INVOLUTED THYMUS

Left: The thymus of a 3-month-old male with Down syndrome weighed only 1 g. The lobular architecture of the thymus is maintained. Hassall corpuscles are prominent and large, probably due to coalescence. Marked diminution of the cortex consists of loss of corticomedullary demarcation, marked reduction in number of lymphocytes, loss of fat cells, and fibrosis of interlobular tissue.

Right: High-power view. (Courtesy of Dr. Junichi Hata, Tokyo, Japan.)

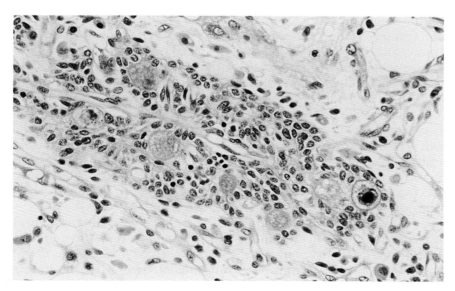

Figure 9-6

SEVERE THYMIC ATROPHY

The thymic lobule in a 54-year-old man with hemophilia A and acquired immunodeficiency syndrome (AIDS) is greatly reduced in size, with a marked reduction in the number of lymphocytes. There is a cell with a cytomegalovirus inclusion body in the right lower corner. (Courtesy of Dr. Morio Koike, Tokyo, Japan.)

Table 9-2

MAJOR IMMUNODEFICIENCY DISORDERS
ASSOCIATED WITH AN ABNORMAL THYMUS GLAND[a]

Syndrome	Thymic Morphology	Inheritance
Congenital thymic hypoplasia (DiGeorge syndrome)	Dysplasia	S[b]
Severe combined immunodeficiencies (SCID)		
Reticular dysgenesis	Dysplasia	AR
Nezelof syndrome	Dysplasia	XL/AR
Adenosine deaminase deficiencies	Dysplasia	AR
Purine nucleoside phosphorylase deficiency	Dysplasia	AR
Ataxia telangiectasia	Dysplasia	AR
MHC[c] antigen deficiency	Atrophy	AR
Wiskott-Aldrich syndrome	Atrophy	XL
Acquired immunodeficiency syndrome (AIDS)	Atrophy	S
Immunodeficiency to Epstein-Barr virus	Atrophy	XL/AR
Graft versus host disease	Atrophy	S

[a]Table 2-2 from Fascicle 21, Third Series.
[b]S = sporadic; AR = autosomal recessive; XL = X-linked recessive.
[c]MHC = major histocompatibility complex.

Table 9-3

WEIGHT AND VOLUME OF
NORMAL HUMAN THYMUSES[a]

Age (years)	Number	Weight (g) Mean	Weight (g) SD	Volume (cm³) Mean	Volume (cm³) SD
0-1	6	27.3	16.4	26.8	16.1
1-4	4	28.0	19.3	27.9	10.4
5-9	7	22.1	9.2	21.5	8.8
10-14	5	21.5	6.1	21.1	6.4
15-19	9	20.2	10.3	19.3	10.1
20-24	18	21.6	9.5	23.0	10.6
25-29	9	23.1	11.8	23.7	11.9
30-34	5	25.5	9.9	27.6	11.2
35-44	17	21.9	9.2	22.2	10.5
45-54	14	24.8	12.8	26.5	12.4
55-64	15	21.3	9.5	23.5	10.4
65-84	17	23.8	16.1	25.6	17.0
85-90	5	18.2	5.4	20.4	6.8
91-107	5	12.4	6.9	13.4	7.2

[a]Modified from Table 2 from Suster S, Rosai J. Thymus. In Sternberg SS, ed. Histology for pathologists. New York: Raven Press; 1992:274.

must be made to standard weight charts of the normal thymus for comparison. The first extensive studies on the normal weights of the thymus were made in fresh autopsy specimens by Hammar in 1906 (15). These figures have been updated, most comprehensively by Steinmann (16) who studied the weight and volume of human thymuses in 136 healthy individuals (Table 9-3). Whether there is any ethnic or geographic difference in thymic weight is not known, and therefore, using data from a single study may be misleading. The pathogenesis and significance of true thymic hyperplasia are unknown.

Thymic hyperplasia has been recognized in several instances as a complication of chemotherapy for Hodgkin lymphoma and germ cell tumors, and has been interpreted as the expression of an immunologic "rebound" phenomenon (fig. 9-7) (17). A similar enlargement of the thymus has been reported in children recovering from thermal burns and in infants following cessation of the administration of corticosteroids. A

case of pure red cell aplasia associated with true thymic hyperplasia was reported in a 35-year-old woman (14). The thymus was found to be enlarged not on chest X-ray examination, but on computerized tomography (CT). Thymectomy for the enlarged thymus was performed and was followed rapidly by full hematologic recovery.

Lymphoid Hyperplasia

In contrast to true thymic hyperplasia, lymphoid hyperplasia of the thymus is usually not associated with enlargement of the thymus but refers to the presence of an increased number of lymphoid follicles (figs. 9-8, 9-9) (12,15,17). Since lymphoid follicles are a normal constituent of the thymus, it is difficult to establish diagnostic criteria for lymphoid hyperplasia. Lymphoid follicles arise at the corticomedullary junction and within the extrathymic perivascular spaces, and are structurally similar to those of peripheral lymphoid tissues (17).

Lymphoid hyperplasia of the thymus is most commonly associated with myasthenia gravis but has also been observed in a number of immunologically mediated disorders including

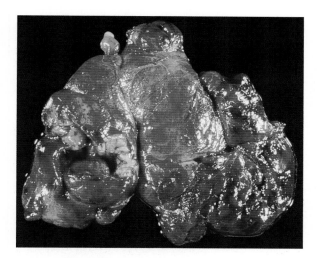

Figure 9-7

HYPERPLASTIC THYMUS

This thymus was excised from a 5-year-old boy and weighed 75 g. An "anterior mediastinal tumor," which proved to be a hyperplastic thymus, was detected 2 years 3 months after resection of a testicular germ cell tumor and postoperative chemotherapy.

Above: Grossly, the normal configuration of the thymus is preserved. The incised surface shows prominent lobulation.

Right: Histologically, thymic cortices and medullae are well defined. Interstitial connective tissue is delicate with rare fat cells. There are no germinal centers.

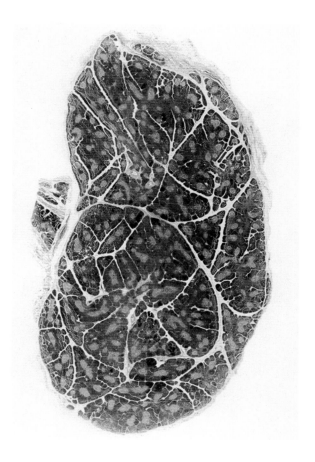

systemic lupus erythematosus, rheumatoid arthritis, scleroderma, allergic vasculitis, and thyrotoxicosis (12,15,17). The pathogenesis of myasthenia gravis has been a topic of interesting but controversial debates (18). Discovery of circulating antibody against postsynaptic acetylcholine receptor (AChR) has led to an extensive study of the thymic microenvironment responsible for the production of anti-AChR antibody. Immunocytochemical evaluation has demonstrated that the myoid cells in myasthenic thymuses are in close contact with antigen-presenting interdigitating cells (13). The relatively large number of AChR-specific autoimmune T cells (CD4 positive, CD8 negative) in myasthenic thymuses are capable of helping AChR-specific B cells in the lymphoid follicles produce pathogenic autoantibodies.

A variant of lymphoid hyperplasia was seen in a patient with thymic enlargement and features of Castleman disease. The patient was a 53-year-old woman who had myasthenia gravis

for 23 years. The symptoms progressed despite medical treatment, and the patient was found to have a soft tissue density in the anterosuperior mediastinum on chest roentgenogram and CT scan, which obscured the aortic arch. The preoperative diagnosis was stage II invasive thymoma, and the patient underwent total thymectomy, Grossly, the thymus showed diffuse enlargement, retaining the shape of the thymus (fig. 9-10A). Histologically, abnormal lymph follicles with germinal centers were frequent, as were Hassall corpuscles and aggregates of hyperplastic small thymic epithelial cells, somewhat resembling features of micronodular thymoma with lymphoid stroma (fig. 9-10B,C) (see fig. 2-62BC). Germinal centers contained a few small blood vessels entering from perifollicular tissue rich in vascularity and were surrounded by concentrically arranged small lymphoid cells (figs. 9-10B-D). Similar lymph follicles were seen in lymph nodes adjacent to the thymus (fig. 9-10E).

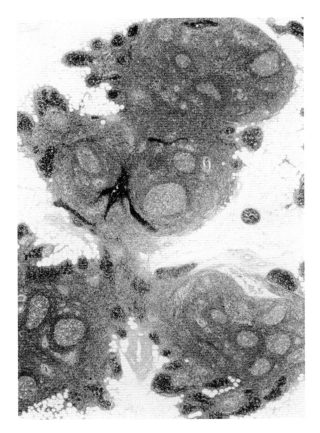 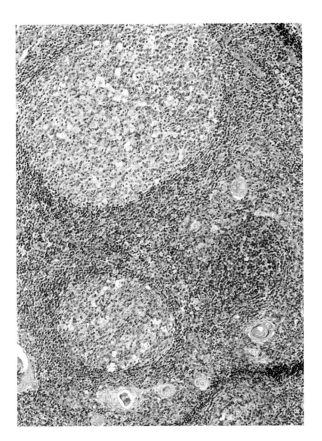

Figure 9-8

LYMPHOID HYPERPLASIA OF THE THYMUS

Left: At low-power, the thymus of a 21-year-old woman with myasthenia gravis shows the absence of involution, many lymphoid follicles with germinal centers in the medulla, and moderate compression of the cortex.

Right: High-power view shows frequent lymph follicles compressing the cortex. (Courtesy of Dr, Norikazu Tamaoki, Isehara, Japan.)

Figure 9-9

LYMPHOID HYPERPLASIA OF THYMUS

A characteristic germinal center with a cuff of small lymphocytes in a patient without myasthenia gravis.

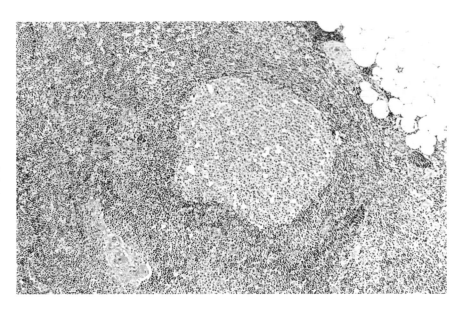

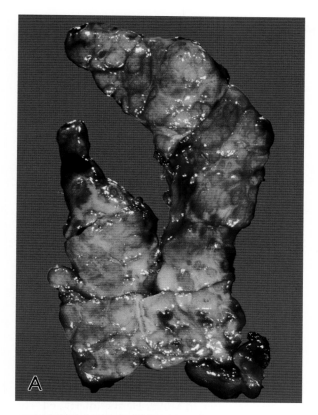

Figure 9-10

LYMPHOID HYPERPLASIA WITH FEATURES OF CASTLEMAN DISEASE IN A MYASTHENIC PATIENT

A: Grossly, the thymus is irregular and diffusely enlarged but retains the original shape.

B: Low magnification reveals thymic lobules bordered by dense collagenous tissue and containing frequent lymph follicles with germinal centers.

C: Medium-power view shows a lymph follicle with a prominent germinal center surrounded by variably sized nests of hyperplastic thymic epithelial cells with Hassall corpuscles. The nests of thymic medullary epithelial cells on the right are reminiscent of epithelial nodules of micronodular thymoma with lymphoid stroma.

D: Small lymphocytes are concentrically arranged around the small germinal center with a prominent central blood vessel. The perifollicular region is vascular. Small thymic epithelial cell nests are seen on the right.

E: A lymph follicle with a prominent blood vessel in the germinal center entering from the perifollicular region is seen in a lymph node adjacent to the thymus. (Courtesy of Dr. Morio Koike, Tokyo, Japan.)

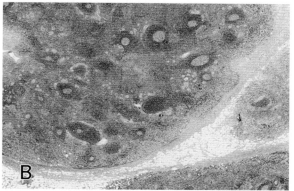

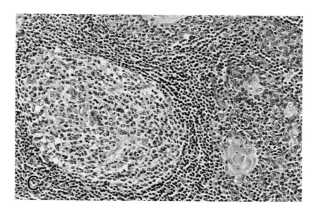

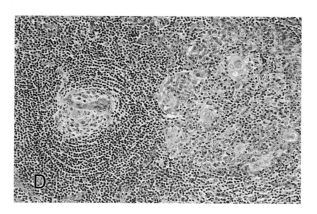

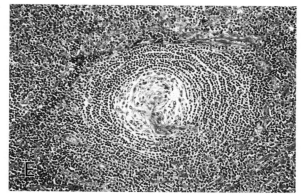

REFERENCES

Thymus in Immunodeficiency

1. Aita M, Amantea A. Distribution of anti-keratins and anti-thymostimulin antibodies in normal and in Down's syndrome human thymuses. Thymus 1991;17:155-65.
2. Buckley RH. Immunodeficiency diseases. JAMA 1992;268:2797-806.
3. Griffith RC. Thymus gland. In Kissane JM, ed. Anderson's pathology, 9th ed. St. Louis: CV Mosby; 1990:1493-516.
4. Larocca LM, Lauriola L, Ranelletti FO, et al. Morphological and immunohistochemical study of Down syndrome thymus. Am J Med Genet 1990;7(Suppl):225-30.
5. Levin S, Schlesinger M, Handzel Z, et al. Thymic deficiency in Down's syndrome. Pediatrics 1979;63:80-7.
6. Nezelof C. Thymic pathology in primary and secondary immunodeficiencies. Histopathology 1992;21:499-511.
7. Ratech H, Hirschhorn R, Greco MA. Pathologic findings in adenosine deaminase deficient-severe combined immunodeficiency. II. Thymus, spleen, lymph node, and gastrointestinal tract lymphoid tissue alterations. Am J Pathol 1989;135:1145-56.
8. Rosen FS, Cooper MD, Wedgwood RJ. The primary immunodeficiencies. N Engl J Med 1995;333:431-40.
9. Seemayer TA, Bolande RP. Thymic involution mimicking thymic dysplasia: a consequence of transfusion-induced graft versus host disease in a premature infant. Arch Pathol Lab Med 1980;104:141-4.
10. Suster S, Rosai J. Thymus. In Mills SE, ed. Histology for pathologists, 3rd ed. New York: Lippincott, Williams & Wilkens; 2007:503-25.
11. van Baarlen J, Schuurman HJ, Huber J. Acute thymus involution in infancy and childhood: a reliable marker for duration of acute illness. Hum Pathol 1988;19:1155-60.

Thymic Hyperplasia

12. Griffith RC. Thymus gland. In Kissane JM, ed. Anderson's pathology, 9th ed. St. Louis: CV Mosby; 1990:1493-516
13. Kirchner T, Hoppe F, Shalke B, Müller-Hermelink HK. Microenvironment of thymic myoid cells in myasthenia gravis. Virchows Arch B Cell Pathol 1988;54:295-302.
14. Konstantopoulos K, Androulaki A, Aessopos A, et al. Pure red cell aplasia associated with true thymic hyperplasia. Hum Pathol 1995;26:1160-2.
15. Rosai J, Levine GD. Tumors of the thymus. Atlas of Tumor Pathology, 2nd Series, Fascicle 13, Washington, DC: Armed Forces Institute of Pathology; 1976.
16. Steinmann GG. Changes in the human thymus during aging. In Müller-Hermelink HK, ed. The human thymus. Histophysiology and pathology. Berlin: Springer-Verlag; 1986:43-88.
17. Suster S, Rosai J. Thymus. In Mills SE, ed. Histology for pathologists, 3rd ed. New York: Lippincott, Williams & Wilkens; 2007:503-25.
18. Wekerle H. The thymus in myasthenia gravis. Ann NY Acad Sci 1993;681:47-55.

10 ECTOPIC TISSUE AND TUMORS IN THE ANTEROSUPERIOR MEDIASTINUM

THYROID LESIONS

Thyroid tissue can be found anywhere between the tongue and the aortic arch due to the abnormal migration of this tissue during embryogenesis (7). In the thorax, not only the anterosuperior mediastinum but also the posterior mediastinum may be involved by thyroid lesions, although involvement of the former is much more frequent.

The majority of *mediastinal goiters* are substernal extensions of cervical goiter involving the eutopic thyroid gland. Such extension is often seen in the goiter zones. Goitrous lesions arising in ectopic mediastinal thyroid are rare. According to Lindskog and Malm (7), among 1,486 operations for goiter, 46 patients (3.1 percent) showed mediastinal extension of goiter and in 7 (0.5 percent), the entire goiter was situated within the thorax without connection to a cervical goiter.

Histologically, thyroid lesions have the features of colloid or nodular (adenomatous) goiter or those of solitary adenoma (figs. 10-1, 10-2). Carcinoma arising in the ectopic thyroid gland is extremely rare (4). For detailed gross and microscopic descriptions of such lesions, the reader is referred to the Atlas of Tumor Pathology, *Tumors of the Thyroid Gland* (9).

PARATHYROID LESIONS

Because of the likely common origin of the thymus and the inferior parathyroid glands from the third branchial pouch, *ectopic parathyroid glands* may be found in the anterosuperior mediastinum, adjacent to or within the thymus (fig. 10-3). Mediastinal parathyroid tumors were found in 64 (22 percent) of 285 patients who underwent surgery for hyperparathyroidism, and in 20 (38 percent) of 53 patients requiring repeat surgery for persistent or recurrent hyperparathyroidism (1). Of these parathyroid tumors, 52 were situated in the anterior mediastinum and 12 in the posterior mediastinum; in 4 patients the

mediastinal tumor was a fifth histologically documented parathyroid gland. For clinical signs, diagnostic approaches, and gross and histologic findings of mediastinal parathyroid lesions, readers are referred to Atlas of Tumor Pathology, *Tumors of the Parathyroid Gland* (3). Wick and Rosai categorize mediastinal parathyroid adenoma and carcinoma as neuroendocrine neoplasms because of the presence of "generic" neuroendocrine markers such as neuron-specific enolase and

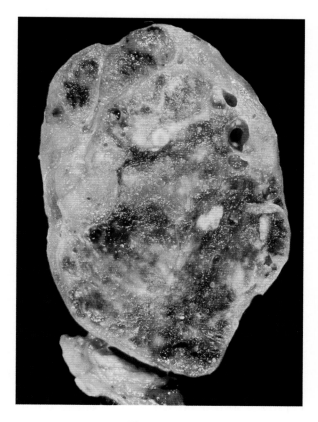

Figure 10-1

MEDIASTINAL GOITER

The cut surface of the roughly oval, encapsulated tumor is nodular, semitranslucent, and brown. Areas of hemorrhage, fibrosis, and microcystic degeneration are present. There was no connection with the thyroid gland of the neck.

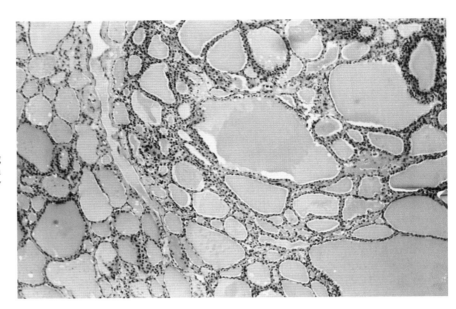

Figure 10-2

MEDIASTINAL GOITER

Follicles vary in size, tending to be large, and contain thin colloid. The follicles are lined by flat epithelium.

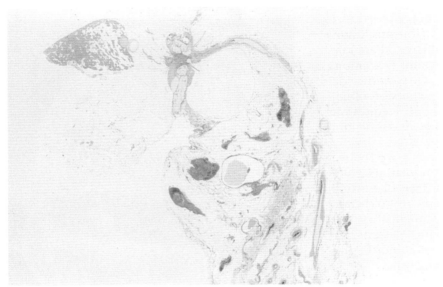

Figure 10-3

MEDIASTINAL PARATHYROID GLAND

A parathyroid gland of normal size and appearance is seen in the left upper corner. Microcystic change is seen in the thymus.

chromogranin A, and the production of parathyroid hormone, a neuropeptide (10).

The following is an illustrative case of a parathyroid lesion in the mediastinum. The patient, a 29-year-old woman, had three parathyroid glands (bilateral upper and left lower) removed and a brown tumor of the femur curetted because of hyperparathyroidism. The three parathyroid glands were reported to be normal or slightly hyperplastic. Since hypercalcemia persisted postoperatively, a right thyroid lobectomy and dissection of the superior mediastinum were done 6 months later, but no parathyroid gland was found. Approximately 1 year later, a ^{201}T1 scintigram revealed uptake in the anterosuperior mediastinum and a 2.2 x 1.5 cm tumor located in the superior portion of the right lobe of the thymus was removed. The tumor was well defined but showed questionable invasive growth. Histologically, it consisted of nests, trabeculae, small follicles, and tubules made up of small polygonal cells, with or without clear cytoplasm, and a few small groups of oncocytic cells. The diagnosis was parathyroid adenoma (fig. 10-4). The postoperative course was uneventful.

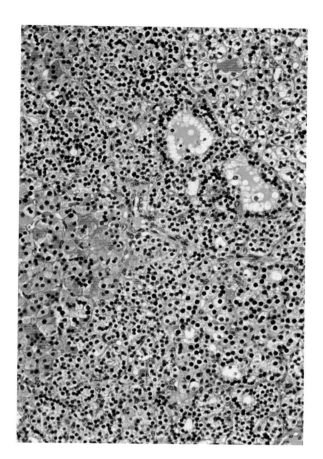 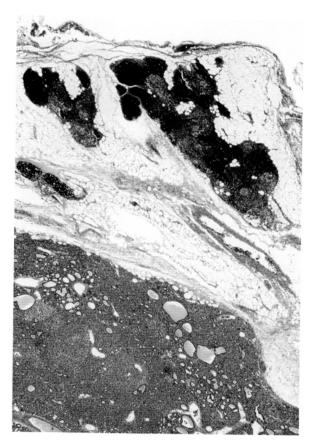

Figure 10-4

MEDIASTINAL INTRATHYMIC PARATHYROID ADENOMA

Left: The parathyroid adenoma, which is composed of sheets, nests, trabeculae, tubules, and follicles made up of chief cells, a few water-clear cells, and small clusters of oncocytic cells, is bordered by thymic tissue.
Right: High-power view.

Because of histologic similarities of *parathyroid hyperplasia* and *adenoma*, distinguishing these two lesions is often difficult, if not impossible, if only a single gland is available for examination. Enlargement of two or more parathyroid glands is usually evident in primary parathyroid hyperplasia, while most adenomas involve a single gland, and thus the presence of a single enlarged gland together with the finding of three normal-sized glands is virtually diagnostic of adenoma (3). If information on the three other parathyroid glands is unavailable, a diagnosis of "parathyroid proliferative disease" is considered to be most appropriate (10).

Parathyroid carcinoma is a rare tumor, which is reported sporadically (2,5,6). The histology varies from mildly atypical, resembling adenoma, to obviously anaplastic, showing thick fibrous bands, capsular and/or vascular invasion, and increased mitotic activity (3). In one case, marked immunoreactivity of tumor cells for p53 protein and absence of nuclear immunoreactivity for retinoblastoma tumor-suppressor protein were reported (6). A rare nonsecretory parathyroid carcinoma arising in the anterosuperior mediastinum was reported by Murphy et al. (8).

REFERENCES

1. Clark OH. Mediastinal parathyroid tumors. Arch Surg 1988;123:1096-100.
2. Delaney SE, Wermers RA, Thompson GB, Hodgson SF, Dinneen SF. Mediastinal parathyroid carcinoma. Endocr Pract 1999;5:133-6.
3. DeLellis RA. Tumors of the parathyroid gland. Atlas of Tumor Pathology, 3rd Series, Fascicle 6, Washington, DC: Armed Forces Institute of Pathology; 1993.
4. Dominguez-Malagon H, Guerrero-Medrano J, Suster S. Ectopic poorly differentiated (insular) carcinoma of the thyroid. Report of a case presenting as an anterior mediastinal mass. Am J Clin Pathol 1995;104:408-12.
5. Hara H, Oyama T, Kimura M, et al. Cytologic characteristics of parathyroid carcinoma: a case report. Diagn Cytopathol 1998;18:192-8.
6. Hofbauer LC, Spitzweg C, Arnholdt H, Landgraf R, Heufelder AE. Mediastinal parathyroid tumor: giant adenoma or carcinoma? Endocr Pathol 1997;8:161-6.
7. Lindskog BI, Malm A. Diagnostic and surgical considerations on mediastinal (intrathoracic) goiter. Dis Chest 1965;47:201-7.
8. Murphy MN, Glennon PG, Diocee MS, Wick MR, Cavers DJ. Nonsecretory parathyroid carcinoma of the mediastinum. Light microscopic, immunohistochemical, and ultrastructural features of a case, and review of the literature. Cancer 1986;58:2468-76.
9. Rosai J, Carcangiu ML, DeLellis RA. Tumors of the thyroid gland. Atlas of Tumor Pathology, 3rd Series, Fascicle 5. Washington, DC: Armed Forces Institute of Pathology; 1992.
10. Wick MR, Rosai J. Neuroendocrine neoplasms of the mediastinum. Semin Diagn Pathol 1991;8:35-51.

11 MESENCHYMAL AND NEUROGENIC TUMORS OF THE MEDIASTINUM EXCLUDING THE HEART AND GREAT VESSELS

MESENCHYMAL TUMORS

Mesenchymal tumors, either benign or malignant, are rare in the mediastinum, constituting less than 2 percent of mediastinal tumors and tumor-like lesions (see Table 2-4). When invasive tumors occupy the anterior mediastinum, it may be difficult to determine whether they arise in the thymus or extrathymic tissue. Many types of mesenchymal mediastinal tumors have been reported (Table 11-1), but symptoms and signs are similar to those of other benign and malignant mediastinal tumors. The pathologic features are similar to similarly named tumors of the soft tissue occurring at other sites. Readers should refer for details to related literature (7,7a,11,13,23).

Benign Mesenchymal Tumors and Tumor-Like Lesions

Lymphangioma. *Lymphangioma* is a benign tumor of neoplastic or hamartomatous nature, composed of proliferating lymphatic vessels lined by endothelial cells. Interconnecting vessels contain chylous material and vary in size, grossly appearing cystic or spongy. Lymphangioma occurs in any compartment of the mediastinum but is most frequent in the anterosuperior mediastinum. In children, *cystic hygroma* of the neck may extend into the mediastinum.

Histologically, lymphangioma resembles hemangioma, and may contain smooth muscle fibers. Lymphocytic infiltration that is not bloody, unless hemorrhage occurs, is frequently noted in the interstitium (figs. 11-1, 11-2). Factor VIII-related antigen cannot be demonstrated immunohistochemically. Recently, antibodies that recognize lymphatic endothelium have become available; these include D2-40 and antipodoplanin.

Lymphangiomatosis is a systemic disorder in children. *Lymphangioleiomyomatosis* involves the lung parenchyma and mediastinal lymph nodes of young women.

Table 11-1

MESENCHYMAL TUMORS OF THE MEDIASTINUM[a]

Tumors of lymph vessels
  Lymphangioma
  Lymphangiomatosis
  Lymphangiomyoma

Tumors of blood vessel origin
  Hemangioma
  Hemangioendothelioma
  Hemangiomatosis
  Epithelioid hemangioendothelioma
  Malignant hemangioendothelioma (angiosarcoma)

Tumors of pericyte origin
  Hemangiopericytoma

Tumors and tumor-like fibrohistiocytic lesions
  Fibromatosis
  Fibrosarcoma
  Malignant fibrous histiocytoma

Tumors of adipose tissue
  Lipoma
  Lipomatosis
  Lipoblastomatosis
  Liposarcoma

Tumors of muscle origin
  Rhabdomyoma
  Rhabdomyosarcoma
  Leiomyoma
  Leiomyosarcoma

Tumors of pluripotential mesenchyme
  Benign mesenchymoma
  Malignant mesenchymoma
  Synovial sarcoma

Tumors of skeletal tissues
  Chondroma
  Osteogenic sarcoma
  Chondrosarcoma

Other tumors and tumor-like conditions
  Solitary fibrous tumor
  Myxoma
  Meningioma
  Chordoma
  Granular cell tumor
  Extramedullary hematopoiesis
  Histiocytosis X
  Amyloid tumor

[a]Modified from Table 4-1 from Fascicle 21, Third Series; data from reference 13.

285

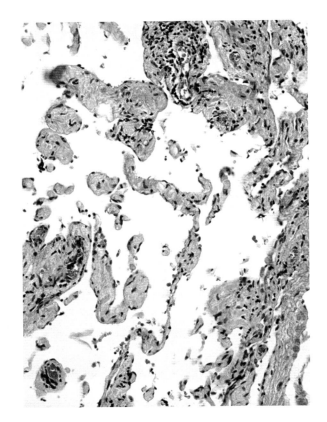

Figure 11-1

LYMPHANGIOMA

A spongy tumor somewhat resembles emphysematous lung. It consists of interconnecting channels lined by flat endothelial cells. The wall is variably fibrotic and focally infiltrated by lymphocytes.

Hemangioma. *Hemangioma* is subdivided into capillary, cavernous, and venous types by the size and structure of the blood vessels, as in hemangiomas at other locations. In the mediastinum, cavernous hemangiomas (fig. 11-3) are more common than other types. During the past 50 years, 61 cases of mediastinal hemangioma were reported in Japan (26). Despite a frequently large size, an often infiltrating appearance, and sporadic mitotic activity, follow-up studies demonstrate the benign nature of mediastinal hemangiomas (14).

Fibromatosis. *Fibromatosis* rarely involves the mediastinum. Two cases possessing some features suggestive of mediastinal fibromatosis were encountered at the National Cancer Center Hospital, Tokyo. One patient was a 23-year-old female who developed extensive fibrosis of

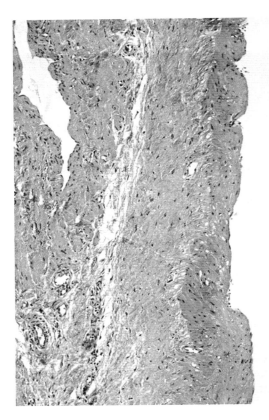

Figure 11-2

**PROBABLE HAMARTOMATOUS
CYSTIC LYMPHANGIOMA**

An approximately 5-cm cystic lesion was attached to the right upper pole of the thymus. Its inner surface was smooth but trabeculated. Histologically, the cyst is lined by flat endothelial cells, beneath which are bundles of smooth muscle. Smaller lymphatic vessels with smooth muscle are present around the cyst. The lining cells were positive for vimentin but negative for cytokeratin and factor VIII-related antigen. Since the histology of the cyst wall resembles that of the thoracic duct, the lesion was considered to be a cystic lymphangioma of hamartomatous nature.

the anterior and middle mediastinum which extended into the right upper lobe of the lung, left main bronchus, pericardium, epicardium, and diaphragm. The patient died of respiratory failure after 6 years of therapy (fig. 11-4, top). An unusual feature in this case was the extensive hyalinization of the lesion recognized at autopsy, which may have been due to radiotherapy. There were no epithelioid granulomatous lesions but scant chronic inflammatory cells were seen around blood vessels (fig. 11-4, bottom). No fungi were demonstrated. These

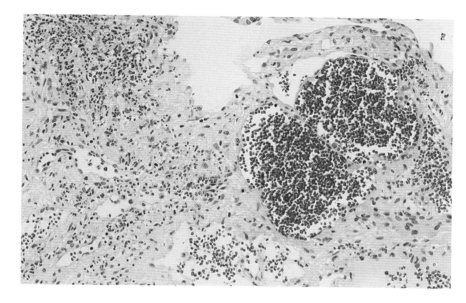

Figure 11-3

CAVERNOUS HEMANGIOMA

Variously sized lumens contain blood and are lined by flat endothelial cells. The walls are fibrous. This tumor measured 1.7 x 1.4 x 1.0 cm and was located in the posterior mediastinum.

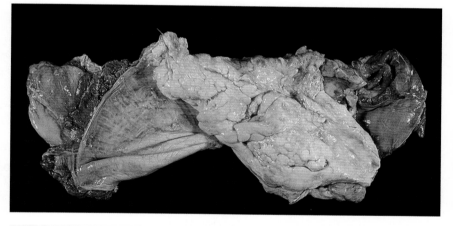

Figure 11-4

MEDIASTINAL FIBROSIS

Top: A plate-like fibrous tumor with a nodular surface is attached to the anterior portion of the diaphragm. It involved the lung, bronchi, pericardium, and epicardium.

Bottom: A needle biopsy of the tumor discloses a proliferation of fibroblasts with collagenization and a mild inflammatory cell reaction around slit-like blood vessels.

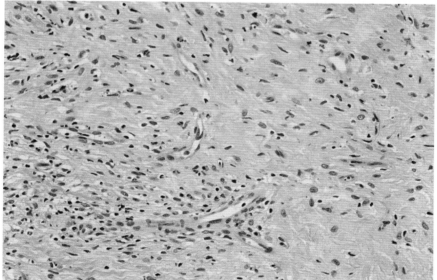

findings may indicate end-stage mediastinal fibrosis (fibrous or sclerosing mediastinitis, granulomatous mediastinitis) of unknown etiology (5,16).

The other patient was a 71-year-old man. The primary site of the fibromatosis was probably the right chest wall, rather than the mediastinum, involving the 1st to 4th ribs, and extending into the mediastinum and neck. The patient has been free of recurrence for 5 years after repeated surgical removal and radiotherapy extending over a 3.5-year period. Histology showed a typical desmoid tumor with fibroblastic proliferation, collagenization, and slit-like vessel proliferations (fig. 11-5).

Other Benign Mesenchymal Tumors. These include *lipoma, leiomyoma, chondroma, granular cell tumor,* and *rhabdomyoma* (17). The last should be differentiated from rhabdomyomatous thymoma (see fig. 2-61).

Mesenchymal Tumors of Intermediate Malignancy

Hemangiopericytoma. *Hemangiopericytoma* is either benign or malignant. The occurrence of true hemangiopericytoma in the mediastinum is extremely rare (23). If the histology of a mediastinal tumor is suggestive of hemangiopericytoma, features characteristic of thymoma should be carefully sought, since a hemangiopericytoma-like thymoma is more common.

Solitary Fibrous Tumor. Previously called benign localized mesothelioma of the fibrous type or localized fibrous tumor of the pleura, *solitary fibrous tumor* is another benign or malignant mesenchymal tumor. This neoplasm shows nodular growth within the thymus or mediastinum, with or without connection to the pleura or pericardium (fig. 11-6). Solitary fibrous tumors were originally described as pleural lesions, but immunohistochemical and ultrastructural studies indicated that the tumors are not of mesothelial cell origin but are derived probably from submesothelial connective tissue cells (6,25). It is now accepted that solitary fibrous tumors occur at a variety of extrapleural sites including abdominal cavity, retroperitoneum, mediastinum, orbit, upper respiratory tract, and soft tissue. Extrathoracic tumors are as common as thoracic lesions, and

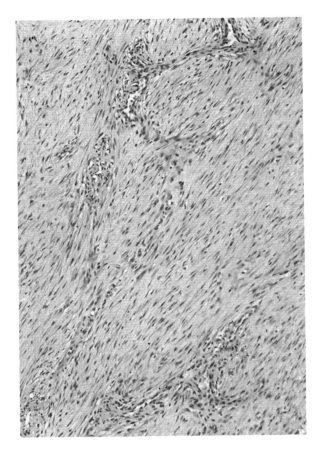

Figure 11-5

FIBROMATOSIS (DESMOID TYPE) INVOLVING CHEST WALL AND MEDIASTINUM

The fibroblasts with a mild degree of collagenization are associated with a proliferation of slit-like blood vessels.

the general consensus favors a (myo)fibroblastic histogenesis (9).

Solitary fibrous tumors are variably cellular and composed of spindle cells arranged in a "patternless pattern," often aligned like strings of beads in a somewhat myxoid matrix or between collagen bundles, or arranged in bundles in cellular areas (fig. 11-7). Immunohistochemically, tumor cells are negative for cytokeratin, muscle-specific actin, and glial fibrillary acidic protein, and positive for vimentin and CD34 (fig. 11-8) (8–10,22). In one study, the tumor cells in some cases were focally positive for desmin and negative for CD34 (10). CD34 antigen, originally described as a marker for human hematopoietic stem cells, is expressed in a diverse group of neoplasms including leukemia,

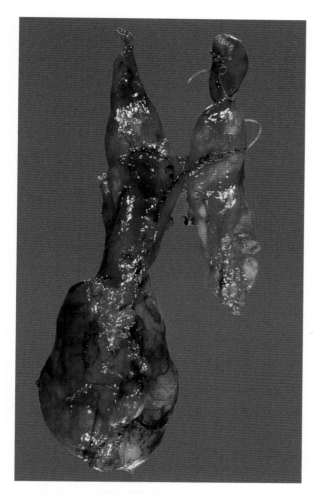

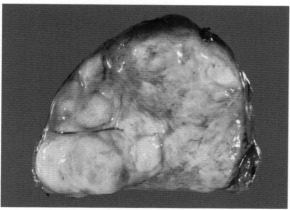

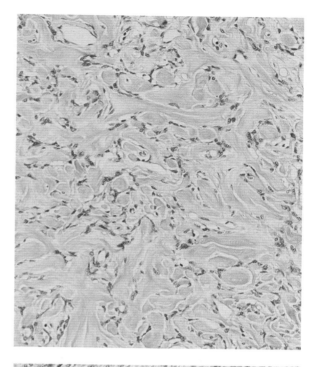

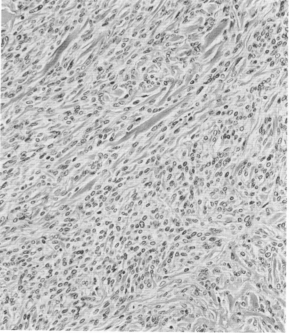

Figure 11-6

SOLITARY FIBROUS TUMOR

Top: The encapsulated tumor is elastic, firm, and adherent to the inferior pole of the right lobe of the thymus.

Bottom: The cut surface is solid, nodular, and bulging, with no signs of necrosis or hemorrhage.

Figure 11-7

SOLITARY FIBROUS TUMOR

Top: Fibroblast-like tumor cells with oval nuclei are aligned like strings of beads or a rosary-like configuration around collagen fibers.

Bottom: In highly cellular areas, tumor cells are arranged in bundles or haphazardly. Collagen is scanty.

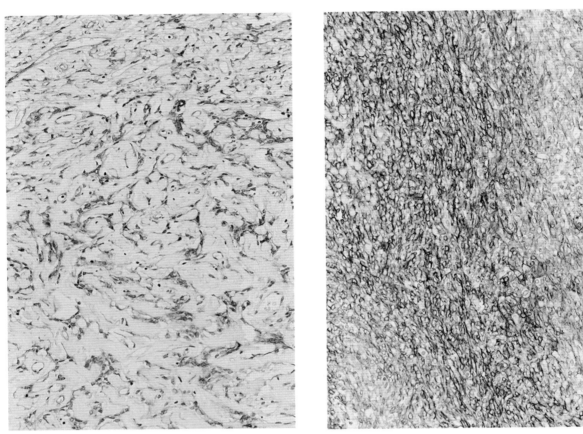

Figure 11-8

SOLITARY FIBROUS TUMOR

The tumor cells stain for CD34 in both less cellular (left) and highly cellular (right) areas.

vascular tumor, hemangiopericytoma, nerve sheath tumor, epithelioid sarcoma, smooth muscle tumor, and solitary fibrous tumor. Reaction with CD34 antibodies can be diagnostically helpful since CD34 antigen tends to be absent from many common tumors such as carcinoma, melanoma, lymphoma, and most types of sarcoma (22). About half of solitary fibrous tumors are positive for CD99 and bcl-2 (9,11).

Recently, a cytokeratin-positive (by AE1/AE3) malignant solitary fibrous tumor was reported (3). The primary tumor arising in the pleura was strongly positive for vimentin, CD34, bcl-2, and CD99, but only a few scattered tumor cells were positive for cytokeratin. In the recurrent tumor, however, cytokeratin-positive cells increased to 70 percent. The authors believed that the increase in cytokeratin-positive tumor

cells was not surprising, since cytokeratin can be expressed in a variety of sarcomas, sometimes when they dedifferentiate or recur.

Solitary fibrous tumor usually behaves in a benign manner but infrequently displays local recurrence or distant metastasis. The biologic behavior does not consistently correlate with atypical histologic features (9). Histologically, malignant solitary fibrous tumor with hypercellularity, some proliferative activity, and foci of coagulation necrosis is rare (fig. 11-9), and always poses a diagnostic problem. Immunohistochemistry may be of help diagnostically (9,10,22). Of 14 patients with solitary fibrous tumor of the mediastinum reported by Witkin and Rosai (25), 2 had accompanying hypoglycemia. Eleven tumors were in the anterosuperior mediastinum, one arose on a pedicle from the thymus, and

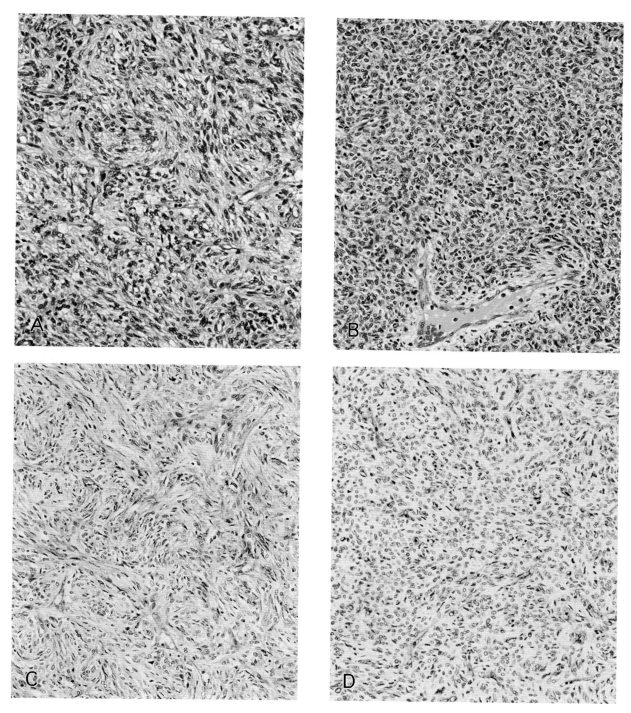

Figure 11-9

HISTOLOGICALLY MALIGNANT SOLITARY FIBROUS TUMOR

A: Elongated tumor cells are arranged in interwoven bundles in small areas.

B: In other areas, the tumor is highly cellular and shows diffuse growth of haphazardly arranged short spindle cells with slightly pleomorphic nuclei, scanty cytoplasm, and occasional mitotic figures.

C,D: Immunostaining for CD34 is positive in tumor cells arranged in interwoven bundles (C) and negative in highly cellular areas, where only vascular endothelial cells are positive (D).

another had entrapped thymic elements. Eight tumors were highly cellular and mitotically active, many behaving aggressively, with occasional recurrence and rare distant metastasis.

The differential diagnosis of solitary fibrous tumor includes spindle cell thymoma, synovial sarcoma, and peripheral nerve tumors.

Malignant Mesenchymal Tumors

Malignant mesenchymal tumors are rare in both the thymus and other mediastinal structures. They include liposarcoma, synovial sarcoma, epithelioid hemangioendothelioma, angiosarcoma, rhabdomyosarcoma, leiomyosarcoma, and others.

One case each of angiosarcoma, malignant fibrous histiocytoma, mesenchymal chondrosarcoma, and liposarcoma of the mediastinum were seen at the National Cancer Center Hospital in Tokyo (4,12,15).

Liposarcoma. A large *liposarcoma,* 17 x 9 x 6 cm, was incompletely removed from a 71-year-old man who had complained of hoarseness for 2 years. It was situated in the anterosuperior mediastinum, extending into the right supraclavicular fossa (fig. 11-10A). Histologically, this tumor was composed of areas of well-differentiated liposarcoma and other areas with a malignant fibrous histiocytoma-like growth pattern. The lipomatous nature of the neoplasm could still be recognized in the malignant fibrous histiocytoma-like areas (fig. 11-10B,C). Liposarcoma is the most common sarcoma in the anterior mediastinum, and the tumor recurs in about one third of patients. Both lipoma and liposarcoma also arise from the thymus.

Synovial Sarcoma. Witkin et al. (24) reported four cases of a biphasic tumor of the mediastinum with features of *synovial sarcoma* (fig. 11-11). The tumors were located in the superior and middle compartments of the mediastinum, and frequently adhered to the pericardium or pleura but did not appear to arise from a mesothelial surface. Three patients followed clinically died of the tumor within 4 years of diagnosis. This neoplasm is considered to originate from pluripotent mesenchyme and should be distinguished from biphasic mesothelioma, thymoma with glandular features (see fig. 2-46), and malignant peripheral nerve sheath tumor with glandular differentiation. Detection of *SYT-SSX*

chimeric RNA transcripts, resulting from the t(X;18) translocation, is useful for the diagnosis of synovial sarcoma (1,21).

Recently, Suster and Moran (18) reported 15 cases of primary synovial sarcoma of the mediastinum. The ages of the patients ranged from 3 to 83 years with a male to female ratio of 2 to 1. The tumors were located in the anterior (9 cases) and posterior mediastinum (6 cases); they were biphasic in 5 cases and monophasic in 10. Immunohistochemically, the tumor cells were focally positive for cytokeratin and/or epithelial membrane antigen, strongly positive for vimentin and bcl-2, and focally positive for CD99 in some cases.

Rhabdomyosarcoma. Suster et al. (20) reported four *rhabdomyosarcomas,* unassociated with germ cell teratomatous or thymic carcinomatous components, in young adults (three men and one woman of 19 to 27 years of age). Histologically, two tumors were alveolar rhabdomyosarcoma, one an embryonal rhabdomyosarcoma, and one a pleomorphic rhabdomyosarcoma. All of the tumors were highly aggressive, and recurrence and metastases developed within 6 months after diagnosis. A case of rhabdomyosarcoma with glycogen-rich clear cells was reported by Bëgin et al. (2). This entity should be differentiated from more commonly encountered clear cell tumors seen in the mediastinum.

Epithelioid Hemangioendothelioma. Suster et al. (19) described 12 patients with *epithelioid hemangioendothelioma* of the anterior mediastinum: 3 women and 9 men, aged 19 to 62 years. The tumors were either encapsulated or locally infiltrative. Some displayed the histologic features of classic low-grade epithelioid hemangioendothelioma seen at other locations and others showed increased cellular atypia and mitotic activity. Five patients developed metaplastic bone formation and osteoclast type giant cells, and 4 tumors had a prominent intravascular papillary endothelial component in some areas. The authors concluded, however, that "despite their ominous clinical, radiological and pathological features, epithelioid hemangioendotheliomas of the anterior mediastinum appear to behave as low-grade malignant neoplasms that may be adequately controlled in most instances by surgery alone."

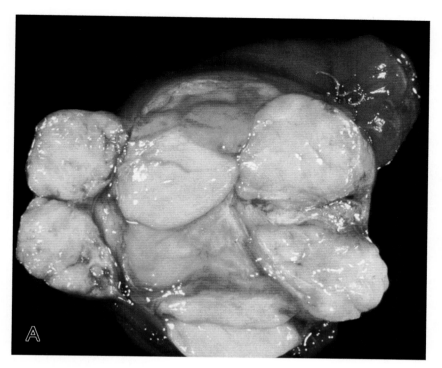

Figure 11-10

LIPOSARCOMA

A: The large, nodular tumor has a bulging, bright yellow to ivory cut surface.

B: The tumor consists in part of mature fat cells and scattered lipoblasts with bizarre nuclei and focal myxoid matrix.

C: In other areas, the tumor is cellular and consists of bundles of elongated cells with moderately atypical nuclei. Fatty droplets can still be seen in the cytoplasm at higher magnification, however.

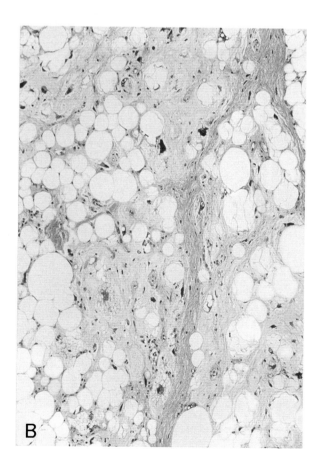

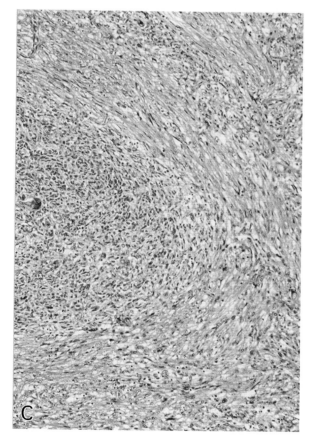

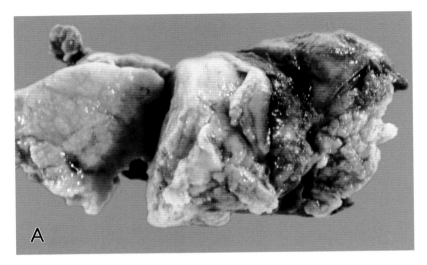

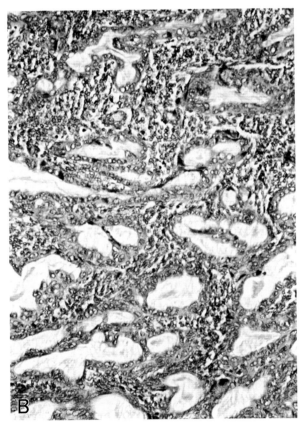

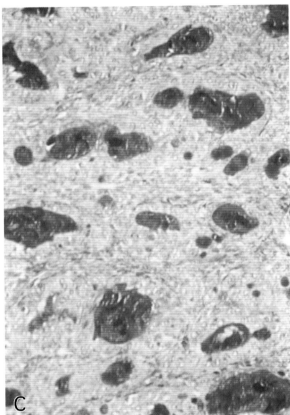

Figure 11-11

BIPHASIC TUMOR WITH FEATURES OF SYNOVIAL SARCOMA

A: The external and cut surfaces of the tumor are tan and friable. (Fig. 1 from Witkin GB, Miettinen M, Rosai J. A biphasic tumor of the mediastinum with features of synovial sarcoma: a report of four cases. Am J Surg Pathol 1989;13:491.)

B: Glandular spaces and clefts are intermixed with a monomorphic plump to spindled sarcomatous component.

C: Periodic acid–Schiff (PAS)-positive, diastase-resistant material is in the glandular lumens. (B and C are from fig. 3 of Witkin GB, Miettinen M, Rosai J. A biphasic tumor of the mediastinum with features of synovial sarcoma: a report of four cases. Am J Surg Pathol 1989;13:494.)

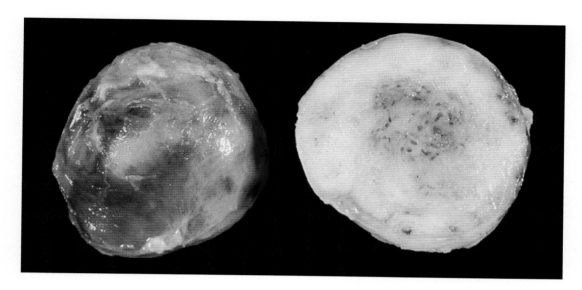

Figure 11-12

SCHWANNOMA

The outer and cut surfaces of a roughly spherical tumor reveal encapsulation and central microcystic degeneration.

NEUROGENIC TUMORS AND TUMORS OF PARAGANGLIA

According to Marchevsky and Kaneko (38), neurogenic tumors account for 19 to 39 percent of mediastinal tumors. They occur most frequently in the posterior mediastinum, arising from sympathetic ganglia, paraganglia, and peripheral nerves. A variety of neurogenic tumors, both benign and malignant as seen in other parts of the body, occur in the mediastinum, particularly the posterior mediastinum. Concerning details of clinical findings, gross and microscopic features, and the outcome of patients, textbooks, monographs, and atlases on tumors of the peripheral nerves and paraganglia should be consulted (35,38,47,52).

Schwannoma. Among neurogenic tumors, *schwannoma (neurilemmoma, neurinoma)* is the most frequent in the mediastinum. It occurs not only in the posterior mediastinum but also in the anterior mediastinum. It is connected with a peripheral nerve, and is solitary in most cases. Multiple schwannomas are often associated with von Recklinghausen disease.

Patients with schwannoma are asymptomatic in most cases and the tumor is generally found incidentally on chest X-ray examination, but may cause symptoms due to compression of nearby organs by a large tumor. The tumor is spherical to oval and encapsulated. The cut surface is milky white or pale yellow, homogeneous, and partly myxomatous or cystic (fig. 11-12).

Histologically, the diagnosis is usually established with ease, but in longstanding tumors it may be difficult to find the characteristic features of Antoni types A and B tissues due to extensive degenerative changes. Scanty tumor tissue of viable appearance and dilated vessels with a hyalinized wall point to a correct diagnosis of schwannoma (figs. 11-13, 11-14). Malignant transformation of schwannoma is almost nonexistent and thus patients can be observed clinically even when the tumor is incompletely removed because of its particular location, such as near nerve roots.

Melanocytic schwannoma is a rare pigmented variant. It may be dumbbell shaped and extend from the posterior mediastinum to the spinal canal. A common origin of Schwann cells and melanocytes from the neural crest would explain this variety.

Neurofibroma. *Neurofibroma* follows schwannoma in frequency in the mediastinum. It presents as a single or multiple tumors (as in neurofibromatosis associated with von Recklinghausen disease). It grows within the nerve and frequently is fusiform in shape. In contrast to schwannoma, it is not encapsulated or cystic. In many cases, neurofibroma

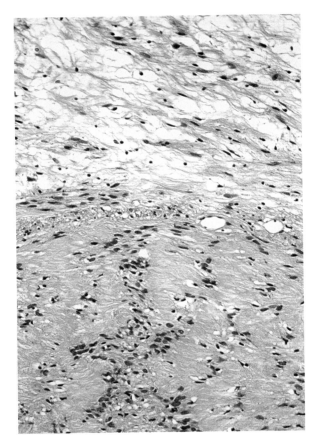

Figure 11-13

SCHWANNOMA

Antoni type A cells are seen at the bottom and Antoni type B at the top.

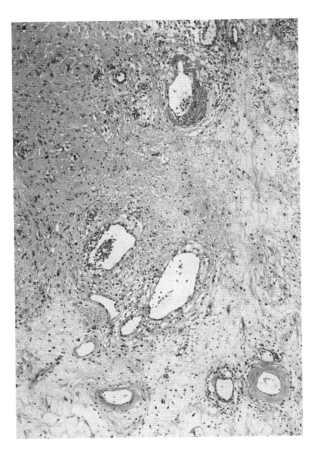

Figure 11-14

SCHWANNOMA

An area of degeneration reveals edematous tissue with dilated blood vessels, whose walls show hyalinization or fibrin deposition. Viable tumor tissue is evident in a small area.

is diagnosed easily by its characteristic features (fig. 11-15), but it may be difficult to differentiate from schwannoma because of mixed histologic patterns. This probably results from the constituent cells of the former: fibroblasts, Schwann cells, and neurites. Solitary neurofibroma rarely shows malignant transformation and surgical resection leads to cure. It occasionally occurs in association with neurofibromatosis.

Neurofibromatosis. This is an autosomal dominant congenital disease in which the abnormality is in chromosome 17q11.2 (*NF1* tumor suppressor gene) (30,37). In the mediastinum, the vagus nerve and sympathetic chains are often involved, frequently showing plexiform neurofibromatosis. Neurofibromatosis involving the mediastinum is categorized as *peripheral neurofibromatosis (neurofibromatosis type 1)* and is often associated with café-au-lait spots. It may be complicated by a variety of tumors such as schwannoma, ganglioneuroma, pheochromocytoma, medullary carcinoma of the thyroid, and nephroblastoma, but rarely by central nervous system tumors.

Malignant Peripheral Nerve Sheath Tumor. Spindle cell malignant tumors of the nerve are variously designated as neurofibrosarcoma, neurogenic sarcoma, malignant schwannoma, and malignant tumor of nerve sheath origin, but *malignant peripheral nerve sheath tumor* is the preferred designation. This tumor is rare in the mediastinum, but is more frequent in the posterior mediastinum than in the other compartments. It is often large and causes symptoms when detected, compressing, displacing, or invading the intrathoracic

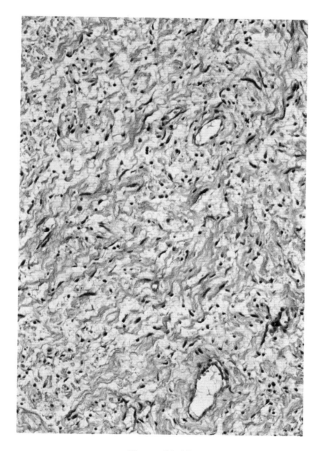

Figure 11-15

NEUROFIBROMA

Wavy elongated cells are in an edematous matrix. Some collagenization is present.

organs and thoracic wall. The prognosis is less favorable in patients with neurofibromatosis than in those with a solitary lesion.

Tumors of Sympathetic Ganglia in the Posterior Mediastinum. These include benign ganglioneuroma and malignant ganglioneuroblastoma and neuroblastoma. *Ganglioneuroma* occurs in the retroperitoneum and posterior mediastinum. It arises de novo, but may result from maturation of neuroblastoma, and is seen in children and adults. It is often large and encapsulated. The cut surface bulges, and is pale tan and faintly trabeculated (fig. 11-16).

Ganglioneuroma is subdivided into maturing and mature types in the International Neuroblastoma Pathology Classification (31). It is composed of abundant Schwann cell–like cells and small foci of immature ganglions or scattered mature ganglion cells. Mature ganglion cells possess Nissl granules and are supported by satellite cells in some areas (fig. 11-17). Granular calcified materials may be scattered.

Neuroblastoma is the most common malignant tumor of early childhood, occurring most frequently in the adrenal medulla. It also occurs in the extraadrenal sympathetic ganglia of the retroperitoneum and posterior mediastinum, although less frequently. There were only 2 neuroblastomas among 67 surgically resected mediastinal neurogenic tumors during a 31-year period at the National Cancer Center Hospital in Tokyo (see Table 2-4). Neuroblastoma may be

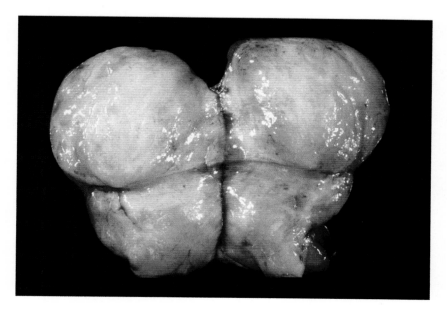

Figure 11-16

GANGLIONEUROMA

The tumor is encapsulated and its cut surface bulges. It is pale tan and faintly trabeculated.

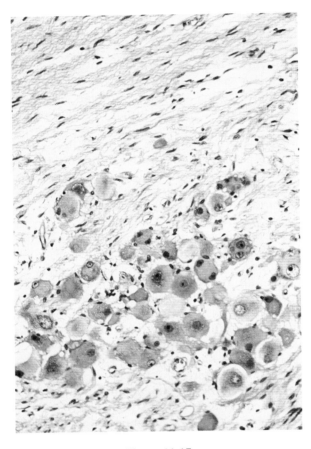

Figure 11-17

GANGLIONEUROMA

The tumor consists of mature ganglion cells with some satellite cells, nerve fibers, and Schwann cells.

congenital: about half of the patients are under 2 years of age, and most tumors are detected before 5 years of age. Three neuroblastomas arising within the thymus of elderly patients were reported by Argani et al. (28). One tumor was associated with the syndrome of inappropriate secretion of antidiuretic hormone, and such an association was also reported in an adult with ganglioneuroblastoma of the adult thymus (29).

Neuroblastoma is associated with loss of heterozygosity for chromosome 1p, which probably occurs at an early stage of tumor development, and amplification of the oncogene N-*myc* at an advanced stage (33,46,48,50).

Patients with mediastinal neuroblastoma often present with symptoms due to compression of neighboring structures by tumor, and experience Horner syndrome as a result of sympathetic nerve damage. Elevated plasma and urinary levels of catecholamines and elevated urinary vanillylmandelic acid (VMA) levels have diagnostic value. The latter are used for screening newborns and infants for this tumor.

Neuroblastoma is often large, encapsulated, and soft, with areas of hemorrhage on cut sections (fig. 11-18). Histologically, it is divided into three subtypes in the International Neuroblastoma Pathology Classification (31): undifferentiated, poorly differentiated, and differentiating. The undifferentiated type consists of small and medium-sized, immature and undifferentiated neuroblasts without overt

Figure 11-18

NEUROBLASTOMA

The tumor is encapsulated and soft. The cut surface bulges, and is nodular or lobulated, with areas of hemorrhage.

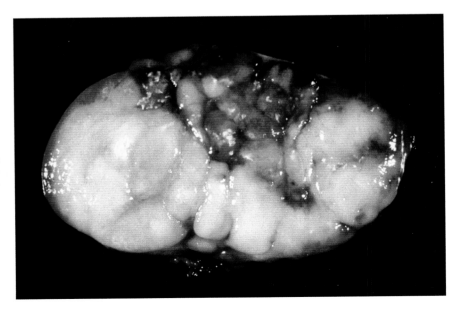

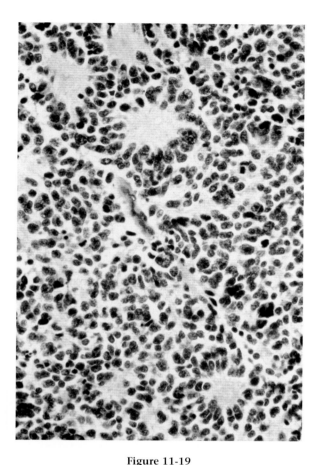

Figure 11-19

POORLY DIFFERENTIATED NEUROBLASTOMA

There is diffuse growth of small hyperchromatic cells (neuroblasts) and frequent rosettes of Homer-Wright type.

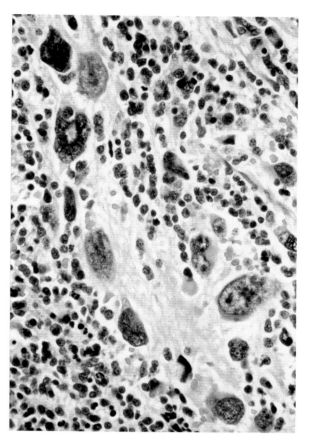

Figure 11-20

NEUROBLASTOMA

Small hyperchromatic cells growing diffusely contain a cluster of immature ganglion cells with neuropil. Depending upon the percentage of tumor cells differentiating toward ganglion cells, the tumor is called either poorly differentiated neuroblastoma or differentiating neuroblastoma.

neuropil. In poorly differentiated tumors, definite neuropil can be found among tumor cells, and cells differentiating toward ganglion cells are present. Ganglion cells occupy less than 5 percent of the tumor areas, and Homer-Wright type rosettes are frequently seen (figs. 11-19, 11-20). Differentiating neuroblastoma is composed largely of immature neuroblasts. Tumor cells that appear to differentiate toward ganglion cells occupy more than 5 percent of the tumor areas. The presence of neuropil is a prominent feature and S-100 protein–positive Schwann-like cells are frequently seen around the blood vessels. Cells that appear to differentiate toward ganglion cells are defined as those with a moderate amount of eosinophilic cytoplasm that is more than double the area of the eccentric nuclei.

Ganglioneuroblastoma is composed of neuroblastoma in a nodular arrangement in the background of ganglioneuroma or ganglioneuroblastoma. The schwannian stromal component occupies more than 50 percent of the tumor area (31). Ganglioneuroblastoma occurs not only in children but also in adults. Some ganglioneuroblastomas arise in the anterior mediastinum and appear to be derived from thymic tissue (42,49). The histogenesis of neuroblastomas and ganglioneuroblastomas includes malignant transformation of a mediastinal teratoma, aberrantly located sympathetic ganglia, neuroectodermal cells native to the normal thymus, and precursors of thymic epithelial cells that have differentiated along neural lines (28). A case of immature teratoma with small foci suggestive of neuroblastoma is shown in figure 5-18. As described before, ganglioneuroblastoma associated with the syndrome of inappropriate secretion of antidiuretic hormone was reported (29).

The prognosis of patients with neuroblastoma is poor, in spite of aggressive treatment, and the overall 2-year survival rate is said to be 60 percent (32). However, survival rates depend on a number of factors including the age of the patient at the time of diagnosis, stage of the disease, location and degree of histologic differentiation of the tumor, DNA ploidy, N-*myc* gene amplification, and other factors (32,50,52). Age and stage are two independent variables and are also the two most important prognostic factors.

Favorable prognostic factors in patients with neuroblastomas are: a young age (less than 1.5 years), favorable histologic type (ganglioneuroma and ganglioneuroblastoma at any age), no N-*myc* amplification, hyperdiploidy, and a mitosis karyorrhexis-index of less than 2 percent (less than 100/5,000 neuroblastoma cells) (31,52). The better prognosis of patients with mediastinal neuroblastoma compared to those with retroperitoneal or adrenal tumors is probably due to an earlier tumor stage at detection. Although rare, spontaneous regression of neuroblastoma has been reported, showing maturation into ganglioneuroma. The prognosis of patients with ganglioneuroblastoma is much better than that of neuroblastoma, although it depends on the degree of differentiation of the neuroblastoma component (31). The 5-year actuarial survival rate is 88 percent (27).

Primitive Neuroectodermal Tumor. *Primitive neuroectodermal tumor* (PNET) is rare in the mediastinum. Wick (53) reported two cases: one in the anterior mediastinum and one in the posterior mediastinum in an adolescent and a young adult. PNET must be differentiated from poorly differentiated neuroblastoma.

Ependymoma. An extremely rare *mediastinal ependymoma* was found in the paravertebral region (44). It was not in continuity with the spinal canal. Histologically, there was palisading of elongated tumor cells around fibrovascular cores and ciliated cells in gland-like structures. The diagnosis was confirmed by positive immunohistochemical staining for glial fibrillary acidic protein and by electron microscopic detection of cilia within intracytoplasmic vacuoles.

Pigmented Neuroectodermal Tumor of Infancy (Melanotic Progonoma or Retinal Anlage Tumor). This tumor, which involves the jaws of infants, also occurs in the mediastinum (39). It was originally thought to be benign, but is now considered malignant because of recurrence and metastasis in some cases (45).

Mediastinal Paraganglioma. This tumor originates from aorticopulmonary paraganglia present in the superior and middle mediastinum and from aorticosympathetic (paravertebral) paraganglia in the posterior mediastinum. Histologically, it is characterized by zellballen of polygonal tumor cells bordered by capillaries (fig. 11-21). Moran et al. (41) reviewed 16 cases of mediastinal paraganglioma collected from the files of the Armed Forces Institute of Pathology. Features included stromal hyalinization, a prominent spindle cell component, and granular cell changes in the cytoplasm of tumor cells in some cases. The reviewers concluded that the only parameters that correlated with aggressive behavior were the extent of circumscription and local infiltration of the tumor at initial resection. They recommended regular follow-up of patients due to the metastatic potential of the tumor. A review of the world literature documented 79 cases of anterior and middle mediastinal paraganglioma (36). There was a high local recurrence rate of 56 percent with a true metastatic capacity of 27 percent, and overall survival of 62 percent. The authors recommended complete surgical resection of the tumor. In contrast, partial encapsulation is more frequently evident in paravertebral paragangliomas than aorticopulmonary paragangliomas, and the former rarely invade extensively or metastasize, resulting in a better prognosis for the patients (54).

A case of aorticopulmonary paraganglioma was reported, and nine other cases reported in Japan were reviewed by Otake et al. (44a). The former tumor was multicystic, adherent to the pericardium, and surrounding the large vessels. It was incompletely resected.

A single case each of pigmented paraganglioma in the anterior mediastinum (40) and gangliocytic paraganglioma in the superior mediastinum (51) were reported. Both of these

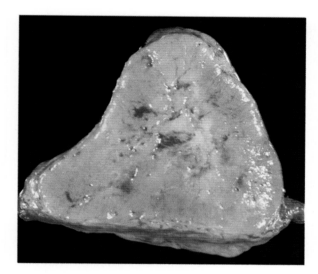

Figure 11-21

PARAGANGLIOMA

Above: The cut surface of this 3.9 x 3.5 x 2.5 cm, triangular tumor bulges at the periphery and is somewhat fibrotic in the center. It was surrounded by the heart, left lower lobe of the lung, aorta, esophagus, and diaphragm, and had been 1.8 cm in diameter 7 years before.

Right: The tumor is composed of zellballen bordered by capillaries. Individual cells were positive on Grimelius staining.

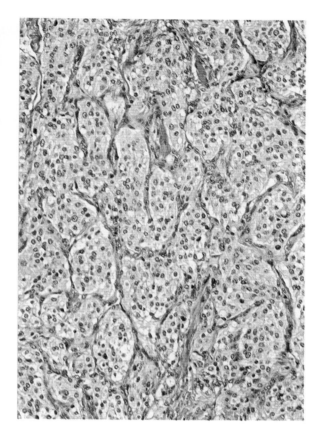

tumor types are very rare, and the latter was accompanied simultaneously by the same tumor in the mid-distal esophagus.

Immunohistochemistry of Neurogenic Tumors and Paraganglioma

Neuron-specific enolase (NSE) can be demonstrated in neurogenic tumors. Neural cell adhesion molecule (NCAM, CD56) is positive in almost all neurogenic and neuroendocrine tumors (34). Schwannoma and neuroblastoma can be differentiated by their staining for S-100 protein and synaptophysin, respectively (43). Catecholamines can be detected by formalin-induced fluorescence. According to Wirnsberger et al. (55), NSE, chromogranins and related proteins (HISL 19), dopamine beta-hydroxylase, protein gene product (PGP) 9.5, neurofilaments, and endocrine granule constituents (EGC) are

excellent markers for neuroblastic tumors since they are present in most cases. S-100 protein is present in ganglioneuroblastomas and ganglioneuromas.

Moran et al. (41) found immunoreactive chromogranin A and S-100 protein in most paragangliomas, and leu-enkephalin and neurofilament protein in about half. To distinguish paragangliomas from well-differentiated neuroendocrine carcinomas (carcinoid tumors), cytokeratin is used, since it is negative in the former and positive in the latter. Both paragangliomas and well-differentiated neuroendocrine carcinomas are Grimelius positive and stain immunohistochemically for chromogranin and in some cases for S-100 protein. Other immunopositive substances in well-differentiated neuroendocrine tumors include a variety of amine and peptide hormones.

REFERENCES

Mesenchymal Tumors

1. Argani P, Zakowski MF, Klimstra DS, Rosai J, Ladanyi M. Detection of the SYT-SSX chimeric RNA of synovial sarcoma in paraffin-embedded tissue and its application in problematic cases. Mod Pathol 1998;11:65-71.

2. Begin LR, Scherch W, Lacoste J, Hiscott J, Melnychuk DA. Glycogen-rich clear cell rhabdomyosarcoma of the mediastinum. Potential diagnostic pitfall. Am J Surg Pathol 1994;18:302-8.

3. Cavazza A, Rossi G, Agostini L, Roncella S, Ferro P, Fedeli F. Cytokeratin-positive malignant solitary fibrous tumor of the pleura: an unusual pitfall in the diagnosis of pleural spindle cell neoplasms. Histopathology 2003;43:606-8.

4. Chetty R. Extraskeletal mesenchymal chondrosarcoma of the mediastinum. Histopathology 1990;17:261-78.

5. Dunn EJ, Ulicny KS Jr, Wright CB, Gottesman L. Surgical implications of sclerosing mediastinitis. A report of six cases and review of the literature. Chest 1990;97:338-46.

6. England DM, Hochholzer L, McCarthy MJ. Localized benign and malignant fibrous tumors of the pleura. A clinicopathologic view of 223 cases. Am J Surg Pathol 1989;13:640-58.

7. Fletcher CD. Soft tissue tumors. In Fletcher CD, ed. Diagnostic histopathology of tumors, 2nd ed, vol 2. London: Churchill Livingston; 2000:1473-540.

7a. Fletcher CD, Unni KK, Mertens F, eds. World Health Organization Classification of Tumours. Pathology and genetics of tumours of soft tissue and bone, Lyon: IARC Press; 2002.

8. Flint A, Weiss SW. CD-34 and keratin expression distinguishes solitary fibrous tumor (fibrous mesothelioma) of pleura from desmoplastic mesothelioma. Hum Pathol 1995;26:428-31.

9. Graadt van Roggen, Hogendoorn PCW. Solitary fibrous tumours: the emerging clinicopathologic spectrum of an entity and its differential diagnosis. Curr Diagn Pathol 2004;10:229-35.

10. Hanau CA, Miettinen M. Solitary fibrous tumor: histological and immunohistochemical spectrum of benign and malignant variants presenting at different sites. Hum Pathol 1995;26:440-9.

11. Kempson RL, Fletcher CD, Hendrickson MR, Sibley RK. Tumors of the soft tissue. AFIP Atlas of Tumor Pathology, 3rd Series, Fascicle 30, Washington, DC: American Registry of Pathology; 1998.

12. Klimstra DS, Moran CA, Perino G, Koss MN, Rosai J. Liposarcoma of the anterior mediastinum and thymus. A clinicopathologic study of 28 cases. Am J Surg Pathol 1995;19:782-91.

13. Marchevsky AM, Kaneko M. Surgical pathology of the mediastinum, 2nd ed. New York: Raven Press; 1992.

14. Moran CA, Suster S. Mediastinal hemangiomas: a study of 18 cases with emphasis on the spectrum of morphological features. Hum Pathol 1995;26:416-21.

15. Morshuis WJ, Cox AL, Lacquet LK, Mravunac M, Barentsz JO. Primary fibrous histiocytoma of the mediastinum. Thorax 1990;45:154-5.

16. Schowengerdt CG, Suyemoto R, Main FB. Granulomatous and fibrous mediastinitis. A review and analysis of 180 cases. Thorac Cardiovasc Surg 1969;57:365-79.

17. Shaffer K, Pugatch RD, Sugarbaker DJ. Primary mediastinal leiomyoma. Ann Thorac Surg 1990;50:301-2.

18. Suster S, Moran CA. Primary synovial sarcomas of the mediastinum: a clinicopathologic, immunohistochemical, and ultrastructural study of 15 cases. Am J Surg Pathol 2005;29:569-78.

19. Suster S, Moran CA, Koss MN. Epithelioid hemangioendothelioma of the anterior mediastinum. Clinicopathologic, immunohistochemical, and ultrastructural analysis of 12 cases. Am J Surg Pathol 1994;18:871-81.

20. Suster S, Moran CA, Koss MN. Rhabdomyosarcomas of the anterior mediastinum: report of four cases unassociated with germ cell teratomatous or thymic carcinomatous components. Hum Pathol 1994;25:349-56.

21. Trupiano JK, Rice TW, Herzog K, et al. Mediastinal synovial sarcoma: report of two cases with molecular genetic analysis. Ann Thorac Surg 2002;73:628-30.

22. van de Rijn M, Rouse RV. CD34: a review. Applied Immunohistochem 1994;2:71-80.

23. Weiss SW, Goldblum JR. Enzinger and Weiss's soft tissue tumors, 4th ed. St. Louis: Mosby; 2001.

24. Witkin GB, Miettinen M, Rosai J. A biphasic tumor of the mediastinum with features of synovial sarcoma. A report of four cases. Am J Surg Pathol 1989;13:490-9.

25. Witkin GB, Rosai J. Solitary fibrous tumor of the mediastinum. A report of 14 cases. Am J Surg Pathol 1989;13:547-57.

26. Yamazaki A, Miyamoto, H, Saito Y, Matsuzawa H, Sakao Y, Anami Y. Cavernous hemangioma of the anterior mediastinum: case report and 50-year review of Japanese cases. Jpn J Thorac Cardiovasc Surg 2006;54:221-4.

Neurogenic Tumors and Tumors of Paraganglia

27. Adam A, Hochholzer L. Ganglioneuroblastoma of the posterior mediastinum: a clinicopathologic review of 80 cases. Cancer 1981;47:373-81.

28. Argani P, Erlandson RA, Rosai J. Thymic neuroblastoma in adults: report of three cases with special emphasis on its association with the syndrome of inappropriate secretion of antidiuretic hormone. Am J Clin Pathol 1997;108:537-43.

29. Asada Y, Marutsuka K, Mitsukawa T, Kuribayashi T, Taniguchi S, Sumiyoshi A. Ganglioneuroblastoma of the thymus: an adult case with the syndrome of inappropriate secretion of antidiuretic hormone. Hum Pathol 1996;27:506-9.

30. Cawthon RM, Weiss R, Xu GF, et al. A major segment of the neurofibromatosis type 1 gene: cDNA sequence, genomic structure, and point mutations. Cell 1990;62:193-201.

31. Committee on Histological Classification of Childhood Tumors, the Japanese Society of Pathology. Peripheral neuroblastic tumors and pheochromocytoma: International Pathology Classification. Histological classification and color atlas of tumors in infancy and childhood, Vol. 2. Tokyo: Kanehara Shuppan; 2004. [Japanese.]

32. Evans AE, D'Angio GJ, Propert K, Anderson J, Hann HW. Prognostic factors in neuroblastoma. Cancer 1987;59:1853-9

33. Fong CT, Dracopoli NC, White PS, et al. Loss of heterozygosity for the short arm of chromosome 1 in human neuroblastomas: correlation with N-myc amplification. Proc Natl Acad Sci U S A 1989;86:3753-7.

34. Hirano T, Hirohashi S, Kunii T, Noguchi M, Shimosato Y, Hayata Y. Quantitative distributions of cluster 1 small cell lung cancer antigen in cancerous and non-cancerous tissues, cultured cells and sera. Jpn J Cancer Res 1989:80:348-55.

35. Lack EE. Tumors of adrenal and extra-adrenal paraganglion system. Atlas of Tumor Pathology, 3rd Series, Fascicle 19, Washington, DC: Armed Forces Institute of Pathology; 1997.

36. Lamy AL, Fradet GJ, Luoma A, Nelems B. Anterior and middle mediastinal paraganglioma: complete resection is the treatment of choice. Ann Thorac Surg 1994; 57:249-52.

37. Legius E, Marchuk DA, Collins FS, Glover TW. Somatic deletion of the neurofibromatosis type 1 gene in a neurofibrosarcoma supports a tumor suppressor gene hypothesis. Nat Genet 1993;3:122-6.

38. Marchevsky AM, Kaneko M. Surgical pathology of the mediastinum, 2nd ed. New York: Raven Press; 1992.

39. Misugi K, Okajima H, Newton WA Jr, Kmetz DR, deLorimier AA. Mediastinal origin of a melanotic progonoma or retinal anlage tumor: ultrastructural evidence for neural crest origin. Cancer 1965;18:477-84.

40. Moran CA, Albores-Saavedra J, Wenig BM, Mena H. Pigmented extraadrenal paragangliomas. A clinicopathologic and immunohistochemical study of five cases. Cancer 1997;79:398-402.

41. Moran CA, Suster S, Fishback N, Koss MN. Mediastinal paragangliomas. A clinicopathologic and immunohistochemical study of 16 cases. Cancer 1993;72:2358-64.

42. Nagashima Y, Miyagi Y, Tanaka Y, et al. Adult ganglioneuroblastoma of the anterior mediastinum. Pathol Res Pract 1997;193:727-33.

43. Nakajima T, Watanabe S, Sato Y, Kameya T, Hirota T, Shimosato Y. An immunoperoxidase study of S-100 protein distribution in normal and neoplastic tissues. Am J Surg Pathol 1982;6:715-27.

44. Nobles E, Lee R, Kircher T, Mediastinal ependymoma. Hum Pathol 1991;22:94-6.

44a. Otake Y, Aoki M, Imamura N, Ishikawa M, Hashimoto K, Fujiyama R. Aortico-pulmonary paraganglioma: case report and Japanese review. Jpn J Thoracic Cardiovasc Surg 2006;54:212-6.

45. Pettinato G, Manivel LC, d'Amore ES, Jaszcz W, Gorlin RJ. Melanotic neuroectodermal tumor of infancy. A reexamination of a histogenetic problem based on immunohistochemical, flow cytometric, and ultrastructural study of 10 cases. Am J Surg Pathol 1991;15:233-45.

46. Seeger RC, Brodeur GM, Sather H, et al. Association of multiple copies of the N-myc oncogene with rapid progression of neuroblastomas. N Engl J Med 1985;313:1111-6.

47. Scheithauer BW, Woodruff, JM, Erlandson RA. Tumors of the peripheral nervous system. Atlas of Tumor Pathology, 3rd Series, Fascicle 24, Washington, DC: Armed Forces Institute of Pathology; 1999.

48. Shimada H. Neuroblastoma: pathology and biology. Acta Pathol Jpn 1992;42:229-41.

49. Talerman A, Gratama S. Primary ganglioneuroblastoma of the anterior mediastinum in a 61-year-old woman. Histopathology 1983;7:967-75.

50. Tsuda H, Shimosato Y, Upton MP, et al. Retrospective study on amplification of N-myc and c-myc genes in pediatric solid tumors and its association with prognosis and tumor differentiation. Lab Invest 1988;59:321-7.

51. Weinrach DM, Wang KL, Blum MG, Yeldandi AV, Laskin WB. Multifocal presentation of gangliocytic paraganglioma in the mediastinum and esophagus. Hum Pathol 2004;35:1288-91.

52. Weiss SW, Goldbrum JR. Enzinger and Weiss's soft tissue tumors, 4th ed. St. Louis: Mosby; 2001.

53. Wick MR. The mediastinum. In Mills SE, ed. Sternberg's diagnostic pathology, 4th ed. New York: Lippincott Williams & Wilkins; 2004:1253-1321.

54. Wick MR, Rosai J. Neuroendocrine neoplasms of the mediastinum. Semin Diagn Pathol 1991;8:35-51.

55. Wirnsberger GH, Becker H, Ziervogel K, Hofler H. Diagnostic immunohistochemistry of neuroblastic tumors. Am J Surg Pathol 1992;16:49-57.

12 MEDIASTINAL CYSTS (OTHER THAN THYMIC CYST)

The various cysts in the mediastinum can be divided into two main categories: congenital and acquired (Table 12-1). Thymic cysts, both congenital and acquired, have been described separately. Mediastinal cysts are uncommon, comprising 10 to 27 percent of all mediastinal space-occupying lesions according to Marchevsky and Kaneko (2). Of the surgically resected mediastinal lesions in a 30-year period at the National Cancer Center Hospital in Tokyo, only 39 (12 percent) were cysts (see Table 2-4).

The majority of patients with mediastinal cysts and cystic lesions have no symptoms and the cysts are found incidentally on chest X-ray examination performed routinely or for other purposes. Solid and cystic lesions, however, cannot be differentiated by plain chest roentgenograms. Computerized tomography (CT) scans, without and with contrast medium, help distinguish cystic from solid lesions in many but not all cases. Ultrasound is also helpful for diagnosis.

The most effective approach for diagnosing cystic lesions is percutaneous or transbronchial needle aspiration of the cyst contents and cytologic examination of the aspirated fluid. This method, together with the location of the lesion, can determine not only the type of process, either cystic or solid, but also the nature of the lesion, in most cases. For example, straw-colored clear fluid is obtained from celomic cysts and some congenital thymic cysts, mucinous cloudy fluid from bronchogenic cysts, chylous fluid from thoracic duct cysts, and muddy or grumous material from mature cystic teratomas. Cytologic examination establishes the nature of the cystic lesion as either benign or malignant and often determines the cell type or cell of origin as either mesothelial, squamous, or respiratory.

BRONCHOGENIC CYST

Bronchogenic cyst is the most common congenital cyst of the mediastinum. While it can be found at any age, it is more frequently found in young adults. It results from the abnormal branching of the tracheobronchial tree during embryonic development. Patients are asymptomatic in many cases but an enlarged cyst may produce symptoms due to compression of the surrounding structures such as the trachea, bronchi, and esophagus.

Bronchial cysts are frequently located in the anterior mediastinum and are often connected by fibrous tissue with the trachea or bronchi. They may be present in other parts of the mediastinum and within the lung parenchyma. The cysts are spherical and usually unilocular, but may be multilocular. They are thin-walled with a smooth outer surface and faintly trabeculated inner lining (fig. 12-1)

The bronchial cyst is lined with respiratory epithelium (fig. 12-2), that is, pseudostratified ciliated columnar epithelium, which may show squamous metaplasia or be denuded. Tracheobronchial

---

Table 12-1

MEDIASTINAL CYSTS AND CYST-LIKE LESIONS[a]

Cysts
  Congenital
    Bronchogenic
    Esophageal
    Tracheoesophageal
    Gastroenteric
    Celomic (pericardial, mesothelial)
    Thymic
  Acquired
    Thoracic duct
    Lymphangioma

Cyst-Like Lesions
  Hematoma
  Parasitic
  Cystic changes in:
    Thymic hyperplasia
    Thymoma
    Thymic carcinoma
    Mature teratoma (dermoid cyst)
    Germinoma
    Low-grade B-cell lymphoma of MALT[b]
    Hodgkin lymphoma

[a]Table 4-2 from Fascicle 21, Third Series.
[b]MALT = mucosa-associated lymphoid tissue.

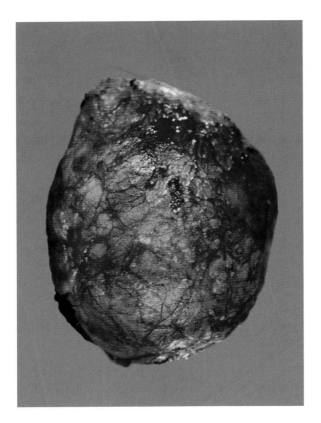
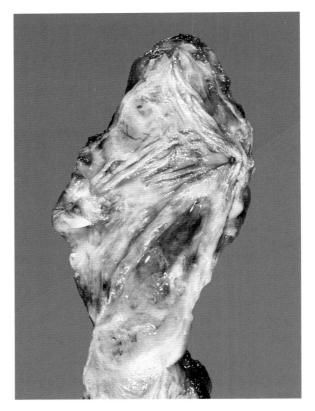

Figure 12-1

BRONCHOGENIC CYST

Left: This thin-walled cyst was present in the posterior mediastinum. It is distended with slightly cloudy, somewhat mucinous fluid.

Right: The inner surface is smooth and trabeculated in areas. (Fig. 4-19 from Fascicle 21, Third Series.)

Figure 12-2

BRONCHOGENIC CYST

The cyst is lined by pseudo-stratified ciliated columnar epithelial cells. The wall contains accessory glands, layers of smooth muscle, and cartilage. (Fig. 4-20 from Fascicle 21, Third Series.)

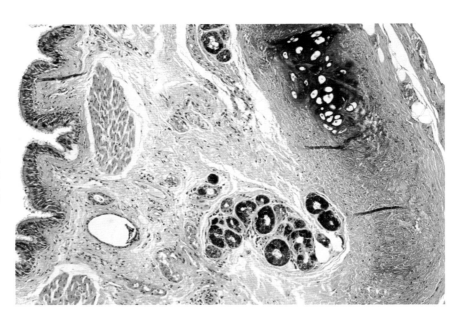

glands are present in the lamina propria, at times even outside the smooth muscle layer of the cyst wall. Cartilage may also be present.

Surgical removal is the treatment of choice for cysts causing symptoms. Percutaneous needle aspiration of the contents is indicated for symptomatic relief. In such cases, the content should be examined cytologically.

ESOPHAGEAL CYST

Esophageal cysts are much less common than bronchogenic cysts. They present within the wall of, or in close association with, the esophagus. They are spherical and unilocular, and lined by stratified squamous epithelium, with or without foci of ciliated columnar epithelium. The epithelium is supported by the lamina propria, which contains esophageal glands, and is surrounded by a double layer of smooth muscle, the lamina muscularis propria. These cysts are differentiated from bronchogenic cysts by location, absence of cartilage, and presence of muscularis propria. The nature of the cyst cannot be determined at times because of the absence of characteristic features.

Tracheoesophageal cysts are rare. They have the combined features of bronchogenic and esophageal cysts.

GASTROENTERIC CYST

Gastroenteric cysts are rare developmental unilocular cysts found in the posterior mediastinum, frequently connected to the vertebral column with fibrous tissue. They are found often in infants as well as adults. Gastroenteric cysts are reported to be frequently associated with malformations of the cervical and thoracic vertebrae such as hemivertebrae, posterior spina bifida, and scoliosis (2,4). Patients are symptomatic when diagnosed and present with pain due to compression of nerves, peptic ulceration of the lining mucosa and wall of the cyst, and other symptoms due to involvement of surrounding mediastinal structures.

The gastroenteric cyst is lined by either gastric mucosa with parietal and chief cells; duodenal, small intestinal, or large intestinal mucosae; or squamous or ciliated columnar epithelium. Outside the lamina propria mucosae are lamina muscularis mucosae, submucosa, and lamina muscularis propria.

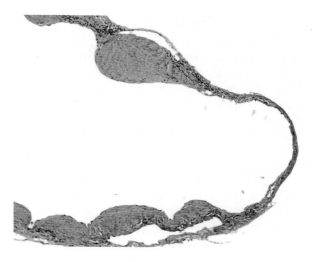

Figure 12-3

PERICARDIAL CYST

A thin-walled cyst is lined by a single layer of flat cells. Focal thickening is seen in a thin fibrous wall. (Fig. 4-21 from Fascicle 21, Third Series.)

Peptic digestion of the cyst wall produces sinuses and fistulae into the chest wall and thoracic organs, and can be fatal. The development of adenocarcinoma of the colonic type in gastroenteric cyst has been reported (2). Also reported was a case of high-grade neuroendocrine carcinoma, of probable large cell type from the authors' description, which arose from a foregut cyst of the posterior mediastinum, most likely a gastroenteric cyst (6).

CELOMIC CYST (PERICARDIAL CYST AND MESOTHELIAL CYST)

Celomic cysts are occasionally seen in the mediastinum, either attached to the pericardium (*pericardial cyst*) or in other parts of the mediastinum (*mesothelial cyst*). Patients are often asymptomatic, and the cysts are detected incidentally at the time of chest X-ray examination, or there are symptoms due to compression of the mediastinal structures by the cyst. Celomic cysts are spherical, unilocular, and thin walled. The cyst content is watery clear or straw colored. They are lined by a single layer of flat to cuboidal mesothelial cells supported by loose connective tissue (fig. 12-3). Celomic cysts can be treated surgically or by percutaneous aspiration of the cyst content.

THORACIC DUCT CYST

Thoracic duct cysts are rare, although sub-diaphragmatic cisterna chyli cysts are common. Tsuchiya et al. (5) reported a case of thoracic duct cyst diagnosed before thoracotomy. The patient was a 49-year-old woman who began to experience eructation. The left lateral chest roentgenogram revealed an ovoid density behind the hilus of the lung. The lesion was cystic and enclosed by, but not connected with, bronchi, esophagus, vertebrae, and descending aorta as assessed by CT, barium swallow, and aortography. Therefore, the cyst was considered to be associated with the thoracic duct. It was proven to be so by lymphangiography taken 24 hours after injection of iodized oil into the lymphatic vessel of the patient's foot. It was a thin-walled unilocular cyst containing chylous fluid and a clotted substance. The internal surface was trabeculated and lined by flat endothelial cells.

CYST-LIKE LESIONS OTHER THAN TRUE CYSTS

Hematoma is often the result of trauma, but may be spontaneous. *Hydatid cyst*, described in the second series of this Fascicle, is found in endemic areas (3). On rare occasions, seminoma and Hodgkin lymphoma of the thymus undergo extensive cystic change to the point of obscuring the true nature of the process (3). The cystic changes in thymoma and thymic carcinoma were described in previous chapters. Low-grade marginal zone B-cell lymphoma of the thymus may also become cystic (see fig. 6-9A) (1).

REFERENCES

1. Isaacson PG, Chan JK, Tang C, Addis BJ. Low-grade B-cell lymphoma of mucosa-associated lymphoid tissue arising in the thymus. A thymic lymphoma mimicking myoepithelial sialadenitis, Am J Surg Pathol 1990;14:342-51.
2. Marchevsky AM, Kaneko M. Surgical pathology of the mediastinum, 2nd ed. New York: Raven Press; 1992.
3. Rosai J, Levine GD. Tumors of the thymus. Atlas of Tumor Pathology, 2nd Series, Fascicle 13. Washington, DC: Armed Forces Institute of Pathology; 1976.
4. Salyer DC, Salyer WR, Eggleston JC. Benign developmental cysts of the mediastinum. Arch Pathol Lab Med 1977;101:136-9.
5. Tsuchiya R, Sugiura Y, Ogata T, Suemasu K. Thoracic duct cyst of the mediastinum. J Thorac Cardiovasc Surg 1980;79:856-9.
6. Yamashita A, Marutsuka K, Moriguchi S, et al. Neuroendocrine carcinoma of the posterior mediastinum arising from a foregut cyst. Pathol Int 2005;55:285-9.

13 OTHER MEDIASTINAL TUMOR-LIKE CONDITIONS

CASTLEMAN DISEASE

Castleman disease, also commonly referred to as *angiofollicular or giant lymph node hyperplasia,* was initially described as a solitary lesion in the mediastinum, which is the most common site of involvement (8). It has now been reported in many other locations including the abdominal cavity, pulmonary parenchyma, neck, axillary regions, and skeletal muscle. Castleman disease involving the mediastinum consists of a well-circumscribed, round nodule (usually in the anterosuperior portion), with a tendency to be on one side of the midline at a lung root, around one of the great vessels, or close to an interlobar fissure (fig. 13-1).

Two forms of Castleman disease have been identified: the much more common localized type and the less common multicentric type (1,8). Although the latter has histologic features similar to the former, the multicentric type develops in older patients, is consistently a peripheral rather than central nodal disease, and has a more aggressive clinical course often associated with the development of malignancies. It is beyond the scope of this chapter to discuss the details of the multicentric type. Description here is restricted to the localized type.

Involvement of the thymus by Castleman disease, either in the multicentric or solitary form, is extremely rare. Multicentric Castleman disease with prominent thymic involvement was reported by O'Reilly et al. (5) in a 12-year-old girl and a localized form of the disease involving the thymus was reported by Karcher et al. (2). The latter was associated with nephrotic syndrome and myelofibrosis. Thymic involvement was thought to be secondary due to the proximity of the primary nodal site of Castleman disease.

The localized or solitary lesions of Castleman disease are usually rounded masses varying from 1.5 to 16.0 cm in diameter. Histologically, two major types have been described: hyaline-vascu-

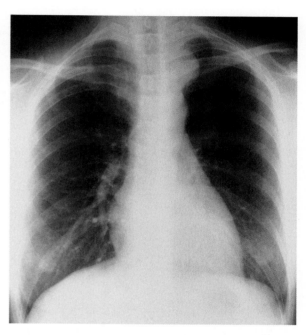

Figure 13-1

CASTLEMAN DISEASE

A chest X ray reveals a well-defined tumorous lesion that projects toward the left thoracic cavity. (Fig. 4-22 from Fascicle 21, Third Series.)

lar type and plasma cell type (1,6,7,8). Intermediate and mixed types have also been reported. The hyaline-vascular type is much more common than the plasma cell type, comprising 90 percent of the cases in a large series (3). The two types differ considerably in their histologic appearance and clinical presentation. Patients with the hyaline-vascular type are mostly asymptomatic, unless the mass causes pressure symptoms by compressing adjacent structures such as the trachea or bronchi. Patients with the plasma cell type often present with systemic symptoms and abnormal laboratory data (8). Following total excision of the mass, the symptoms disappear and laboratory data return to normal.

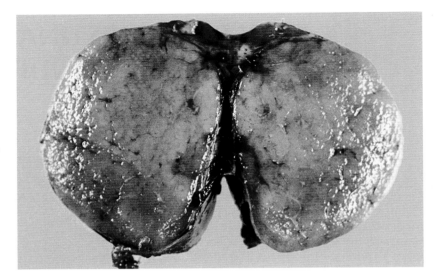

Figure 13-2

CASTLEMAN DISEASE

The cut surface bulges and is finely granular.

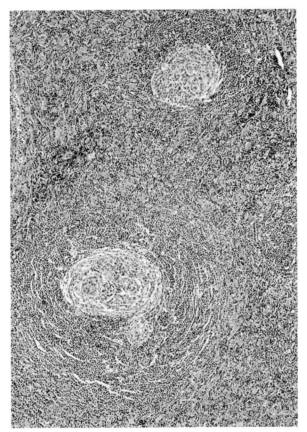

Figure 13-3

CASTLEMAN DISEASE, HYALINE-VASCULAR TYPE

The follicles have atrophic germinal centers surrounded by a wide mantle zone of concentrically arranged lymphocytes. The interfollicular areas are highly vascular, with a network of small blood vessels.

Hyaline-Vascular Type Castleman Disease

This type may occur in children as well as adults (median age of 33 years in one series [8]). This is also true for the plasma cell type (median age of 22 years). There is no gender predilection. Macroscopically, the lesion consists of a single encapsulated mass. The cut surface is solid, homogeneous, gray, finely granular or nodular, and sometimes hemorrhagic (fig. 13-2).

The main histologic features include abnormal lymph follicles and a striking interfollicular vascularity. The latter feature causes significant bleeding if the lesion is incised during surgery. The follicles often have expanded mantle zones composed of small lymphocytes surrounding abnormal germinal centers, which range in size from medium to barely recognizable (fig. 13-3). Most of the germinal centers are small, although large abnormal ones are also present. The follicles contain one or more small blood vessels that enter from the perifollicular tissue (fig. 13-4). Only vessels in the germinal centers are hyalinized, which superficially resemble Hassall corpuscles or splenic white pulp (8). The former can be mistaken for thymoma, and the latter for ectopic spleen. Some of the germinal centers are surrounded by greatly expanded, concentrically arranged ("onion skin"), small mantle zone lymphocytes which may completely obscure the germinal centers. When these histologic features predominate, the lesion is referred as the *lymphoid variant of the hyaline-vascular type*. Another characteristic finding is the presence of

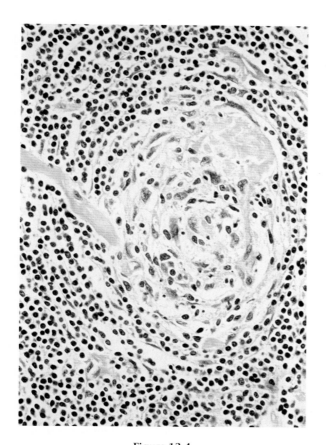

Figure 13-4

CASTLEMAN DISEASE, HYALINE-VASCULAR TYPE

An atrophic germinal center contains a small blood vessel entering from the perifollicular tissue.

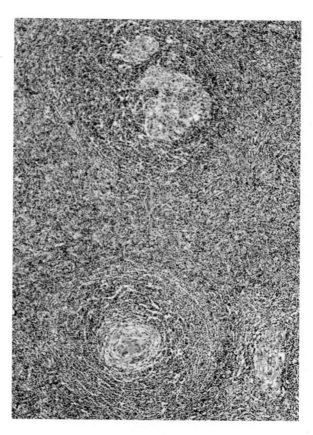

Figure 13-5

CASTLEMAN DISEASE, HYALINE-VASCULAR TYPE

One of two follicles contains two atrophic germinal centers.

more than one small germinal center within a single follicle (fig. 13-5).

The interfollicular areas contain varying numbers of small blood vessels, which may be extremely numerous. Most are lined by flat endothelium, but some have prominent endothelial cells and resemble postcapillary venules (fig. 13-6). Small lymphocytes are the predominant cells between vessels. A small number of plasma cells and rare immunoblasts may be present as well. Large fibrotic masses, which often surround large vessels, are often scattered in the interfollicular zones. The normal lymph node architecture, such as sinuses, is often seen at the periphery of the lesion.

Fine needle aspiration cytology of two cases disclosed a mature, small lymphoid population associated with large atypical cells consistent with follicular dendritic cells. This pattern is suggestive of Castleman disease. The diagnosis was confirmed by the identification of a polytypic B-cell population by flow cytometry and immunohistochemistry (4).

The hyaline-vascular type of germinal center is not specific for Castleman disease. It is occasionally seen as a single follicle in nonspecific reactive lymph nodes, and it has also been reported in lymph nodes of patients with acquired immunodeficiency syndrome (AIDS) and AIDS-related complexes, and in patients with angioimmunoblastic lymphadenopathy (8).

Plasma Cell Type Castleman Disease

The lesions of the plasma cell type of Castleman disease range from 3 to 15 cm in diameter and are composed of several discrete, matted nodes or a mass with adjacent smaller nodes. Patients may have systemic symptoms and signs

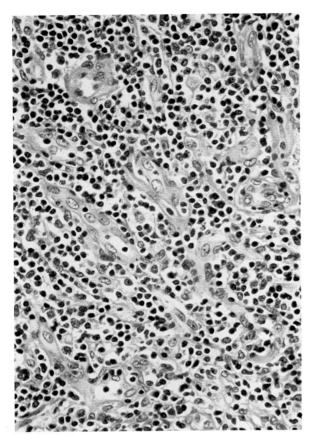

Figure 13-6

CASTLEMAN DISEASE, HYALINE-VASCULAR TYPE

The interfollicular area is rich in blood vessels.

(8), including anemia, polyclonal gammopathy, elevated erythrocyte sedimentation rate, bone marrow plasmacytosis, and thrombocytosis. Following complete excision of the mass, the symptoms disappear and laboratory data return to normal. The plasma cell type is most commonly found in the abdomen, usually in the mesentery of the small intestine. Fewer cases of the plasma cell type are located in the mediastinum and yet fewer in the peripheral lymph nodes.

Histologically, the nodal architecture is relatively well preserved. Interfollicular areas are densely infiltrated by plasma cells, and sometimes accompanied by numerous Russell bodies (fig. 13-7). The germinal centers are numerous but the hyaline-vascular changes are inconspicuous or absent. The overall appearance is reminiscent of that seen in the lymph nodes of patients with rheumatoid arthritis.

Immunohistochemically, the peripheral areas of the abnormal follicles are composed of small lymphocytes expressing the phenotype of mantle zone lymphocytes, and usually, CD5 (1). The central regions of the follicles show an abundance of follicular dendritic cells. Plasma cells produce polyclonal immunoglobulin but several reports have documented a monoclonal plasma cell component, either diffusely replacing the interfollicular area or forming a recognizable nodule (1).

Castleman disease has been considered to be a hamartoma or neoplasm, but it is now regarded as a peculiar hyperplastic lymphoid process. The histogenesis of Castleman disease is not fully understood. There is little information regarding the hyaline vascular type. In this type, proliferation of follicular dendritic cells is suggested to be the core of the disease process. Atypical or neoplastic proliferation of follicular dendritic cells within this lesion has been documented. On the other hand, the plasma cell type seems a peculiar form of lymphoid hyperplasia. This type may be solitary or multicentric. The latter is often associated with systemic symptoms, one example being the POEMS (polyneuropathy, organomegaly, endocrinopathy, M-proteins, skin lesions) syndrome. Participation of human herpesvirus-8 (HHV-8) in the development of the plasma cell type has been suggested. The genome of HHV-8 contains a gene homologous to the human *IL-6* gene. The product of this gene, together with human IL-6, is thought to cause the clinicopathologic manifestations of multicentric Castleman disease (1).

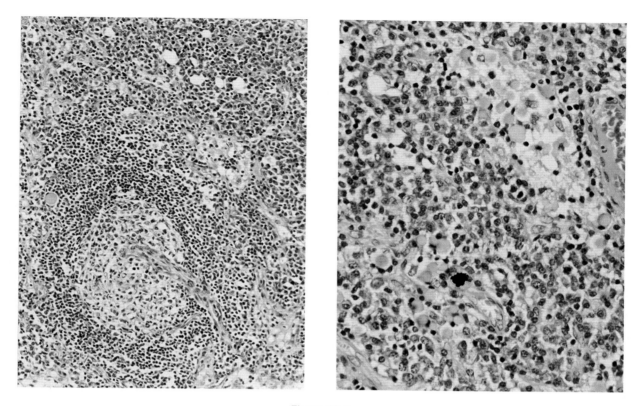

Figure 13-7

CASTLEMAN DISEASE, PLASMA CELL TYPE

Left: The interfollicular tissue is crowded with mature plasma cells. Prominent vascularization is also seen. A follicle with a germinal center is on the right.

Right: Higher-power magnification of the interfollicular tissue shows the cytologic appearance of the plasma cells, many of which contain Russell bodies.

REFERENCES

1. Frizzera G. Atypical lymphoproliferative disorders. In Knowles DM, ed. Neoplastic hematopathology, 2nd ed. Philadelphia: Lippincott Williams & Wilkins; 2001:569-622.
2. Karcher DS, Pearson CE, Butler WM, Hurwitz MA, Cassell PF. Giant lymph node hyperplasia involving the thymus with associated nephrotic syndrome and myelofibrosis. Am J Clin Pathol 1982;77:100-4.
3. Keller AR, Hochholzer L, Castleman B. Hyaline-vascular and plasma cell types of giant lymph node hyperplasia of mediastinum and other locations. Cancer 1972;29:670-83.
4. Meyer L, Gibbons D, Ashfaq R, Vuitch F, Saboorian MH. Fine-needle aspiration findings in Castleman's disease. Diagn Cytopathol 1999;21: 57-60.
5. O'Reilly PE Jr. Joshi VV, Holbrook CT, Weisenburger DD. Multicentric Castleman's disease in a child with prominent thymic involvement: a case report and brief review of the literature. Mod Pathol 1993;6:776-80.
6. Rosai J. Lymph nodes. In Rosai J, ed. Rosai and Ackerman's surgical pathology, 9th ed. St. Edinburgh, London, New York: Mosby; 2004:1905-8.
7. Rosai J, Levine GD. Tumors of the thymus. Atlas of Tumor Pathology, Fascicle 13, 2nd Series. Washington, DC: Armed Forces Institute of Pathology; 1976.
8. Schnitzer B. Reactive lymphadenopathies. In Knowles DM, ed. Neoplastic hematopathology, 2nd ed. Philadelphia: Lippincott Williams & Wilkins; 2001:537-68.

Index*

A

Acquired immunodeficiency syndrome (AIDS), 274
Acquired multilocular thymic cyst, 263
    differentiation from mucosa-associated
      lymphoid tissue lymphoma (MALT), 264
Adenocarcinoma, 131
Adenoid cystic carcinoma-like thymic carcinoma, 135
Adenosquamous carcinoma, 129
Adrenocorticotrophic hormone (ACTH) in car-
    cinoid tumor, 172
Anaplastic large cell lymphoma, 241
Anatomy, normal, 1, 3
    mediastinum, 1
    thymus gland, 1
Angiofollicular hyperplasia, 309
Angiomatoid carcinoid tumor, 167
Angiosarcoma, 292
Aorticopulmonary ganglioma, 300
Aplastic anemia and thymoma, 97
Atrophy, *see* Thymic atrophy
Atypical carcinoid tumor, 148, **158**, 176
    differentiation from thymic carcinoma, 148
Atypical (type B3) thymoma, 53

B

B-cell follicle, 13
B-cell lymphomas, 225
    primary mediastinal large B-cell lymphoma,
      225, *see also* Primary mediastinal large B-cell
      lymphoma
    thymic extranodal marginal zone B-cell lympho-
      ma of mucosa-associated lymphoid tissue
      (MALT), 230, *see also* Thymic extranodal
      marginal zone B-cell lymphoma of mucosa-
      associated lymphoid tissue
B lymphocytes, 13
Basaloid carcinoma, 127
    from thymic cysts, 127
Biphasic metaplastic thymoma, 64
Biphasic thymoma, of mixed polygonal and
    spindle cell type, 64
Bronchogenic cyst, 305

C

Carcinoid tumor, 99, 148, **157**
    and multiple endocrine neoplasia, 159
    association with Cushing syndrome, 159, 168
    association with paraneoplastic syndrome, 168
    association with Zollinger-Ellison syndrome, 159
    atypical carcinoid tumor, 148, **158**, 176
    clinical findings, 159
    combined with thymoma, 186
    cytologic findings, 168
    differential diagnosis, 176; differentiation from
      thymoma, 99; from thymic carcinoma, 148
    ectopic ACTH production, 172
    gross findings, 160
    histogenesis, 158
    immunohistochemical findings, 168
    microscopic findings, 160
    molecular findings, 176
    nonfunctional, 159
    treatment and prognosis, 177
    ultrastructural findings, 168
    variants, 166
      angiomatoid, 167
      oncocytic carcinoid, 167
      pigmented carcinoid, 166
      spindle cell carcinoid, 166
      with amyloid stroma, 167
      with mucinous stroma, 167
      with sarcomatous changes, 167
Carcinoid tumor with amyloid stroma, 167
Carcinoid tumor with mucinous stroma, 167
Carcinoid tumor with sarcomatous changes, 167
Carcinoma, thymic, *see* Thymic carcinoma
Carcinoma with t(15;19) translocation, 139
Carcinoma with thymus-like differentiation
    (CASTLE), 260
Carcinosarcoma, 138
Castleman disease, 26, 276, **309**
    association with lymphoid hyperplasia, 276
    hyaline-vascular type, 310
    lymphoid variant, 310
    plasma cell type, 311
Celomic cyst, 307

*In a series of numbers, those in boldface indicate the main discussion of the entity.

mesothelial cyst, 307
pericardial cyst, 307
Chondroma, 288
Chondrosarcoma, 292
Choriocarcinoma, 193, 201, **212**
Classification, thymic tumors, 19, 45, 48, 53, 55,
    102, 103, 144, 216
    clinical staging of Masaoka, 102
    comparison of classification systems, 45
    controversies surrounding classifications
      systems, 56
    histogenetic classification of Müller-Hermelink,
      19, **55**, 68, 84
    TNM classification, 102, 103, **144**, 216
    traditional classification, 53
    World Health Organization (WHO) histologic
      classification, *see* World Health Organization
      histologic classification
    Yamakawa-Masaoka system, 103
Clear cell carcinoma, 97, **135**
    differentiation from thymoma, 97
Clear cell thymoma, 59
Combined small cell carcinoma, 182
Combined thymic epithelial tumor, 185
Composite thymoma-thymic carcinoma, 185
Congenital thymic cyst, 262
Cortical, lymphocyte-predominant (type B1)
    thymoma, 53
Cortical, mixed lymphocytic/epithelial (type B2)
    thymoma, 53
Cortical thymic epithelial cells, 10, 45, 77
Cortical (type B2) thymoma, 53, **56**
Cushing syndrome, and carcinoid tumor, 159, 172
Cystic hygroma, 285
Cystic thymoma, 59
Cysts, 262, **305**
    bronchogenic, 305
    celomic, 307, *see also* Celomic cyst
    esophageal, 307
    gastroenteric, 307
    thoracic duct cyst, 308
    thymic, 262, *see also* Thymic cyst
    tracheoesophageal, 307
Cytokeratins, 5, 11, 85
    in thymoma, 85

D

Dendritic cell tumors, 246
    follicular dendritic cell tumor/sarcoma, 246
    interdigitating dendritic cell tumor/sarcoma, 246
Dermoid tumor, 208
Down syndrome, 273
Dysplasia, *see* Thymic dysplasia

E

Ectopic hamartomatous thymoma, 260
    carcinoma with thymus-like differentiation
      (CASTLE), 260
    spindle cell epithelial tumor with thymus-like
      differentiation (SETTLE), 260
Ectopic parathyroid tissue, 281
Ectopic thyroid tissue, 281
Embryology, normal thymus gland, 2
Embryonal carcinoma, 201, **211**
Encapsulated thymoma, 29
Endodermal sinus tumor, *see* Yolk sac tumor
Ependymoma, 300
Epithelial cell thymoma, 41, 77
    classification systems, 45
    cortical epithelial cell, 45
    cytology, 77
    medullary epithelial cell, 45
    polygonal epithelial cell, 41
    spindle epithelial cell, 45
    subtype and stage, 45
Epithelial cell-predominant (type B3) thymoma, 53
Epithelial cells, **4**, 41, 77, 84
    antibody analysis, 10
    cytology, 77
    immunohistochemistry, 10, 84
    in thymoma, 41
    morphology, 10
    subtypes, 41
    ultrastructure, 89
Epithelioid hemangioendothelioma, 292
Epstein-Barr virus, 101, 150
    and thymic carcinoma, 150
    and thymoma, 101
Esophageal cyst, 307
Extramedullary acute myeloid leukemia, 247
Extrathyroidal medullary carcinoma, 167

F

Fibromatosis, 286
Follicular dendritic cell tumor/sarcoma, 246
Foxn1, 142

G

Ganglioneuroblastoma, 299
Ganglioneuroma, 297
Gastroenteric cyst, 307
Genetic abnormalities, thymoma, 94
Germ cell tumors, 193, *see also under individual tumors*
    association with hematologic malignancies, 194
    association with Klinefelter syndrome, 194
    choriocarcinoma, 212
    classification, 193
    clinical features, 193
    diagnostic techniques, 196
    differentiation from thymic carcinoma, 148,
        196; from thymoma, 201
    embryonal carcinoma, 211
    histologic variants, 201
    incidence, 193
    malignant germ cell tumors, 216
    mixed cell tumors, 212
    molecular findings, 216
    seminoma, 208
    staging, 216
    teratoma, 201
        pure, 216
        with nongerminal malignant tumor, 212
    treatment and prognosis, 216
    yolk sac tumor, 211
Germ cell tumors, malignant, 216
Germinal centers, 13
Germinoma, *see* Seminoma
Giant lymph node hyperplasia, 309
Glandular thymoma, 59
Goiters, mediastinal, 281
Graft versus host disease, 274
Granular cell tumor, 288
Granulocytic sarcoma, 247

H

Hassall corpuscles, normal, 9
Hemangioma, 286
Hemangiopericytoma, 288
Hematoma, 308

Hematopoietic neoplasms, 225
Histiocytic cell tumors, 245
    histiocytic sarcoma, 246
    Langerhans cell histiocytosis and sarcoma, 246
Histiocytic sarcoma, 246
Histogenetic classification of Müller-Hermelink, 19,
    55, 68, 84
Histogenetic thymoma subtypes, 55
Histologic thymoma subtypes, 48, 58
Histology and malignancy, 67
Hodgkin lymphoma, 98, **241**
    differentiation from thymoma, 98, 243
Hormones, thymus, 10
Hyaline-vascular Castleman disease, 310
Hydatid cyst, 265, 308
Hydatidosis, 265
Hyperplasia, *see* Thymic hyperplasia
Hypogammaglobulinemia and thymoma, 101

I

Immature teratoma, *see* Teratoma
Immunodeficiency, 271
    associated syndromes, 276
    in primary immunodeficiencies, 272
    in secondary immunodeficiencies, 274
    thymic atrophy, 271
    thymic dysplasia, 271
Inflammatory pseudotumor, 265
Interdigitating dendritic cell tumor/sarcoma, 246
Interdigitating reticulum cells, 13
Invasive thymoma, 115
Involucrin, 11, 85
    in epithelial cells of thymoma, 85
Involution, 16

K

Klinefelter syndrome, and germ cell tumors, 194

L

Langerhans cell histiocytosis and sarcoma, 246
Langerhans cells, 13
Large cell carcinoma, 137
Large cell lymphoma, differentiation from un-
    differentiated carcinoma, 146
Large cell neuroendocrine carcinoma, 178
Leiomyoma, 288
Lipofibroadenoma, 67

Lipoma, 288
Liposarcoma, 260, **292**
    differentiation from thymolipoma, 260
Lipothymoma, 257
Low-grade metaplastic carcinoma, 64
Lung carcinoma, differentiation from thymic car-
    cinoma, 198, *see also* Pulmonary carcinoma
Lymphangioma, 285
Lymphangiomatosis, 285
Lymphangioleiomyomatosis, 285
Lymphocyte-predominant (type B1) thymoma, 53
Lymphocyte-rich (type B1) thymoma, 53
Lymphocytes, normal, 10, *see also* Thymocytes
    antibody analysis, 10
    B lymphocytes, 13
    T lymphocytes, 13
Lymphocytes, thymoma, 46, 89, 93
Lymphocytic (type B1) thymoma, 53
Lymphoepithelioma-like carcinoma, 97, **135**, 145
    and Epstein-Barr virus, 150
    and squamous cell carcinoma, 135
    differentiation from thymoma, 97
Lymphoid hyperplasia, 60, **276**
    and micronodular thymoma, 60
Lymphoma, 84, 98, **225**
    B-cell lymphomas, 225, *see also* B-cell lymphomas
    differentiation from thymoma, 84
    Hodgkin lymphoma, 98, **241**, *see also* Hodgkin
      lymphoma
    T-cell lymphomas, 237, *see also* T-cell lymphomas

M

Macrophages, normal, 13
Malignancy and thymoma, 67
Malignancy-associated factors, thymic carcinoma, 144
    cell atypia, 145
    histologic type, 144
    immunohistochemical factors, 146
    nuclear DNA content, 146
    TNM/stage, 144
Malignant fibrous histiocytoma, 292
Malignant germ cell tumors, 216
    infants and young children, 216
    adolescents and adults, 216
Malignant histiocytosis, 246
Malignant lymphoma, *see* Lymphoma
Malignant melanoma, 262
Malignant peripheral nerve sheath tumor, 296

Malignant thymoma, 115
MALT lymphoma, *see* Mucosa-associated lymphoid
    tissue lymphoma
Masaoka staging system, 102
Mature teratoma, *see* Teratoma
Mediastinal giant lymph node hyperplasia, 26
Mediastinal goiter, 281
Mediastinal paraganglioma, 300
Mediastinal tumor types, 23
Mediastinum, normal, 1
Medullary epithelial cells, 6, 45, 77
Medullary (type A) thymoma, 45, **48**, 55, 58, 59,
    63, 100
Melanocytic schwannoma, 295
Melanoma, malignant, 262
Melanotic progonoma, 300
Mesenchymal tumors, 285, *see also individual tumors*
    epithelial hemangioendothelioma, 292
    fibromatosis, 286
    hemangioma, 286
    hemangiopericytoma, 288
    liposarcoma, 292
    lymphangioma, 285
    rhabdomyosarcoma, 292
    solitary fibrous tumor, 288
    synovial sarcoma, 292
Mesothelial cyst, 307
Mesothelioma, 255
Metaplastic carcinoma, 62
Metaplastic thymoma, 62
Metastatic carcinoma, 146, **253**
    differentiation from thymic carcinoma, 146
    differentiation of thymic and pulmonary
      carcinomas, 254
    from lung, 253
    from ovary, 253
Metastasizing thymoma, 115
Microcystic, pseudoglandular thymoma, 59
Micronodular thymoma, 60
    and mucosa-associated lymphoid tissue (MALT)
      lymphoma, 62
    with lymphoid B-cell hyperplasia, 60
Microscopic thymoma, 64
Mixed germ cell tumor, 201, **212**
Mixed lymphocyte and epithelial thymoma, 53
Mixed neuroendocrine carcinoma and thymoma, 185
Mixed (type AB) thymoma, 38, **48**, 56, 59
Morphologic classification, thymoma, 53

Mucoepidermoid carcinoma, 97, **127**, 131
    differentiation from thymoma, 97
Mucosa-associated lymphoid tissue (MALT)
        lymphoma, 62, 98, **231**, 265
    and micronodular thymoma, 62
    differentiation from acquired multilocular
        thymic cyst, 264; from thymoma, 98
Müller-Hermelink histogenetic classification, 19,
        55, 68, 84
Multilocular thymic cyst, 9, *see also* Acquired
        multilocular thymic cyst
Multiple endocrine neoplasia, and carcinoid
        tumor, 159
Myasthenia gravis, 24, 97, 99, 257, *see also* Para-
        neoplastic syndromes
    association with thymolipoma, 257
    association with thymoma, 99
Myeloid sarcoma, 247
Myoid cells, 13, 89
    immunohistochemistry, 89
    in thymoma, 89
    ultrastructure, 93

N

Neurilemmoma, 295
Neurinoma, 295
Neuroblastoma, 297
Neuroendocrine carcinomas, 157
    combined with thymoma, 185
    poorly differentiated neuroendocrine carcinoma,
        148, 157, **178**, *see also* Poorly differentiated
        neuroendocrine carcinoma
    well-differentiated neuroendocrine carcinoma,
        157, *see also* Carcinoid tumor
Neurofibroma, 295
Neurofibromatosis, 296
Neurogenic tumors, 295, *see also individual tumors*
    ependymoma, 300
    ganglioneuroblastoma, 299
    ganglioneuroma, 297
    immunohistochemistry, 301
    malignant peripheral nerve sheath tumor, 296
    neuroblastoma, 297
    neurofibroma, 295
    neurofibromatosis, 296
    paraganglioma, 300
    pigmented neuroectodermal tumor of infancy, 300
    primitive neuroectodermal tumor, 300

schwannoma, 295
NK-cell lymphoma, 241
Non-Hodgkin large cell lymphomas, 225
Nuclear DNA content, 95, 146
    carcinoma, 146
    thymoma, 95

O

Oncocytic carcinoid tumor, 167
Organoid (type B1) thymoma, **53**, 56

P

p53 gene, 143
Paraganglioma, 300
Paraneoplastic syndromes, 97, 168
    association with carcinoid tumor, 168
    association with thymoma, 97
    differentiation from thymoma, 97
Parathyroid adenoma, 283
Parathyroid carcinoma, 283
Parathyroid hyperplasia, 283
Parathyroid lesions, 281
Pericardial cyst, 307
Peripheral neurofibromatosis, 296
Pigmented carcinoid tumor, 166
Pigmented neuroectodermal tumor of infancy, 300
Pigmented thymoma, 64
Plasma cell-rich thymoma, 64
Plasma cell type Castleman disease, 311
Pleomorphic large cell lymphoma, 230
Polygonal epithelial cells, 45, 77
Poorly differentiated neuroendocrine carcinomas,
        148, 157, **178**
    cytologic findings, 184
    differential diagnosis, 185; differentiation from
        carcinoid tumor, 176
    histogenesis, 184
    immunohistochemical findings, 184
    large cell neuroendocrine carcinoma, 178
    malignancy-associated factors, 185
    molecular findings, 185
    small cell neuroendocrine carcinoma, 179
        combined with large cell carcinoma, 182
        combined with squamous cell carcinoma, 182
    treatment and prognosis, 185
Precursor T-lymphoblastic leukemia/lymphoblastic
        lymphoma, 237
    differentiation from thymoma, 98, 239

Predominantly cortical (type B1) thymoma, **53**, 56
Predominantly epithelial lymphoma, 53
Primary immunodeficiency diseases, 272
Primary mediastinal large B-cell lymphoma, 225
    clinical features, 225
    cytologic findings, 228
    differential diagnosis, 228
    general features, 225
    gross findings, 225
    immunohistochemical findings, 228
    microscopic findings, 228
    molecular findings, 228
    prognosis, 230
Primitive neuroectodermal tumor, 300
Prognostic indicators for thymic carcinoma, 144
    cell atypia, 145
    histologic type, 144
    immunohistochemical factors, 146
    nuclear DNA content, 146
    TNM stage, 144
Pseudoglandular thymoma, 59
Pulmonary carcinoma, 148, 159, 177, 254
    association with carcinoid tumor, 159
    differentiation from thymic carcinoma, 148,
        254; from thymic carcinoid, 177
Pure teratoma, 216

R

Red cell aplasia and thymoma, 100
Retinal anlage tumor, 300
Rhabdomyoma, 288
Rhabdomyomatous thymoma, 60
Rhabdomyosarcoma, 292

S

Sarcomatoid carcinoma, 138
    carcinosarcoma, 138
    spindle cell carcinoma, 138
Schwannoma, 295
    melanocytic schwannoma, 295
Sclerosing thymoma, 64
Secondary carcinoma, *see* Metastatic carcinoma
Secondary immunodeficiency disease, 274
Secondary thymic carcinoma, 253
Seminoma, 193, 199, **208**, 228
    differential diagnosis, 208; differentiation from
        primary mediastinal large B-cell lymphoma,
        228

Sjögren syndrome, and thymic extranodal
    marginal B-cell lymphoma, 232
Small cell carcinoma, neuroendocrine type, 179
Small cell lymphoma, differentiation from
    thymoma, 98
Solitary fibrous tumor, 288
Spindle cell carcinoid tumor, 166
Spindle cell carcinoma, 138
Spindle cell epithelial tumor with thymus-like
    differentiation (SETTLE), 260
Spindle cell thymoma, 45, **48**, 55, 58, 63, 100
Spindle epithelial cells, 45, 77
Spindle/oval cell (type A) thymoma, **48**, 100
    and associated diseases, 100
Squamoid (type B3) thymoma, 53
Squamous cell carcinoma, 97, **120**, 182
    and small cell neuroendocrine carcinoma, 182
    and thymoma, 121
    differentiation from thymoma, 97
    in thymic cyst, 121
    less-differentiated, 120
    well-differentiated, 120
Staging systems, thymoma, 102
    Masaoka, 102
    TNM, 102, *see also* TNM classification and
        staging systems
    World Health Organization, 102, *see also* World
        Health Organization histologic classification
    Yamakawa-Masaoka staging, 103
Staging systems, carcinoma, 144
Striated cells, 13
Subcapsular epithelial cells, 84
Synovial sarcoma, 292

T

T lymphocytes, 13
T-cell deficiency diseases, 273
T-cell lymphomas, 237
    anaplastic large cell lymphoma, 241
    precursor T-lymphoblastic leukemia/lympho-
        blastic lymphoma, 237
Teratoma, 194, **201**
    classification, 204
    cystic, 194
    malignant transformation, 208
    immature, 201, 216
    mature, 201, 216
    with nongerminal malignant tumor, 212

Terminal deoxynucleotidyltransferase, 13, 47, 54, 60, 141
  in thymic carcinoma, 141
  in thymoma, 47, 54, 60
Thoracic duct cyst, 308
Thymic atrophy, 271
Thymic carcinoma, 56, 84, 97, **115**, 185, 196, 253, *see also individual tumors*
  and pulmonary carcinoma, 254
  clinical features, 116
  combined with thymoma, 185
  cytologic findings, 139
  differential diagnosis, 146; differentiation from thymoma, 84, 97; from germ cell tumors, 148, 196
  Epstein-Barr virus association, 150
  general features, 115
  gross findings, 118
  histologic subtypes, 118
    adenocarcinoma, 131
    adenoid cystic carcinoma-like, 135
    adenosquamous carcinoma, 129
    basaloid carcinoma, 127
    carcinoma with t(15;19) translocation, 139
    clear cell carcinoma, 135
    large cell carcinoma, 137
    lymphoepithelioma-like, 135
    mucoepidermoid carcinoma, **127**, 131
    sarcomatoid carcinoma, 138
    squamous cell carcinoma, 120
  immunohistochemical findings, **141**, 144
  malignancy-associated factors, 144, *see also* Malignancy-associated factors
  microscopic findings, 118
  molecular findings, 143
  nuclear DNA content, 146
  prognosis, 150
  prognostic indicators, 144
  secondary, 253
  spread and metastases, 149
  stage, 144
  transition from thymoma, 120
  treatment, 149
Thymic cyst, 262
  acquired multilocular cyst, 263
  congenital cyst, 262
Thymic dysplasia, 271, **272**
Thymic epithelial tumors and Epstein-Barr virus, 150

Thymic epithelial tumor with adenoid cystic carcinoma-like features, 135
Thymic extranodal marginal zone B-cell lymphoma of mucosa-associated lymphoid tissue (MALT), 230
  association with Sjögren syndrome, 232
  differential diagnosis, 237
  general features, 230
  gross findings, 232
  immunohistochemical findings, 232
  microscopic findings, 232
  molecular findings, 232
  prognosis, 237
Thymic hormones, 10
Thymic hyperplasia, 274
  lymphoid hyperplasia, 274
  true thymic hyperplasia, 274
Thymic lymphocytes, *see* Thymocytes
Thymocytes, 10, 15, 89, 93
  involution, 16
  maturation, 15
Thymolipoma, 257
  differentiation from liposarcoma, 260
  disease association, 257
Thymoma, **19**, 146, 177, 185, 196, 239, 243, 260
  associated diseases, 99
  cellular subtypes, 41
    epithelial cell, 41, *see also* Epithelial cell thymoma
    lymphocyte cell, 46
  classification, 19
  clinical features, 24
  coagulation necrosis, 32
  combined with carcinoid tumor, 186
  combined with thymic carcinoma, 185
  cystic changes, 32
  cytologic findings, 80
  diagnostic techniques, 24, 80
  differential diagnosis, 97; differentiation from thymic carcinoma, 84, 97, 146; from carcinoid tumor, 177; from germ cell tumor, 196; from precursor T-lymphoblastic leukemia/lymphoma, 239; from Hodgkin lymphoma, 243
  ectopic hamartomatous, 260
  encapsulated, 29
  epithelial cell subtypes, 41
  frozen section, 77

general features, 23
genetic abnormalities, 94
gross findings, 29
histogenetic subtypes, 55
histology and malignancy, 67
histologic subtypes, 48, 58
immunohistochemical findings, 84
invasive, 27, 31, 33
lymphocyte cell subtypes, 46
malignancy, 67
metastases, 101
microscopic findings, 33
molecular findings, 94
nuclear DNA content, 95
perivascular spaces, 38
proliferative activity, 76
prognosis, 105
staging, 102
transition to carcinoma, 120
treatment, 105
ultrastructural findings, 89
Thymoma with hemangiopericytoma-like features, 59
Thymoma with myoid cells, 59
Thymoma with pseudosarcomatous stroma, 64
Thymoma with rosette-like structures, 58
Thymoma with squamous differentiation, 59
Thymosin, 10
Thymus gland, normal, 1
    anatomy, 3
    embryology, 2
    gross findings, 3
    involution, 15
    microscopic findings, 4
Thyroid transcription factor-1, 148, 177, 254
TNM classification and staging systems, 102, 103,
    144, 216
    germ cell tumors, 216
    thymic carcinoma, 144

Tracheoesophageal cyst, 307
Traditional morphologic classification, thymoma, 53
True thymic hyperplasia, 274
Tuberculosis, 265
Type A thymoma, 45, **48**, 55, 58, 59, 63, 100
Type AB thymoma, 38, **48**, 56, 59
Type B1 thymoma, 53
Type B2 thymoma, 53
Type B1/B2 thymoma, 59
Type B3 thymoma, **53**, 56
Type B2/B3 thymoma, 59
Type II malignant thymoma, 115

U

Undifferentiated carcinoma, 137
    differentiation from large cell lymphoma, 146
Union International Against Cancer, 144

W

Well-differentiated neuroendocrine carcinoma,
    157, *see also* Carcinoid tumor
Well-differentiated thymic carcinoma, **53**, 56
Wiskott-Aldrich disease, 273
World Health Organization histologic classification,
    19, 22, 45, **48**, 53, 71, 102, 118, 157
    comparison with other systems, 45
    controversies, 56
    of thymic tumors, 19, 22, **48**, 53, 102
    of germ cell tumors, 193
    of neuroendocrine tumors, 157
    of thymic carcinoma, 118
    of thymoma, 19, **48**, 71, 102

Y

Yamakawa-Masaoka TNM classification, 103
Yolk sac tumor, 201, **211**